11/29/93

Audition

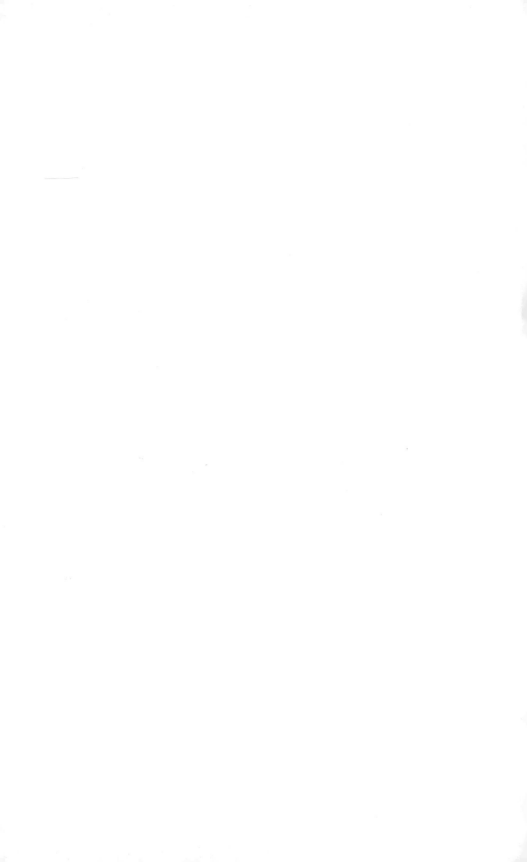

Audition

Pierre Buser and Michel Imbert

Translated by R. H. Kay

A Bradford Book
The MIT Press
Cambridge, Massachusetts
London, England

This book was set in Univers and Palatino by Achorn Graphics Services and was printed and bound in the United States of America.

Library of Congress Cataloging-in-Publication Data

Buser, Pierre A.
  [Audition. English]
  Audition / Pierre Buser, Michel Imbert; translated by R.H. Kay.
    p. cm.
  Translation of: Audition.
  "A Bradford book."
  Includes bibliographical references and index.
  ISBN 0-262-02331-8
  1. Hearing. I. Imbert, Michel, 1935–   . II. Title.
QP461.B9713   1991   91-4438
612.8'5—dc20   CIP

Contents

2

The Auditory Receptor System   110

Preface

Our objective in writing this textbook was to gather into a single volume information on three aspects of hearing that are more often dealt with separately than together. The first section concerns auditory psychophysics, with a brief visit to the science of musical sounds. The second section, on the physiology of the auditory periphery, discusses the influences of morphological and mechanical properties of receptors on their transduction characteristics. The third reviews processing mechanisms in the auditory pathways that are involved in elaborating the coding of neuronal messages as they ascend the auditory pathways from the periphery to the auditory areas of the cerebral cortex.

Naturally, we had to be selective in our choice of material to keep the book to a reasonable length. We chose to emphasize mammalian audition rather than take a broad comparative perspective. The book is intended primarily for upper-level undergraduates and graduate students in basic science courses.

We wish to thank Dr. R. H. Kay, who is responsible for translating the French text. We also thank those who helped us revise the original French edition, notably M. C. Botte and Y. Galifret, and the authors and publishers who allowed us to use some of their material.

P. B., M. I.

TRANSLATOR'S NOTE

Happily, the authors and I agreed that a real translation into current English language scientific usage would be better than a literal word-for-word transform. Liaison across the Channel with Dr. Buser, even over difficulties, has been friendly, and I have enjoyed working across the Atlantic with Fiona Stevens and Katherine Arnoldi of The MIT Press.

R. H. K.

Pierre Buser, Professor of the Université Pierre et Marie Curie, Paris, France, was born in 1921. His major research is concerned with sensorimotor integrative mechanisms of the central nervous system.

Michel Imbert, Professor of the Université Pierre et Marie Curie, Paris, France, was born in 1935. His major research is concerned with the neurophysiology of development in the visual nervous system.

R. H. Kay, Emeritus Fellow of Keble College, Oxford, England, was born in 1921. His major research is in sensory mechanisms, particularly of human hearing.

Audition

The Physiological Psychology of Hearing

1 THE BASIC CHARACTERISTICS OF AUDIBLE STIMULI

1.1 OSCILLATORY STIMULI

The adequate stimulus for hearing comprises a certain range of mechanical oscillations. We begin by briefly examining the properties of such vibratory processes in general terms.

When a small element of volume M_0 situated within a solid, liquid, or gas is acted on by an impulsive force (that generates a rapid displacement of small amplitude) then, as a consequence of collision forces, other similar elements M in the rest of the medium also suffer displacement after a delay that increases with the distance of the element M from M_0. The disturbance is continuously propagated from one place to the next with a finite speed. In the absence of matter (in vacuo), no disturbance can propagate.

Accordingly, if at the point M_0 there should exist a succession of such elementary changes, these will produce continuous elementary compressions and dilatations of the medium around some equilibrium value according to some function of time $x(t)$. M_0 can then become the source of a continuous vibration that propagates at a given speed c and which under certain conditions can be a continuous audible sound.

In a *fluid medium*, liquid or gaseous, the vibration propagates longitudinally along a line perpendicular to the plane of the original disturbance. In a fluid medium each particle oscillates about its equilibrium position along the direction of propagation of this *longitudinal wave*. Two sorts of vibration are mainly considered in acoustics: One is the propagation of a *plane wavefront* that is normal to the direction of propagation and is the result of a planar disturbance at M_0; the other is the propagation of a *spherical wave* surrounding a punctate source of original disturbance at M_0 that spreads out in all directions from its original point of origin in the fluid. In either case it is observed that the speed of propagation c depends only on the nature and physical state of the medium and is independent of the waveform of the disturbance, the function $x(t)$.

In a *solid medium*, in contrast, it is possible to have simultaneous propagation of both longitudinal and transverse vibrations.

WAYS OF DESCRIBING OSCILLATORY PHENOMENA

The vibration at a point M in the body of a fluid can in general be specified from two different, complementary viewpoints (Bendat & Piersol 1966; de Boer 1976; Zwicker & Feldtkeller 1981). *Analysis in the temporal domain* specifies the time variation of one selected characteristic of the displacement of a small particle at M, either of its amplitude a or of its velocity v. Alternatively, the temporal variation of the pressure p that the disturbance is instantaneously exerting at the place M may be specified. In contrast, *analysis in the frequency domain* may be used. This is concerned with breaking down an oscillation, however complex it might be, into a series of harmonically related sinusoidal components, specifying not only their harmonic frequencies but also their individual amplitudes and phase relationships.

In practice, for audible as for other vibrations, it is sometimes useful to categorize the oscillations in other ways too. Some are long lasting. In audition, these are usually called *continuous tones* or, if they are sinusoidal, *pure tones*. In contrast, *transients* are vibrations that last only briefly. It has become the custom to treat these two sorts of disturbance by different analytical methods.

Continuous Oscillations
The simplest continuous vibration is a *pure sine wave*. This is completely specified by its peak amplitude X, its phase Φ, and its frequency f, which can also be specified by one of the equivalent variables, the *period* ($T = 1/f$) or the *angular frequency* ($\omega = 2\pi/T = 2\pi f$). Thus

$$x(t) = X\sin(2\pi ft - \Phi) = X\sin(2\pi t/T - \Phi) = X\sin(\omega t - \Phi).$$

The amplitude or energy versus frequency spectrum of a pure sinusoidal wave has a single peak at its own frequency (figure 1.1A).

A much more commonly encountered situation and a more general case is any vibration that is *periodic*, i.e., that is merely constrained by being a function that repeats itself identically after a time T, called its *period*. In which case

$$x(t + nT) = x(T + t) = x(t)$$
for $n = 2, 3, 4, \ldots$, etc.

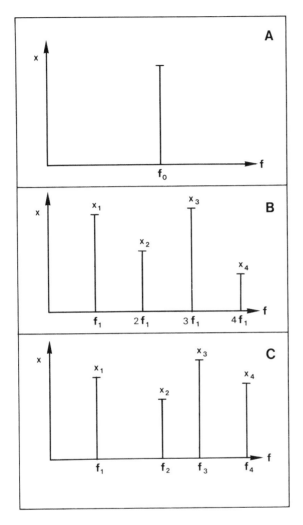

Figure 1.1
Examples of different spectra. Amplitudes x of components of frequency f, for (A) a pure sine wave; (B) a complex periodic function; (C) a pseudoperiodic (quasiperiodic) function. (From Bendat & Piersol 1966)

In general, this function will not be purely sinusoidal. But it is important to realize that, provided it is regularly periodic, it can be broken down and analyzed ("decomposed" is becoming common jargon for the process) into a series of elementary sine waves. However complex the original periodic wave might be, it can be fully described by an algebraic summation of its elementary sinusoidal components.

Each such elementary component has an amplitude x_i and phase Φ_i. Its frequency f_i is a simple integer multiple ($i \times f_1$) of the *fundamental* or *first harmonic component* that has a frequency f_1. The other successive harmonic components for which $i = 2, 3, 4$, etc. are called the *second, third, fourth* etc. *harmonics.*

The complete formal description of this summation, called a *Fourier series* is:

$$x(t) = x_0 + \sum_{n=1}^{n=\infty} (a_n \cos n\omega t + b_n \sin n\omega t)$$

where $a_n = 2/T \int_0^T x(t)\cos n\omega t\ dt$, and $b_n = 2/T \int_0^T x(t)\sin n\omega t\ dt$; for $n = 1, 2, 3$, etc.

Therefore the spectrum of any regularly repeating function can be described either by a single spectral line for a sinusoidal function (figure 1.1A) or by a line spectrum with its individual peaks at the harmonic frequencies f_1, $2f_1$, $3f_1$, etc. (figure 1.1B).

Figure 1.2 (left) shows how by using the inverse process to Fourier analysis one can *synthesize* any regularly repeating periodic function by adding together an appropriate series of simple sine waves that are harmonically related in frequency.

An alternative expression for the Fourier series, equivalent to the above, employs exponentials and (Eulerian) complex number notation:

$\sin x = [\exp(jx) - \exp(-jx)]/2j;$
$\cos x = [\exp(jx) + \exp(-jx)]/2.$

It therefore becomes, by substitution:

$$x(t) = k \sum_{-\infty}^{+\infty} c_k \exp(-j\omega t),$$

where $c_k = 2/T \int_{-T/2}^{T/2} x(t)\exp(-j\omega t)dt$; for $k = 1, 2, 3$, etc.

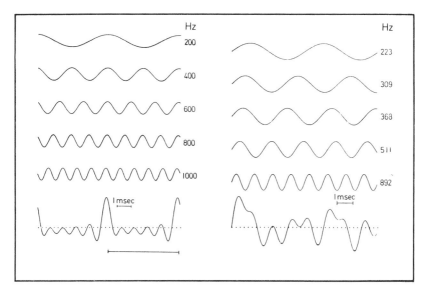

Figure 1.2
Generation of functions by adding pure sine waves (Fourier synthesis). *Left,* The component frequencies (Hz) are a harmonic series; they generate a periodic function of period specified by the horizontal bar. *Right,* Frequencies (Hz) of the components are not in simple ratios; the resulting function is not periodic. (From de Boer 1976)

It is essential in acoustics to distinguish between linear and nonlinear systems. In the above considerations, we have already assumed the following two characteristics of a *linear* system:

• When acted on by a purely sinusoidal disturbance, the system continues to generate a sinusoid of the same frequency, with an output amplitude that is proportional to the input, and introduces no other frequency component.
• When acted on by several different sinusoids, the output will contain the same frequency content as the input.

In contrast, a system is designated *nonlinear* if it behaves differently and generates new outputs. For example, from a sinusoidal input it might generate an output of the same fundamental period but which contains harmonics. If the input comprises two pure sinusoids, intermodulations between the different harmonic distortions of each sinusoid might well generate further frequency components that were not present in the input. Such nonlinear sources of distortion are common in the auditory system and will be considered again later.

Some systems can generate disturbances that, as above, can be specified as the sum of a set of sine waves. But in this case a series of harmonically related sinusoids will not suffice, since some of the component frequencies are not simply related to one another. Oscillations of this sort are called *pseudoperiodic* or *quasiperiodic*. These can be described by an expression of the type

$$x(t) = \sum_{n=1}^{n=\infty} x_n \sin(2\pi f_n t - \Phi_n),$$

where, in this case, n takes integer values that bear simple relationships to one another. Figure 1.1C illustrates the case in which three frequencies are summated and

$$x(t) = X_1 \sin(2t + \Phi_1) + X_2(\sin 3t + \Phi_2) + X_3 \sin(\sqrt{50} \cdot t + \Phi_3).$$

Note that $2/\sqrt{50}$ and $3/\sqrt{50}$ are not rational numbers (Bendat & Piersol 1966).

Figure 1.2 (right) gives an example of a nonperiodic waveform resulting from the summation of sinusoidal signals whose frequencies have a variety of ratios to one another.

A continuous sound can be *amplitude modulated*. Given a constant (angular) frequency (ω_1), and a mean amplitude of the sound around which its amplitude is modulated (X_1), if we specify the *modulation* by its angular frequency ω_{mod} and its own amplitude X_2 (the ratio X_2/X_1 being designated the *modulation index, m*), then such sounds are described by expressions of the form

$$x(t) = X(t)\cos\omega_1 t = (X_1 + X_2\cos\omega_{mod}t)\cos\omega_1 t$$
$$= X_1(1 + m\cos\omega_{mod}t)\cos\omega_1 t.$$

The above expression is easily transformed into the following:

$$x(t) = X_1\cos\omega_1 t + \tfrac{1}{2}X_2\cos(\omega_1 + \omega_{mod})t + \tfrac{1}{2}X_2\cos(\omega_1 - \omega_{mod})t,$$

which allows us to predict that the line spectrum of such a function will be represented by three peaks at $\omega_1 - \omega_{mod}$, ω_1, and $\omega_1 + \omega_{mod}$ (figure 1.3, upper).

Frequency-modulated sounds comprise continuous tones that are modulated in a different way. Here, the amplitude of the sound oscillation is kept constant but its frequency is modulated about some central value f_1. Suppose that the frequency varies by an amount δf

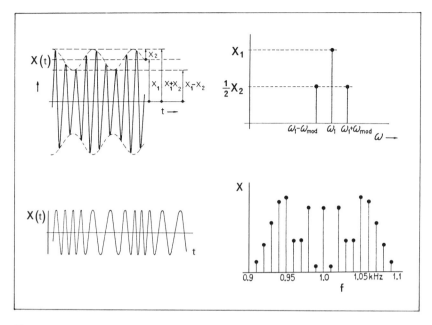

Figure 1.3
Amplitude-modulated and frequency-modulated sounds. *Above,* Amplitude-modulated sound. *Left,* Sound waveform; X_1 = mean amplitude; X_2 = amplitude of modulation. *Right,* Amplitude spectrum of the amplitude-modulated sound (where ω_1 = $2\pi f$ and ω_{mod} = $2\pi \times$ modulation rate); the spectrum comprises three line components at ω_1, $\omega_1 - \omega_{mod}$, $\omega_1 + \omega_{mod}$. *Below,* Frequency-modulated sound. *Left,* Sound waveform $X(t) = f(t)$. *Right,* Amplitude spectrum of such a frequency-modulated sound. The spectrum shown refers to a sound of carrier frequency 1 kHz, modulation frequency 10 Hz, frequency deviation 70 Hz. The modulation index is 7 and the spectral components span 0.920 kHz to 1.080 kHz (see text). (After Zwicker & Feldtkeller 1981)

between the extreme values $f_1 + \delta f$ and $f_1 - \delta f$ and that the frequency of the imposed modulation is f_{mod}, then we can show (Zwicker & Feldtkeller 1981) that the line spectrum generated by such a sound displays a series of peaks around the central frequency, the entire spectrum spreading across a bandwidth $\delta f + f_{mod}$ to either side of the central frequency. (Figure 1.3, lower, shows the waveform of such a frequency-modulated sound and its line spectrum.)

Another important class of oscillations can be regarded as the summation of many, or an essentially infinite number of, elementary sinusoidal waves with varied phase relationships between them. The resulting vibration changes apparently randomly with time. This so-called *noise* signal is best analyzed by the application of statistical methods. These allow the specification of various characteristics such as the *mean frequency,* the *probability density of the amplitude,* and the *power spectral density.*

In acoustics it is usually this last function, the power spectral density, that proves to be of interest because it tells something about the spectral characteristics of the signal. By this means we can specify, in a series of narrow frequency bands (of bandwidth f to $f + \delta f$), the mean square amplitude during a time interval (0 to T). This represents the power developed by the vibration within each elementary frequency band.

$$G_x(f) = \lim_{\delta f \to 0} \lim_{T \to \infty} 1/[\delta f \cdot T] \int_0^T x^2(t,f,\delta f)\,dt.$$

This results in a spectrum for the noise signal that consists not of separate lines but of a smooth, continuous curve that represents the variation of $G_x(f)$ as a function of f.

Figure 1.4 shows examples of the energy spectral density for a sine wave mixed with noise for (1) a narrow (frequency) band noise signal and (2) wide band noise (*white noise*). Essentially, in acoustics, white noise can be regarded as having a uniform power spectral density throughout the whole audible spectrum. White noise filtered by a sharp cut-off low-pass device (that is to say, one that does not attenuate at frequencies lower than the cut-off frequency) is called *low-pass noise* and for the inverse case, mutatis mutandis, *high-pass noise* results.

Roughly speaking, listeners tend to classify sounds subjectively in a similar way; sounds are "musical" or "melodic" when they are truly periodic, whether simple or complex, and "noisy" when they are quasiperiodic or randomly varying. We shall consider the spectral structure of musical sounds in more detail later.

Boundaries between such distinctions nevertheless tend to be blurred in practice. For example, many sounds, particularly sustained natural sounds such as a continuously emitted vowel sound or, notably, a consonant, can simultaneously include amplitude and frequency modulations and, in some circumstances, enharmonic components as well as "noise." All this can result in a very complicated line spectrum upon which continuous spectral distributions may also be superimposed in particular frequency ranges (figure 1.4).

Transients
Acoustically, this widespread class of sounds embraces any brief noise, sounds from percussion instruments of the orchestra (see be-

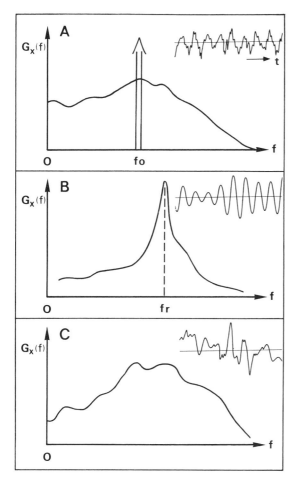

Figure 1.4
Power spectral density. Power spectral density $G_x(f)$ against frequency f ("power spectra"), of three functions (amplitude against time in inset). A, Sine wave + random noise. B, Narrow-band noise. C, Wide-band noise. (From Bendat & Piersol 1966)

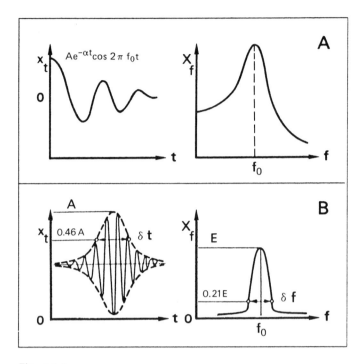

Figure 1.5
Analysis of transients. Examples of transients, amplitude x_t as a function of time, and their spectral composition $X(f)$ as a function of f, i.e., transformation from the temporal domain to the frequency domain. A, Damped sine wave, amplitude decreasing exponentially $(x(t) = A\,e^{-\alpha t}\cos 2\pi f_0 t$ for $t > 0$; $x = 0$ at $t = 0$). B, Gaussian unit tonal impulse. This function can be described by a duration δt, being the width of a rectangle the height of which is A (the amplitude) and which has the same surface area as the function. Computation shows that the bandwidth δf characterizing the curve of energy spectral density is such that $\delta t \times \delta f = 1$. The abscissa (frequency) is in linear coordinates. (A from Bendat & Piersol 1966; B from Blauert 1983)

low), as well as animal vocalizations and human speech. Figure 1.5 (left) shows two examples of transients, a damped sine wave and a gaussian unit impulse tone (Bendat & Piersol 1966; Zwicker & Feldtkeller 1981).

Physicists are faced with a problem when they want to determine the spectrum of a transient, i.e., to transform the signal from the *time domain* to the *frequency domain*. Broadly speaking, the solution is to exploit the *Fourier integral* method rather than attempt to analyze a transient by the Fourier series as described above for treating continuous periodic functions.

If $x(t)$ is the function to be analyzed, its spectrum can be represented by the expression

$X(f) = \int_{-\infty}^{+\infty} x(t)\exp(-j2\pi ft)dt.$

This Fourier spectrum $X(f)$ is generally expressed in the complex form

$X(f) = |X(f)|\exp[-j\Phi(f)],$

where $|X(f)|$ is the modulus and $\Phi(f)$ the argument. The curves of $|X(f)|$ and of $\Phi(f)$ as a function of frequency describe the amplitude and the phase spectra of $x(t)$, respectively.

As for the amplitude spectrum, suffice it to say here that in the case of transients such as these it is very like a noise spectrum, being represented not by a set of discrete lines but by a continuous curve. Figure 1.5 (right) illustrates such spectra ($X(f)$ as a function of f) for a damped sine wave and for a gaussian unit impulse. Note that the latter sound has a limited spread in both the time and frequency domains. This provides a useful stimulus that is something of a compromise between the extreme cases of (1) the infinitely brief pulse that is very well defined in time but poorly delineated in the frequency domain and (2) the pure sine wave, which has a very sharp frequency spectrum but lasts indefinitely.

We are often hard put to find an adequate description of sounds that vary in both frequency and amplitude and also include transients. These are particularly common in animal vocalization and human speech. Ideally, the representation of such sounds should be three dimensional to define how the frequency content varies with time as well as how the amplitude changes at each frequency. Such a display is not easy to arrange. Generally we resort to sonograms in which frequency content, that is, the "instantaneous spectrum," is represented by a set of points on the ordinate with time as the abscissa. We then attempt to represent the third dimension, sound intensity, by simultaneously modulating the blackness (contrast) of the individual points that represent the individual peaks in the instantaneous spectrum. Figures 1.6 and 1.7 give examples of sonograms that different authors have published illustrating different animal calls (Evans & Pick 1972; Winter, Ploog & Latta 1966).

1.2 SOUND INTENSITY: GENERAL CHARACTERISTICS

Having characterized the different oscillations somewhat generally, we can now consider the particular properties of a sound that, after

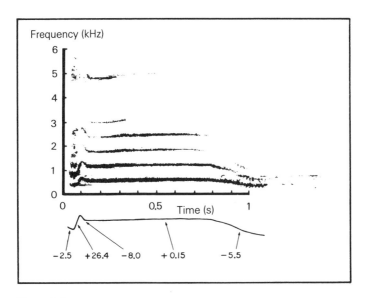

Figure 1.6
Sonogram of a cat vocalization. Note the relatively simple harmonic structure and smooth frequency changes. Relative intensities are indicated by the blackness of the trace (see text). Traced from cat in rut. The bottom curve shows frequency changes in octaves per second. (From Evans & Pick 1972)

transmission from the sound source to the receptors of the inner ear, will contribute to exciting an *audible* sensation. Essential characteristics are the following:

• Its amplitude must exceed a certain minimum value, called the *threshold* or *liminal amplitude*.
• Its frequency (or at least one of its frequency components, if we are concerned with a complex sound) must be sited within the waveband of audible frequencies.

Practically, then, the first problem is how best to quantify the sound intensity I_a. By definition, this is the energy that is propagated by the sound wave in unit time across a unit area normal to the direction of propagation or, in other words, the power P transmitted per unit cross-sectional area ($I_a = P/A$).

When acted on by a certain periodic force per unit area, i.e., by a certain periodic pressure p, a particle in fluid suffers an *instantaneous longitudinal displacement* ξ at an *instantaneous velocity u*, each varying according to the same periodic function.

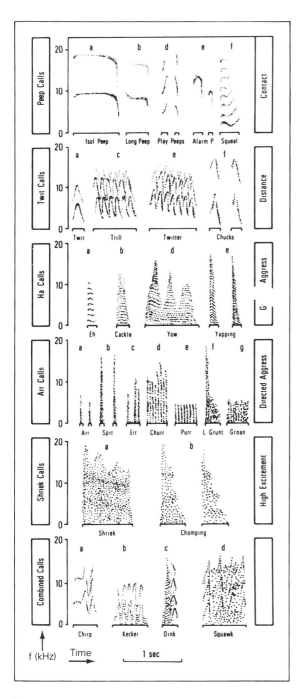

Figure 1.7
Sonograms of squirrel monkey vocalizations (calls). Intensity is indicated by the blackness of the trace. (From Winter, Ploog & Latta 1966)

Table 1.1. Equivalent values of cgs units and SI units

	CGS	SI
Pressure (p)	bar (b)	Pa
Velocity (u)	$cm \cdot s^{-1}$	$m \cdot s^{-1}$
Sound intensity (I_a)	$W \cdot cm^{-2}$	$W \cdot m^{-2}$
Specific acoustic impedance (Z_{sp})	$dynes \cdot s \cdot cm^{-3}$	$Pa \cdot s \cdot m^{-1}$ $N \cdot s \cdot m^{-3}$
Acoustic impedance (Z_a)	$dynes \cdot s \cdot cm^{-5}$	$Pa \cdot s \cdot m^{-3}$ $N \cdot s \cdot m^{-5}$

Note: 1 Pa $= 10 \mu bar = 1 N \cdot m^{-2} = 1.02 \cdot 10^{-5}$ atm $= 750 \cdot 10^{-5}$ torr; 1 bar $= 10^5$ Pa; 1 barye $= 1 \mu bar = 0.1$ Pa $= 1$ dynes $\cdot$ cm; where bar, Pa (pascal), atm (atmosphere), and torr are units of pressure; N (newton) and dynes are units of force.

At any instant, we can define the ratio between the pressure p on the particle on the one hand and its velocity u on the other. The ratio p/u has, by analogy with the corresponding electrical case, been designated as the specific acoustic impedance Z_{sp}. In the case of a surface of cross-sectional area A on which the acoustic pressure p is acting, the acoustic impedance Z_a becomes the ratio between the pressure and the *acoustic-velocity flux* $(u \cdot A)$ across that surface, leading immediately to the relationship $Z_a = Z_{sp}/A$.

All these values (p, u, ξ, Z_{sp}, Z_a) and the acoustic intensity can be expressed in SI units, although in practice the cgs system and other units are still in general use. Table 1.1 shows the dimensions of the various units used in the two most popular systems.

We can show that Z_{sp} is related to the specific mass (density) of the fluid and to the velocity c of the wave's propagation by the expression:

$$Z_{sp} = p/u = \rho \cdot c,$$

and to the elasticity of the fluid by:

$$Z_{sp} = (\rho \cdot S)^{1/2},$$

with S in dynes $\cdot$ cm^{-2}.

Strictly, impedance is represented by a complex number of the form $Z = R + jX$ where R, the "resistive component" (acoustic resistance), is related to frictional forces and X, the "reactive component," is determined by the inertial mass M of the system on the one hand (acoustic inductance) and by its elasticity S on the other (acoustic capacitance). *Acoustic resistance* is independent of frequency. In contrast, *acoustic reactance* is very frequently dependent. *Acoustic inductance*, related to inertia, depends on the mass M of the system and increases with frequency: It is given by the product of the mass and the angular frequency $M\omega = 2\pi fM$. *Acoustic capacitance* results from the effects of the elasticity S or stiffness of the material opposing the action of the applied force: It decreases with frequency and is given by $S/\omega = S/2\pi f$. The complete expression for the modulus of Z is

$$|Z| = \sqrt{\{R_f^2 + [(2\pi fM) - (S/2\pi f)]^2\}},$$

where f is the frequency at which the system is driven. In such a system one needs also to specify the *phase shift*. This is given by

$$\tan \Phi = R/\{2\pi fM - (S/2\pi f)\},$$

since

$$Z = |Z| \exp j\Phi.$$

The reciprocal of the stiffness is called the *compliance*. This refers to the medium's compressibility; air, being more compressible than liquid, has the greater compliance.

Here are some values for Z_{sp} (cgs units): hydrogen 11.4; air 42; fresh water 145,000; sea water 160,000; iron 4,000,000; wood 290,000; glass 1,300,000.

We can see that in the above expressions the factor $2\pi fM$ predominates at high frequencies, whereas the term $S/2\pi f$ is the more significant at low frequencies.

Finally, it is sometimes preferable to use the reciprocal of the impedance, $1/Z$, called the *admittance*.

Let us now calculate the sound intensity I_a. One can show that when sound propagates with a plane or a spherical wavefront the intensity, being the sound power transfer across unit cross-sectional area, is proportional to the square of the vibratory displacement according to the expression

$$I_a = 2\pi^2 \cdot \xi^2 \cdot \rho \cdot f^2 \cdot c,$$

where ξ is the displacement, ρ is the specific mass, f is the frequency, and c is the velocity of propagation of the wave.

The pressure variation p can itself be expressed as

$$p = 2\pi \cdot \xi \cdot \rho \cdot c \cdot f.$$

In other words, sound intensity is proportional to the square of the sound pressure or to the square of the sound amplitude ($I_a = kp^2 = k'\xi^2$).

In the case of a sinusoidal wave, the pressure is of the form $p = p_M \sin\omega t$ and the instantaneous particle velocity $u = uM \sin(\omega t - \Phi)$, where p_M and u_M are the peak pressure and peak velocity, respectively. These considerations lead to the following expression for I_a:

$$I_a = k(p_{eff} \cdot u_{eff} \cos\Phi),$$

where p_{eff} and u_{eff} are the effective values of the pressure and particle velocity (i.e., $p_M/\sqrt{2}$ and $u_M/\sqrt{2}$), and Φ is the phase shift between p and u. Since p and u are proportional to each other (being linked by the value of the impedance) we can write

$$I_a = k \cdot (p_{eff}^2/Z)\cos\Phi,$$

that is to say, I_a will be effectively proportional to the pressure squared, provided that the phase shift Φ can be neglected (i.e., $\cos\Phi$ is close to unity). Experiments show that this is almost invariably so in the case of the mechanical vibrations that we are considering (Bouasse 1926; Bruhat 1940). As a quantitative example, for a sound wave in air of frequency 1000 Hz and a particle displacement amplitude $\xi = 10$ μm, the corresponding pressure variation is 260 μbar, and the sound intensity is $0.810 \ 10^{-4}$ W/cm^2, which corresponds with a sound level of about 120 dB.

The concept of impedance is essential for appreciating the way in which sound is transferred from a medium 1 (impedance Z_{sp1}) into another medium 2 (impedance Z_{sp2}). In fact, when Z_{sp1} is less than Z_{sp2}, by writing the intensity of the incident sound in medium 1 as I_i, we can show that the part of the sound energy transmitted into medium 2 (I_t) and the part reflected back (I_r) are given, respectively, by the expressions

$$I_t = I_i\{4q/(q + 1)^2\},$$
$$I_r = I_i\{(q - 1)^2/(q + 1)^2\},$$

where $q = Z_{sp2}/Z_{sp1}$.

Practically, the sound energy from medium 1 can only be transferred into medium 2 more or less intact when the values of Z_{sp1} and Z_{sp2} are very close (q as nearly as possible unity).

If Z_{sp2} is greater than Z_{sp1}, once again a part of I_i cannot enter medium 2. We shall see below how these considerations are relevant to the transfer of sound in the middle ear.

As a worked example, consider a sound source situated in the air near the surface of the sea. We wish to find out what proportion of the emitted sound is reflected (I_r) from the sea surface and what part is transmitted through it (I_t). From the selection of impedance values given above, the ratio q is $160,000/40 = 4000$; in this case the fraction of energy reflected $I_r/I_i = 999/1000$, and the fraction transmitted $I_t/I_i = 1/1000$ only.

We also need to know how the intensity of a sound vibration varies with the distance from its source. In the (theoretical and limiting) case of propagation of the sound by a plane wave in one particular direction only, there is no loss of intensity. In contrast, in the case of propagation with spherical wavefronts issuing from a point source, it can be shown that in a uniform medium the sound intensity varies inversely as the square of the distance from the source. Real cases of sound propagation are for the most part some mixture of these two extreme theoretical cases.

After all this, one might imagine that all sound intensities are speci-fied in one of the usually employed units of power per unit area, formerly $W \cdot cm^{-2}$, now $W \cdot m^{-2}$, with the sound pressure for its part being expressed appropriately in dynes $\cdot cm^{-2}$ or in Pa, according to the system of units employed (cgs or SI). In fact, a *ratio scale* of inten-sity is preferred, which takes account of the fact that subjectively perceived intensity varies essentially as the logarithm of the objective physical acoustic intensity. A *sound power level* L_P is therefore desig-nated for a sound of physical power P, not absolutely but according to the logarithm of its ratio to a reference magnitude of sound power P_0:

$$L_P = \log_{10} P/P_0.$$

In practice, it is often more convenient to determine a sound pres-sure p corresponding to the power P, leading to the following modi-fication of the above expression for the sound power level (remember that $P = k \cdot p^2$):

$$L_P = \log_{10} (p^2/p_0^2) = 2 \log_{10} (p/p_0),$$

where $\log_{10} (p/p_0)$ is the *sound pressure level* L_p.

Clearly, the values of L_P and L_p are *relative* measures of sound power and sound pressure levels. By definition, the corresponding measure for (relative) sound intensity level is also given by

$$L_P = \log_{10}(I/I_0),$$

since I is proportional to p^2.

We must take care to specify sound pressure level or sound intensity level precisely since the too-frequent use of the term "sound intensity" with no further specification is too vague.

The choice of a reference pressure p_0 can vary. When 1 μbar is employed, levels are specified "re 1 μbar." Sometimes the pressure that represents approximately the usual level of the threshold sound pressure for human hearing at 1 kHz is chosen as reference: 2.10 μbar or 20 μPa. This latter reference pressure ("re 20 μbar") is the most frequently used in audition and corresponds with a sound power reference level $P_0 = 1$ pW. The sound intensity at this reference level is therefore $I_0 = 1$ pW/m^2.

When using either reference level, L is normally specified in bels (B) or more frequently—since the bel is often too large a unit in studies of audition—in decibels (dB). The decibel is defined thus:

$$L\text{ (dB)} = 20\log_{10}(p/p_0) = 10\log_{10}(P/P_0) = 10\log_{10}(I/I_0).$$

Table 1.2 compares different ratios of p and P and their expression in decibels. Table 1.3 lists several absolute values of p and P and their decibel levels re 20 μPa.

It is also necessary to specify sound levels for noise signals and to quantify their intensity. In this case we are dealing with a band of many different frequencies that may be a wide or a narrow one.

To attack this problem, let us begin with the expression $L = 10\log_{10}(I/I_0)$ dB, not losing sight of the fact that in this case I is a function of the frequency f.

This necessitates introducing an intensity spectral density function where $R = dI/df$ represents the variation of I with frequency. We then compare each value of R with a reference value R_0 corresponding to the threshold intensity density level I_0/Hz:

$$R_0 = 10^{-12}\,\text{W} \cdot \text{m}^{-2} \cdot \text{Hz}^{-1}.$$

From this, a fraction I_R, called the *sound intensity density level*, can be specified (in decibels) by

$$I_R = 10\log_{10}(R/R_0).$$

Table 1.2. Ratios of sound pressure (p) and power (P) and equivalents in decibels

p/p_0	P/P_0	L (dB)
0.10	0.01	-20
0.50	0.25	-6
0.71	0.50	-3
1.00	1.00	0
1.12	1.26	$+1$
1.41	2.00	$+3$
2.00	4.00	$+6$
3.16	10.00	$+10$
10.00	100.00	$+20$
31.60	1,000.00	$+30$
1,000.00	1,000,000.00	$+60$

Table 1.3. Absolute values of sound pressure and power and their decibel levels (re 20 μPa)

Pressure (p)		Power (P)		
cgs (μbar)	SI (Pa)	cgs (W/cm^2)	SI (pW/m^2)	dB
20000	200	10^{-2}	10^7	140
200	20	10^{-4}	10^6	120
20	2	10^{-6}	10^5	100
2	0.2	10^{-8}	10^4	80
$2 \cdot 10^{-1}$	0.02	10^{-10}	10^3	60
$2 \cdot 10^{-2}$	2000 μPa	10^{-12}	10^2	40
$2 \cdot 10^{-3}$	200 μPa	10^{-14}	10	20
$2 \cdot 10^{-4}$	20 μPa	10^{-16}	1	0

[In industrial physiology there is the problem of assessing the levels of noises in potentially damaging environments such as the workshop. For this purpose, a sound level meter is used to determine the *weighted sound level* for the noise (A) in decibels, which is currently specified as dB(A). The sound level meter normally has a filter incorporated to generate a characteristic such as the 40 phon equal loudness contour. Frequencies in the middle range of audible sounds are thus weighted more than lower or higher frequencies in the meter's output. Thus dB(A) represents hazards to the auditory system better than dB, which are frequency independent.]

Table 1.4. Intensity level of some sounds (dB re 20 μPa)

120	Thunder. Aircraft engine at 10 m
100	Pneumatic road drill at 2 m
90	Symphony orchestra
70–80	Noisy street
60	Cocktail party conversation
50	Quiet music
40	Quiet street
30	Quiet room
20	Recording studio
10	Gentle rustle of leaves

Table 1.4 helps illustrate the range of some real sounds by specifying their intensity level (in decibels re 20 μPa).

1.3 NOTES ON THE VELOCITY OF PROPAGATION (SPEED) OF SOUND WAVES

We can demonstrate that the speed of propagation of a sound wave in a homogeneous medium at a constant temperature is governed by the specific mass (density) of the fluid and by its coefficient of compressibility χ:

$$c = (\chi \cdot \rho)^{-1/2}.$$

In contrast, remember that this velocity is independent of the nature of the function $x(t)$. A clear everyday support for this is that a musical tune remains essentially unchanged with distance from its source (Bouasse 1926; Bruhat 1940).

Both theory and experiment show that for a given *gas*, for example air, the velocity of propagation is independent of the gas pressure but is proportional to the square root of its absolute temperature:

$$c = c_0\sqrt{(1 + \alpha T)},$$

with c in m/s, c_0 being the speed at 0°C and T the absolute temperature.

For dry air, $c_0 = 331.4$ m/s, and between 0°C and 20°C the variation with temperature is about 0.60 m/s/degree (340 m/s at 15°). For gases other than air and assuming that the compressibility coefficient χ remains the same (which is approximately true), the velocity varies inversely as the square root of the gas density, therefore inversely as the square root of the molecular mass also. Table 1.5 gives several examples.

Table 1.5. Density of medium as a determinant of sound velocity

Gas	Relative density	Speed (m/s)
Air	1.0000	331.5
Oxygen	1.1052	316
Nitrogen	0.9675	334
Hydrogen	0.0695	1284
Helium	0.1376	965
Carbon dioxide	1.5290	259

Liquids are much less compressible than gases (the coefficient χ is therefore much smaller), but the specific mass (density) is considerably higher—so much so that in many liquids the velocity of sound is only a few times greater than in air (1435 m/s in fresh water at 8°C, 1500 m/s in sea water at 15°C). However, in *solids* the speed of sound propagation is yet higher: for example, 5850 m/s in iron, 4000 m/s in wood, and 4000 to 5000 m/s in glass.

Apart from being reflected by or transmitted into an object that is encountered, a sound wave can escape around it by *diffraction.* The amount that does is determined by the size of the object relative to the sound's wavelength. Just as in the optical case, a sharp acoustic shadow is blurred in this way when the dimensions of the object are less than the sound wavelength. In other words, diffraction of sound past an object is more likely at low frequencies than at high. When the frequency is low enough, an object might effectively create no sound shadow.

2 AUDITORY THRESHOLDS

When measuring thresholds, particularly the absolute threshold, it is necessary to test monaurally to ensure that one ear only is stimulated (unless otherwise specified).

2.1 THE ABSOLUTE THRESHOLD

The absolute threshold, defined as the just-detectable sound intensity, has been measured in many and various ways but usually by employing simple sinusoidal sounds. One procedure used in measuring the absolute threshold is *automatic audiometry,* which uses a tracking technique devised by von Békésy (von Békésy 1960; Portmann & Portmann 1978; Zwicker & Feldtkeller 1981). Essentially, an apparatus is provided that allows the subject to adjust the sound intensity, by successively closer steps, to his or her own absolute

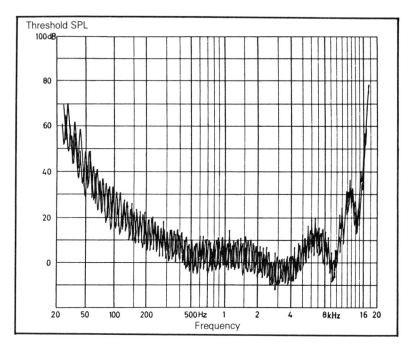

Figure 1.8
Example of a human hearing threshold plot (audiogram) traced by von Békésy audiometer. (From Zwicker & Feldtkeller 1981)

threshold while its frequency is slowly and steadily changed. The
subject continually varies the intensity between "just heard" and
"just not heard." A typical experimental run of this sort would use
a steady frequency change of about 1 octave/min (covering the whole
auditory range in between 4 and 8 min) with the increasing and
decreasing steps of intensity between the criteria being of order 2.5
dB/s (figure 1.8).

Measurements made on a very large population of young subjects
(18 to 25 years old) have established the classic curve of auditory
sensitivity (audiogram) for binaural listening under *free-field* conditions, that is to say, heard without earphones (ISO standard 1961).
It is clear that the minimal audible sound intensity field (figure 1.9)
depends on frequency. Its value passes through a minimum near 3
kHz and rises monotonically toward lower frequencies and in a more
complicated way toward high frequencies, these latter irregularities
being related to diffractions by the body, the external ear, and the
head of the subject. Threshold is considered to be effectively infinite

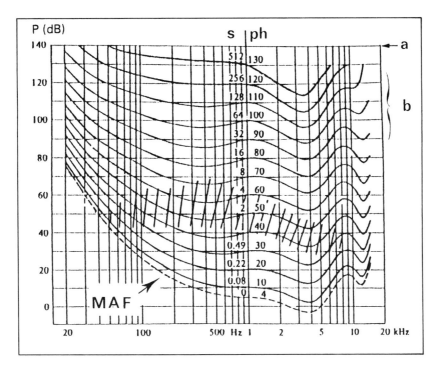

Figure 1.9
Curves of human audibility and equal loudness (free-field listening). Curve MAF is the internationally agreed average minimum audible field, averaged across many young listeners. The curves above the MAF are the internationally agreed contours of equal loudness level. Each curve is designated by the number of phons equal to the sound pressure level (db SPL) at 1 kHz (ordinate Ph). Ordinate S, subjective intensity or "loudness" in sones (see text); ordinate P, sound pressures in dB SPL with respect to $2 \cdot 10^{-4}$ μbar. The sound pressure levels of the frequencies in conversational speech measured in 1/3 octave bands at about 0.3 to 3 m from the speaker are indicated approximately by the shaded area. a, pain region; b, loudness discomfort; abscissa, frequency (log scale). (Modified from Evans 1982a)

below 20 Hz at the low-frequency end of the audiogram, and similarly infinite at the high-frequency end above 20 kHz. These limits at both the infrasonic and ultrasonic ends of the range are somewhat arbitrary; various authors report modifications of these estimates in one direction or the other. In spite of this, one can say that the human audible range comprises 10 octaves (Licklider 1951; Pieron 1945; Zwicker & Feldtkeller 1981; Scharf & Buus 1986; Scharf & Houtsma 1986; see Table 1.6).

Similar measurements have been made through headphones for binaural hearing. Under these conditions the curve for the absolute

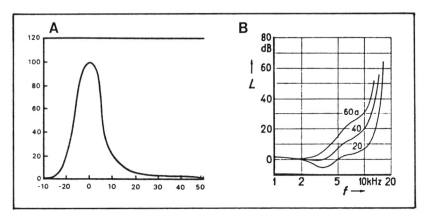

Figure 1.10
Hearing sensitivity as a function of age. *A*, Auditory sensitivity distribution in a 20-
to 29-year-old population. The absolute threshold was measured for 35,589 subjects at
880 Hz. *B*, Deterioration of auditory threshold for the higher frequencies due to age
(indicated as parameter). (*A* from Licklider 1951; *B* from Zwicker & Feldtkeller 1981)

threshold is often expressed as the *minimal audible pressure* at the
tympanic membrane. This method alone does not allow as precise
an estimate of the minimal audible pressure as would stimulating a
single tympanic membrane (under truly monaural conditions), and it
often does not show the irregularities toward the higher frequencies.

Finally, note that a reference minimal audible intensity to allow the
expression of sound levels in decibels has been fixed by the American
Standards Association as 20 μPa SPL (2×10^{-10} bar, corresponding,
as we have noted, to 1 pW $\cdot$ m^{-2} or 10^{-16} W $\cdot$ cm^{-2}; (International
Standards Organization 1966). Referred to a level of 1 μbar, this reference minimal pressure represents -80 dB (figure 1.9).

To make some estimate of deafness in an individual, it is important
to determine the variation of absolute threshold at any given frequency for people of similar age within the population. But it is not
always easy to distinguish between what is normal and abnormal.
For example, there is no clear discontinuity in the absolute threshold
values measured at 880 Hz in a population of 35,589 subjects aged
between 20 and 29 years (figure 1.10A).

In contrast, we know quite well that the greater the age of the
subject and the higher the testing frequency, the more rapidly the
threshold for hearing becomes raised. The curves in figure 1.10B illustrate this increasing deterioration graphically. Below 1 kHz there is

very little change of sensitivity with age, whereas at 10 kHz the auditory threshold at 60 years of age is 40 dB higher than at 20 years old, even when no other causes of deterioration than age, such as workplace noise in particular, have been encountered (Licklider 1951; Scharf & Buus 1986; Scharf & Houtsma 1986).

In most people the absolute threshold is not exactly the same for each ear. The normal interaural differences are somewhat variable and can attain 6 dB.

2.2 DIFFERENTIAL THRESHOLDS

Let us now examine two types of differential threshold that have been investigated extensively. One is the differential threshold for *intensity change*, the other for *frequency change*. In each case we shall consider monaural measurements.

DIFFERENTIAL THRESHOLD FOR INTENSITY

Pure Tones

In principle, change determining this threshold is a simple matter, since it consists in finding the change in intensity level (δL) that is just perceived by a subject (just-noticeable difference, jnd) in a sound of a particular frequency and of a particular intensity level L. In practice, many precautions need to be taken to avoid introducing transients (and therefore extra frequencies) by the process used to change the intensity. One resolution of this problem has been to modulate a sound's amplitude very slowly, the jnd then being specified as the smallest detectable fractional modulation change m_0 (modulation index m was defined earlier in the section on "continuous oscillations").

Suppose that the sound intensity in an amplitude-modulated wave swings between values I_{max} and I_{min} at threshold; then the differential threshold δL can be expressed in terms of the modulation index m:

$\delta L = 10 \log (I_{max}/I_{min})(\text{dB})$,

therefore

$\delta L = 20 \log \{(1 + m)/(1 - m)\}(\text{dB})$.

In practice, over a wide range of values of m (for $m < 0.3$) a good approximation is given by the expression

$\delta L = 17.5 m (\text{dB})$.

In this sort of experiment, one of the parameters concerned is the frequency of modulation. A whole series of preliminary experiments showed that the optimum frequency of modulation for yielding the smallest jnd at low modulation rates was around 4 Hz for humans. All the results that follow are based on a modulation rate near 4 Hz.

If a curve is plotted of δL (dB) as a function of L (dB), its negative slope is clear (figure 1.11). There is a jnd of 2 dB at 15 dB sound intensity, of 1 dB at 30 dB, and of 0.5 dB at 60 to 70 dB. (These data are for an audiofrequency of 1 kHz.) In others words, the jnd for modulation is about 10% (m = 0.1) at 20 dB, falling to 1% (m = 0.01) near 100 dB. Such a function is in no way like a Weber's law relationship, since the differential sensitivity decreases as one approaches lower intensities (Licklider 1951; Zwicker 1976; Zwicker & Feldtkeller 1981; Scharf & Buus 1986; Scharf & Houtsma 1986).

On the other hand, in contrast to its dependence on modulation frequency, the jnd for intensity does not vary very much with the audiofrequency of the sound.

White Noise

When the same sort of experiment is carried out using white noise, that is, a sound with a wide-band continuous spectrum, the practical difficulties are to some extent less, since some of the precautions just mentioned with respect to pure tones are not needed. We can, for instance, employ either a square-wave amplitude modulation (since much of its transient content is masked by the noise) or a sinusoidal amplitude modulation of the noise. In the case of noise, unlike for pure tones, the jnd (in decibels) is highest at low sound intensities then decreases with increasing intensity until attaining (at 30 dB and above) a plateau value of about 0.7 dB.

Figure 1.11 shows that at high sound levels, human hearing is more sensitive to intensity variations of pure tones than of noise and also that the noise sensitivity is relatively better for square than for sinusoidal modulation.

Band-Pass Noise

Let us examine what happens if the passband of the noise signal is not "infinite" as it is for white noise but of a limited extent δf. Assume again that measurements are made at a modulation rate near 4 Hz and at an appropriate sound intensity, such that the variation of jnd with modulation rate is not very great. If the noise bandwidth δf is broad, then the random modulation of the noise itself is rapid, so

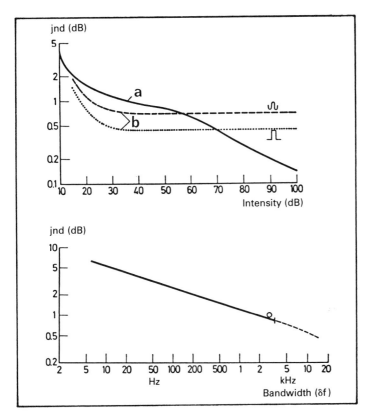

Figure 1.11
Just-noticeable intensity differences. *Above,* Variation of intensity jnd as a function of
intensity level. The full trace (a) is for a pure tone, the interrupted traces (b) are for wide
passband noise; dashes show sinusoidally modulated noise; dots show rectangularly
modulated noise (1 kHz sounds). *Below,* Variation of the intensity jnd for a rectangularly modulated noise as a function of the width δf of the passband measured from 2
Hz to 500 Hz, then from 1 kHz to 20 kHz. The open circle represents the jnd for very
wide bandpass noise. (From Zwicker 1976)

that the unmodulated noise sounds uniform, and a modulation superimposed at 4 Hz is clearly perceived ($m_0 = 4\%$, therefore $\delta L =$
~ 0.7 dB). The more the noise bandwidth is reduced, the more the
random noise modulation itself sounds like a definite audible tone
and the stronger the superimposed 4-Hz modulation needs to be
perceived for what it is. In other words the jnd for intensity increases
with decreasing noise bandwidth. In figure 1.11 (log/log plot), we
can see that the variation of jnd as a function of noise bandwidth δf
is linear with δL (dB) $= -k\delta f$. For $\delta f = 10$ Hz, the modulation needs
to be about 30% ($m = 0.3$) to be audible, equal to a jnd of about 5
dB.

Some authors (see, e.g., Jesteadt, Wier & Green 1977; Scharf &
Buus 1986) have advocated using a different method that is in some
respects more realistic (despite theoretical interpretive difficulties
arising from having to ignore some of the precautions mentioned
above). These researchers have compared, in any one subject, the
detection of separate "tone pips" of different intensities. The results,
although they are mutually self-consistent, do not immediately appear to be easily reconciled with those obtained from using continuous long-lasting modulations. (Comparing brief tones no doubt gives
greater prominence to detectors of the onset of a stimulus. These are
probably less important when the stimulus is present for some time
and is being continually modulated at a finite modulation rate. Maybe
this explains the differences between the results from the two
methods.)

DIFFERENTIAL THRESHOLD FOR FREQUENCY CHANGE

Measuring the differential sensitivity for frequency changes is also
beset by technical difficulties. These have been minimized by using
well-defined modulation waveforms and selecting well-controlled
modulation rates. In practice, workers have looked for the *minimum
detectable frequency swing.* (If the frequency f is modulated between
$f - \delta f$, and $f + \delta f$, the frequency swing in question is $2\delta f$.)

Using such methods it has become clear that δf depends on: (1) the
speed at which the modulation takes place, that is, on the modulation
rate (f_{mod}) and the waveform of the modulation (e.g., sinusoidal or
square); (2) the audiofrequency f of the sound; (3) its intensity level;
and (4) the duration of the stimulus.

As described above, it has been shown that at low modulation
rates the auditory system appears to be most sensitive for detecting

frequency change at an f_{mod} near 4 Hz. Once again, we will confine ourselves in what follows to measurements made near that modulation rate.

We can plot the differential threshold sensitivity for detecting frequency change either as δf as a function of f (figure 1.12) or, perhaps more commonly, the detectable, fractional, differential frequency change $\delta f/f$ as a function of f. In either case it is necessary to control and quote the intensity of the sound, a parameter which can cause the differential threshold to vary (Zwicker 1976; Zwicker & Feldtkeller 1981; Scharf & Buus 1986; Scharf & Houtsma 1986).

To summarize these results:

• For a sound level greater than about 20 dB, the (fractional) jnd $\delta f/f$ decreases between $f = 60$ Hz and $f = 1$ kHz (because in that frequency range the (absolute) jnd in frequency δf is almost constant, of magnitude about 2 to 4 Hz.
• In contrast, above $f = 1$ kHz, the perceptual jnd obeys a Weber-type law, δf increasing in direct proportion to the frequency increase with the result that the fractional jnd $\delta f/f$ remains practically constant at around 0.2 to 0.3 at frequencies up to around 8 kHz.
• Above that frequency, $\delta f/f$ increases once more. These characteristics are particularly clearly distinguished when $\delta f/f$ is plotted as a function of f.

[Values of the differential frequency jnds are of practical importance for deciding the limits of frequency fluctuations at different rates ("wow" and "flutter") that can be tolerated in commercial systems used for recording and playing back sounds.]

Just as in the experiments on intensity discrimination, other ways for determining jnds of frequency have been tried. In contrast to the usual method of exploiting continuous frequency modulation (used since Shower & Biddulph 1931 onward), some recent researchers have preferred to present brief tone pips that differ only in frequency (e.g., Wier, Jesteadt & Green 1977). The results of this sort of experiment are rather different from the above. The tone pip presentations show a constancy of δf only up to 500 Hz, with a smaller absolute differential detection value: Beyond 500 Hz the increase in δf with increasing frequency is steeper and conforms less well with a Weber-type relationship.

In whatever circumstance, the relative constancy of the differential fractional jnd over a wide frequency range ought to be emphasized,

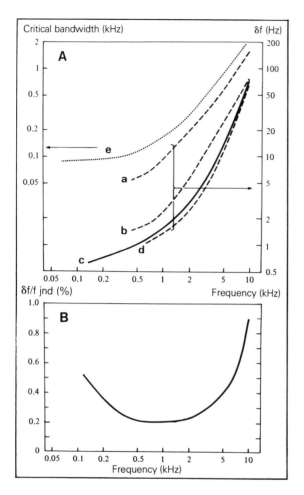

Figure 1.12
Frequency discrimination in humans. *A,* Differential threshold (jnd) for frequency change. The different curves are for different sound intensity levels: (a) 5 dB, (b) 20 dB, (c) 40 dB, and (d) 80 dB. Note that discrimination improves as the intensity increases up to 40 dB, and that the 5-dB curve is close to that of the variation (e) of the "critical bandwidth" with frequency (see text). *B,* Fractional jnd for frequency change δf/f as a function of frequency at 40 dB SL. The relative acuity for frequency change falls below 0.5 kHz and above 2 kHz. (From Evans 1982b)

remembering the importance of frequency *ratios*, particularly in music.

The jnd for frequency changes (for a given frequency) does not vary much with changes in sound intensity level. Generally it tends to be smaller with greater intensity (measured by a variety of experimental procedures); however, sensitivity for detecting a frequency change does deteriorate at very low sound levels. At sound levels between 5 and 20 dB, δf can exceed 10 Hz for a sound of frequency 1 kHz, such that $\delta f/f \approx 3\%$ (contrast 0.2% to 0.3% at higher sound levels).

When a subject is exposed to a *noise* signal, the modulation of its frequency is not very easily perceived when the noise concerned is broad-band white noise but can be heard when the signal is low-pass or high-pass and the cut-off frequency is modulated. It is interesting first of all to compare the action of these two types of signals as a function of intensity level. A high-pass signal behaves like a pure tone; the differential threshold (variation of frequency δf of the low-frequency cut-off at f that is just perceptible) is approximately independent of intensity, except at very feeble sound levels. In contrast, for low-pass signals in which, remember, it is the high-frequency cut-off that varies, the detectability of its frequency change δf deteriorates rapidly with increasing intensity.

As for the variation of the jnd δf as a function of the noise passband's cut-off frequency, it is quite like that for pure tone signals except that the sensitivity of detection is less for the noise signal. At 1 kHz, for example, the jnd δf for a pure tone is 2 Hz, whereas the detectable frequency change δf in the noise cut-off frequency needs to be as much as 20 Hz (the modulation rate being the same in all cases, near 4 Hz; figure 1.13).

The differential threshold for detecting frequency change also depends on the duration of the sound. Essentially, beyond a duration normally around 200 ms, the threshold jnd δf improves appreciably with inceasing duration, d. The relationship between δf and d is thus a function with a negative slope: This slope is steeper at low (≈ -1.5) than at high audiofrequencies (≈ -0.5). An explanation proposed for this difference postulates that different mechanisms for discrimination apply in different frequency ranges, spatial coding being predominant for high frequencies, temporal coding for low (see below).

[All the data in this chapter refer to the human subject. To remedy

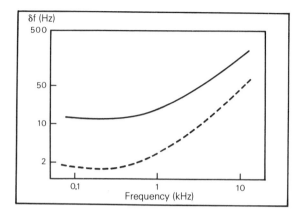

Figure 1.13
Jnds for frequency change. *Solid curve,* jnd for frequency change δf for high pass filtered noise as a function of upper frequency cut-off. Modulation frequency 4 Hz. *Dashed curve,* The curve (a) of figure 1.12 for a pure tone is presented for comparison. (From Zwicker & Feldtkeller 1981)

this to some extent, Table 1.6 lists the auditory ranges for several different vertebrates. Some of the data is inevitably incomplete, approximate, and vulnerable to revision (see, e.g., Fay 1988).]

3 SUPRATHRESHOLD HEARING OF PURE TONES

The range of audible intensity of sounds is extensive: 120 dB, a generally accepted upper limit for comfortable hearing, represents a power one million times that at threshold. Outside these limits, sensation stops being purely audible but also becomes a tactile flutter; very low frequencies elicit a tickling sensation, while at 130 to 140 dB the sound pressure level induces intolerable pain (see figure 1.9).

Audible sounds, though they can be specified purely objectively in physical terms, nevertheless possess subjective attributes, the perception of which needs to be studied also. It has long been recognized that *loudness* is related to intensity and *pitch* to frequency.

3.1 SCALES OF LOUDNESS AND SOUND INTENSITY

It is clear from examination of the plot of absolute threshold against frequency that sounds of the same physical intensity can have subjective sound levels that vary greatly with frequency. We shall now look at studies of the suprathreshold regions designed to quantify such differences (Licklider 1951; Zwicker 1976; Zwicker & Feldtkeller 1981).

Table 1.6. Approximate ranges of hearing in different species

Species	Low	High (kHz)
Human	20 Hz	20
Chimpanzee	100 Hz	20
Rhesus monkey	75 Hz	25
Squirrel monkey	75 Hz	25
Cat	30 Hz	50
Dog	50 Hz	46
Chinchilla	75 Hz	20
Rat	1 kHz	60
Mouse	1 kHz	100
Guinea pig	150 Hz	50
Rabbit	300 Hz	45
Bats	3 kHz	120
Dolphin (*Tursiops*)	1 kHz	130
Galago	250 Hz	45
Tupaia	250 Hz	45
Sparrow	250 Hz	12
Pigeon	200 Hz	10
Turtle	20 Hz	1
Frog	100 Hz	3
Goldfish	100 Hz	2
Ostariophysi	50 Hz	7
Other teleosts	50 Hz	1

Data taken from Fay 1988

THE SCALE OF EQUAL LOUDNESS

A first approach is to trace curves, point by point, obtained by asking subjects to match the loudness of tones that have different frequencies. Selecting a sound of 1 kHz and n dB, the examiner asks the subject to decide at what sound intensity each sound at one of many other frequencies, near or far, excites a sensation of the same subjective intensity (loudness). *Equal loudness* curves can thus be obtained in a quantitative way. From these can be specified a dimensionless unit, the *phon,* such that a sound or a noise is said to have an equal loundness level of n phons when it has been judged by a normally hearing subject to be as loud as a pure tone of frequency 1 kHz of n dB sound pressure level. The sounds should ideally arrive at the subject face on and have plain wavefronts. Very roughly, equal loudness curves constitute a family of curves that are approximately parallel to the curves of absolute thresholds (figure 1.9). Notice that in figure 1.9, the regions concerned with the perception of speech and music are indicated within this family of curves.

THE SCALE OF DIFFERENT LOUDNESS LEVELS: THE SONE

Experiment shows that the scale of phons is not itself satisfactory for estimating the loudness of one tone with respect to another. Various researchers have therefore designed experiments in which subjects are asked to make "vertical" estimates of loudness ratios rather than the ("horizontal") direct comparisons of equality just described. Typically, the subject's task in this sort of study is to set one tone at, for example, double or half the loudness of a reference tone of the same frequency.

The essential problem has therefore been to establish a scale of relative loudness, specified as values N with the unit designated the *sone*, and to try to compare the results from this sort of experiment with the (perhaps more objectively established) scale of equal loudness in phons.

All experiments lead to the following conclusion: at a given frequency, the subjective loudness of a sound doubles when its intensity is increased by 10 phons (provided the sound level is above 40 dB). In other words, the subjective loudness of a 1-kHz tone doubles when its intensity level is increased by 10 dB.

A loudness reference point is needed and has been internationally established by giving the loudness value of 1 sone to a sound of 1 kHz when delivered at a level of 40 phons and heard under free-field conditions (International Standards Organization 1961, 1966).

In this range of intensities N may be defined by

$$N_{\text{sones}} = 2^{0.1(L_N - 40)}$$

where L_N is the equal loudness level in phons, or expressed alternatively, by the (approximate) logarithmic form

$$\log_{10} N = 0.03 (L_N - 40).$$

This formulation in turn may equally well be expressed in terms of relative intensity level I/I_0 or, more often, of the sound pressure ratio p/p_0:

$$N_{\text{sones}} = (I/I_0)^{0.3}/16 = (p/p_0)^{0.6}/16.$$

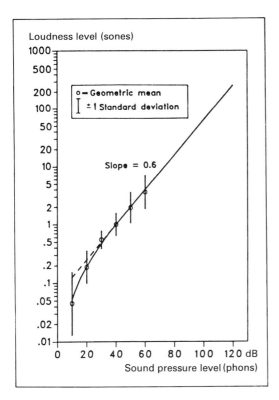

Loudness level (sones)

o = Geometric mean

∓ 1 Standard deviation

Slope = 0.6

Sound pressure level (phons)

Figure 1.14
Loudness of a pure tone. Loudness of a 1 kHz binaural pure tone (sones) as a function of sound level (phons) (log/log scales). As explained in the text, when plotted this way the function has a slope of −0.5 down to 40 dB. The dashed curve represents what would be seen if the same relationship held right down to absolute threshold. In fact, the solid curve inflects below 40 phons, since the subjective loudness then diminishes more quickly than the sound level. (From Scharf & Houtsma 1986)

Expressions of this sort are precisely the type of functions that have been shown, notably by Stevens (reviewed in Buser & Imbert 1982), to apply to the relationships between physical stimulus intensity and its perceptual correlate in a variety of sensory modalities. Figure 1.14 shows that a log/log plot of sones (ordinate) versus sound pressure level (abscissa) is linear (between 40 dB and 80 dB) with a slope of 0.6 (at 1 kHz). This is also illustrated in table 1.7, which shows values obtained by binaural, free-field experiments. We can see that at levels above 40 phons the subjective impression doubles when the sound level increases by 10 phons. In each illustration is it notable that at sound levels above 40 phons, loudness decreases more and more steeply with decreasing sound pressure.

THE LOUDNESS OF NOISE SIGNALS

It is clearly also necessary to consider the loudness of noisy sounds and to what extent it depends on the bandwidth of the noise. To answer this question, measurements have been made while varying

Table 1.7. "Objective" (phons) and "subjective" (sones) scales of relative loudness

Phons	Sones	Phons	Sones
10	0.052		
20	0.190	65	5.66
25	0.305	70	8.00
30	0.460	75	11.3
35	0.700	80	16.0
40	1.00	85	22.6
45	1.41	90	32.0
50	2.00	95	45.3
55	2.83	100	64.0
60	4.00	105	90.5
		110	128
		115	181
		120	256

the bandwidth of the noise and at the same time appropriately ad-justing the intensity spectral density levels so that the overall inten-sity of the noise remains constant. In fact, merely increasing the bandwidth of the noise would cause its total intensity to increase also, thus the need for the adjustment. Figure 1.15 shows how loud-ness varies as a function of the bandwidth, the parameter being the intensity of the sound in decibels. These results show that at all levels the auditory effect of this noise is independent of its bandwidth, provided that this is less than a certain value of δf, called the *critical band* (see also below). In this particular case δf equals 160 Hz. This experiment shows that noise intensity within a critical band can be either concentrated at one particular frequency or spread across the whole critical bandwidth δf. In contrast, when the noise bandwidth is increased beyond this critical value, the impression of loudness increases if the sounds are of moderate or high intensity (40 to 80 dB). On the other hand, the loudness stays pretty much the same or even decreases for feeble sounds on the order of 20 dB (Zwicker 1976; Zwicker & Feldtkeller 1981).

Remarks Concerning the Measurement of Thresholds
The family of curves in figure 1.9 showing the characteristics of an average, young, normally hearing subject was plotted from free-field results; the sounds were presented to the subject through a loud-

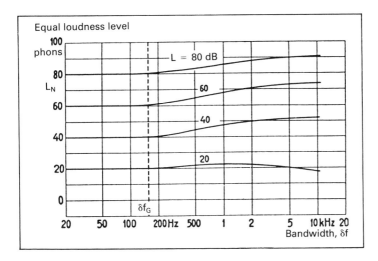

Figure 1.15
Equal loudness level for a noise band of constant overall spectral density as a function of its bandwidth (centered on 1 kHz). The vertical dashed line represents the width of the "critical band," 160 Hz in this case. L, sound level in dB for each curve. (From Zwicker & Feldtkeller 1981)

speaker placed in front of him, and later the sound parameters were calibrated via a microphone placed where the subject had been. The plot of this free-field measurement reveals the beneficial effects of the external and middle ear on sound conduction. They somewhat reinforce sensitivity around 3 kHz, a frequency within the zone of speech signals (see above). In practical audiology, an audiogram is normally plotted from measurements made using earphones and monaural stimulation. The curve of the threshold sound pressure level no longer shows some of the finer aspects that are seen in the free-field curve.

In routine audiology, it is current practice to specify the threshold as a function of frequency, not absolutely but by its ratio (expressed in decibels) to the threshold of a "standard" subject, who is adult, young, and healthy. This normal threshold is therefore designated 0 dB HL (*hearing level*) or 0 dB HTL (*hearing threshold level*). Any hearing loss relative to that in a particular subject is expressed in negative decibels.

In auditory psychophysics, intensities are specified not by their ratio to the threshold of the theoretical standard subject but to the threshold of the real subject who is being investigated. The designation dB SL (*sensation level*) is used by English-speaking investigators.

COMBINATIONS OF SOUNDS OF IDENTICAL OR VERY CLOSE FREQUENCIES

Consider two sinusoidal sounds with identical sound pressure levels and frequencies f_1 and f_2, which can be identical or very close.

When the *frequencies are identical*, if the two sounds are in phase their amplitudes reinforce one another. In contrast, when the sounds are in phase opposition they are antagonistic. This sort of antiphase cancellation is often used as a method for showing up the presence of a certain component in a mixture of different sounds. We shall see some examples of this later.

When the *frequencies are close*, the resulting sound is heard as a sound modulated in amplitude at a rate ($f_1 - f_2$): This phenomenon is usually referred to as *beats*. A rigorous study would show that this combination of sounds produces both amplitude modulation and some frequency modulation in general. This latter is nevertheless not usually easily perceptible.

3.2 A PITCH SCALE FOR PURE TONES

Let us now consider, as a parallel with what we have just discussed with respect to loudness, how the subjective pitch sensation that a sound creates is related to its frequency. It has been possible to achieve such a scale for subjective pitch using a unit called the *mel* for pitch level, such that by definition 500 mels corresponds to the pitch of a 500-Hz tone at 40 dB above threshold. It has proved possible to plot curves of pitch level as a function of frequency in a way analogous to plotting loudness levels as a function of intensity. The curves show clearly that subjective pitch increases less steeply the higher the sound's frequency becomes.

Below 500 Hz the pitch in mels is practically identical with the frequency in hertz; the relationship between the two is linear. At frequencies above this, the pitch begins to increase relatively less steeply, the relationship becoming more or less logarithmic. Thus it is notable that while 131 Hz (the musical note C_3) has a pitch of 131 mels and 500 Hz a pitch of 500 mels, the pitch of 5000 Hz is only 2000 mels and that of 16,000 Hz is merely 2400 mels (figure 1.16). Let us remember in this context that, whereas the auditory range might extend from 20 Hz to 20 kHz, pitch judgments are only reasonably accurate between about 100 Hz and 5 kHz. In fact, the establishment

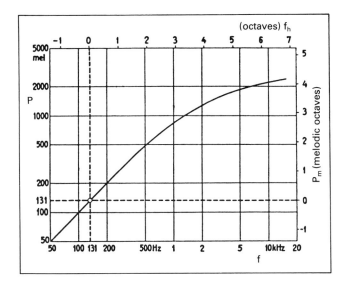

Figure 1.16
Pitch of a pure tone as a function of frequency. Lower abscissa, Frequency f (log
scale). Left ordinate, pitch P in mels (log scale). A reference point (open circle) is at
the coincident values 131 Hz (C_3) and 131 mels (dashed lines). Upper abscissa, octave
frequency scales of harmonic pitch f_h, referred to C_3. Right ordinate, octave scales of
melodic pitch P_m. (From Zwicker & Feldtkeller 1981)

of a scale of pitch as a function of frequency requires, like all estimates
of perceived magnitudes of stimuli, a series of precautions for worthwhile measurements that we do not have the space to discuss here.

HARMONIC PITCH AND MELODIC PITCH
We shall discuss the concept of dividing pitch into octaves in a later
section; for now, we note that frequencies in the ratio 2:1 give an
impression of unison and this ratio constitutes an octave. Therefore
we can construct a scale of octaves in terms of frequency, provided
we fix a reference tone to begin with (the note C_3, for example, 131
Hz). This scale defines the *harmonic pitch* of a tone, H_h, in octaves
against frequency in hertz:

$$H_h = 1/0.31 \cdot \log f/131.$$

Similarly, another scale can be constructed based instead on the
pitch scale in mels, again taking a tone of 131 mels as a base. This
scale defines the *melodic pitch* H_m against Z, the pitch in mels.

$$H_m = 1/0.31 \cdot \log Z/131.$$

These two scales of octaves, harmonic pitch determined by frequency and melodic pitch determined by subjective pitch, are plotted
in figure 1.16. It is clear that while the harmonic pitch can span seven
octaves, the spread of subjective pitch is no more than 4.3 octaves.

PITCH INTERVALS (TONALITY) AND PITCH LEVEL

The attribute of pitch is not necessarily describable in only one way.
First, we could consider pitch in terms of tonality, which recognize
the phenomenon that two notes differing by a fixed frequency ratio
$2:1$ (an octave) are perceived as having a common quality involving
pitch sensation (see below), a sensation that repeats itself for each
successive octave. Alternatively, we could attribute a pitch level to
the fact that a continuous, smoothly changing increase in audiofrequency leads to the sensation of an increasing pitch (Shepard 1982).

PITCH LEVEL AND INTENSITY LEVEL

The fact that the pitch of a pure tone can vary with the sound's
intensity has been known since the nineteenth century and studied
vigorously since then (Stevens 1935; Walliser 1969; Terhardt 1974, to
mention but a few). The method, in essence, consists in presenting
two pure tones in succession to the subject. One sound (the reference
tone) is of fixed frequency and sound pressure level, whereas the
second sound (the comparison tone) has its sound level fixed at a
different level and its frequency is adjustable. The task of the subject
is to adjust the frequency of the comparison tone until its pitch level
is perceived to be the same as the reference tone's.

All in all, the results from different studies are in agreement: An
increase in sound pressure level raises the pitch of high-frequency
sounds, does little to sound perception in the mid-range of pitch
levels, and makes the pitch of low-frequency sounds become even
lower than before. Note, however, that these experimental conclusions are extracted from results that show so wide an individual variation that the rules above are only a matter of statistical probability.
We illustrate the procedure below.

Terhardt (1974) presented his subjects with a reference tone of 40
dB SPL, then immediately afterward with a test tone of 40, 60, or 80
dB (both monaural and binaural listening were investigated). The
subject had to adjust the frequency of the test tone until test and
reference appeared to have the same pitch. The frequency of the
reference tone was one of 0.2, 1, 4, or 6 kHz, and an attempt was
made to determine a ratio (v) to characterize the relative discrepancy

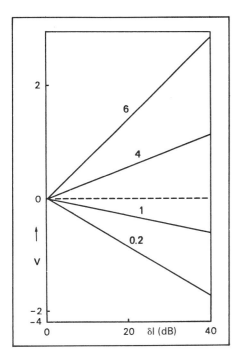

Figure 1.17
Subjective impression of the pitch of pure tones as a function of their intensity. The experiments are described in the text. v, Relative frequency disparity; δI, difference in intensity between the test and reference tones. Parameter: Frequency (kHz). (From Terhardt 1974)

between the reference (f_{40}) and test (f_T) frequencies for an equal pitch sensation:

$$v = (f_{40} - f_T)/f_T$$

In summary:

• At 1 kHz, the effect of intensity on perceived pitch is very feeble.
• At 200 Hz, the higher the intensity the lower the perceived pitch.
• At 4 kHz and still more so at 6 kHz, an increase in intensity brings with it a small increase in pitch level (figure 1.17).

As an aside, let us briefly discuss the question of so-called *absolute pitch*. It is possible to distinguish in the general population those who can make relative judgments of sound quality and those who can make absolute estimates. The former can classify one sound with respect to another and in particular can specify the pitch interval between two tones. Those endowed with absolute pitch (and they are rare) can specify the pitch of a tone without needing any recourse to a comparison tone. In reality, a significant number of these people probably possess only quasi-absolute pitch or learned pitch, which they acquire by exploiting personally convenient clues, such as the highest and lowest notes they can sing or, more generally, by using sensations that are generated when the vocal cords vibrate and are perceived when subjects quietly hum the sound they have heard. People with "true absolute pitch" can recognize a tone very quickly (2 s) and their most frequent errors are concerned with which particular octave the sound occupies. Most other people take much longer than 2 s to make a judgment. There is still doubt whether absolute pitch is inborn or acquired later. One rather old classic study suggests that absolute pitch is often a gift from the genes; it cannot be acquired late in life; it can only be acquired in a subject with an inbuilt predisposition to it; it is acquired more easily by those who are musicians; and it is more often observed in blind people than in the normally sighted. Those who are born blind do in fact tend to be enormously attentive to sounds, to such an extent that the acquisition of absolute pitch becomes more likely in them (Bachem 1937, 1940, 1954).

3.3 MASKING OF SOUNDS AND FREQUENCY RESOLUTION

A low-intensity sound that can be heard in a quiet environment may cease to be audible in noisy surroundings: This illustrates the phenomenon of *masking*. It can also happen that the relative audibility of a particular sound, if not abolished, might be diminished by the presence of another sound (Licklider 1951; Zwicker 1976; Zwicker & Feldtkeller 1981).

Let us identify the test tone (the sound that is masked) by T, its frequency being f_T and its intensity L_T, with the masker M having frequency f_M and intensity L_M. Masking may be total or partial; what is more, it is most clearly demonstrated during monaural testing. A tone applied to one ear can be masked by another applied to the opposite ear, but the effect is always very much less than in the monaural case.

Having outlined the effect, let us examine some of the more important factors that determine masking, such as the intensity of the masking tone, its spectrum, and also the relative frequencies of the masker and the masked tones.

MASKING OF A PURE TONE BY A PURE TONE

One type of experiment, no doubt the best known (Fletcher 1929; Zwicker 1976; Zwislocki 1978), consists in using a masking sound M of fixed frequency f_M (e.g., 1 kHz) and of fixed intensity level L_M

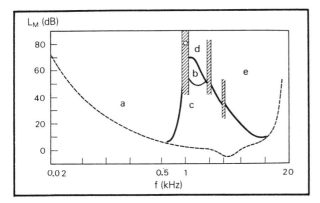

Figure 1.18
Masking of a pure tone by another pure tone. A masking tone M of frequency f_M = 1 kHz is applied at an intensity level L_M = 80 dB (open circle). *Solid curve,* Resulting masking plotted as threshold detectable intensity level L_M of a test tone T as a function of frequency. *Note:* It is possible to hear M and T simultaneously in regions (a) and (e); the tone M and the difference tone are heard in region (b); only M is heard in region (c); tones T, M and difference tone are heard in region (d). The hatched areas are where beats exist. The dotted line shows the audibility of T in the absence of M. (From Zwicker & Feldtkeller 1981)

(e.g., 80 dB), and measuring the value of L_T that is just perceptible at different f_T values (figure 1.18). It can be seen that:

• Masking is more pronounced when the frequency f_T is close to f_M.
• A masking tone is much more effective against sounds of higher frequency ($f_T > f_M$) than against lower-frequency sounds ($f_T < f_M$); in practical cases, therefore, low-frequency sound is more generally disturbing than high.
• A large contribution to masking resides in the monaural component.
• By evaluating how L_T varies as a function of L_M, it becomes clear that the masking effect increases linearly with the masker's intensity, provided f_T and f_M are close but with a relationship that is more complex when they are widely separated (figure 1.19).

In addition, when the intensity of the test tone is such that both the test tone and the masking tone can be heard simultaneously, their joint presence gives rise to complicated phenomena. Beats are heard when f_T is very close to f_M or to one of its higher harmonics. In the range $f_T \neq k \cdot f_M$ (k being a positive integer) the subject hears, depending on the intensities of the sounds, either a mixture of two

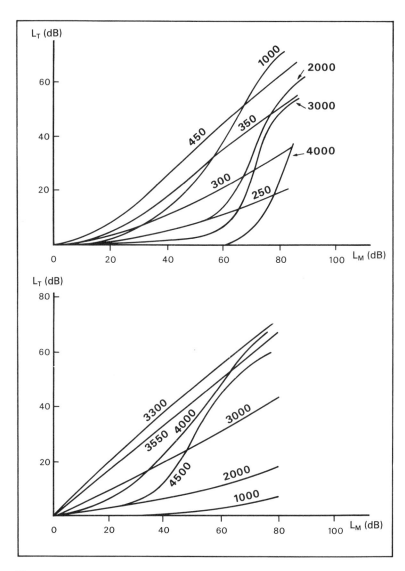

Figure 1.19
Variation of the liminal intensity of a masked tone. Liminal intensity L_T of a masked tone plotted in dB relative to its unmasked threshold, as a function of the intensity L_M of the masking sound. Parameter: Frequency in Hz of the masked sound. Masking frequency: 400 Hz upper diagram; 3.5 kHz lower diagram. (From Licklider 1951, after Fletcher 1929.)

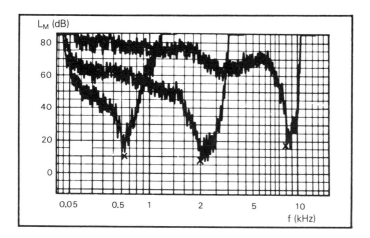

Figure 1.20
Thresholds for masking effects. Masking thresholds for three masked tones of frequencies (from left to right): 630 Hz, 2 kHz, 8 kHz. Sound pressure level L_M of liminal masking sound as a function of its frequency f (see text). (From Zwicker 1974)

tones, some mutual reinforcement, or their *difference tone* ($|f_M - f_T|$) (see below, "Hearing Two Pure Tones Simultaneously").

Another way of attacking this problem uses in some respects the opposite approach (Zwicker 1974), which is to determine what intensity L_M the masking sound must attain to be effective in masking a test sound T that has a fixed frequency and intensity. The intensity L_T is kept very low, on the order of 5 dB above the unmasked threshold. The subject determines the masking intensity L_M that is just needed to mask T at each of a variety of masking frequencies f_M. Curves plotted from these results show that (1) the further f_M is away from f_T the greater L_M needs to be; (2) high frequencies have a feeble or zero masking effect; (3) the curves obtained (in figure 1.20, for f_T 630, 2000, and 8000 Hz) are surprisingly like the profile of single auditory nerve fiber thresholds such as described below in the discussion of vertebrate neuronal analytical mechanisms. These latter are, it must be emphasized, obtained by quite different, neurophysiological methods. Such a similarity between independent psychophysical and neurophysiological data certainly deserves to be inspected. It suggests that an important part of masking might be effectively determined by the properties of the peripheral cochlear mechanisms and does not need much further elaboration in the more central nervous system to explain it.

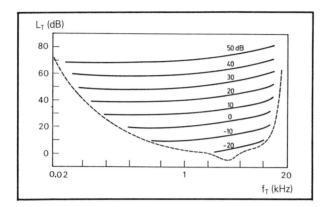

Figure 1.21
Masking of a pure sinusoidal tone (*T*) by white noise (monaural listening). Frequency f_T of tone *T* and the intensity L_T (dB SPL) that *T* must reach to be heard above the noise. Family of curves for different masking noise levels. (From Licklider 1951, after Hawkins & Stevens 1950)

MASKING OF A PURE TONE BY WHITE NOISE

When a masking noise signal has a given intensity I_R, the threshold of audibility of a test tone L_T (the intensity required to be just heard above the noise) as a function of the test tone's frequency demonstrates two regimens (figure 1.21):

• Below 500 Hz the curve is practically horizontal; the threshold for audibility does not vary.
• Above 500 Hz the threshold for audibility rises by 10 dB for each tenfold increase in frequency (by 4 dB per octave).

In contrast, masking rises very steeply as a result of increasing the masker's intensity spectral density. It follows from all this that a noise signal with an intensity spectral density that is made constant up to 500 Hz and is thereafter progressively attenuated in proportion to frequency (at a rate 10 dB per tenfold frequency increase) provides a sound that is a *uniform masker*, affording a pure tone masking curve that is horizontal and independent of the pure tone's frequency.

SIMULTANEOUS, FORWARD, AND BACKWARD MASKING

We now introduce a further parameter in our consideration of masking effects: the time at which the test tone *T* is applied in relation to the masking sound *M*. Apart from *simultaneous masking* (*T* applied

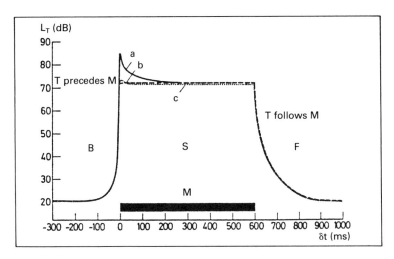

Figure 1.22
Backward and forward masking. Backward masking (B), simultaneous masking (S), and forward masking (F) as demonstrated by the level L_T (dB) of a test signal T (white noise or 2 ms tone pip of 5 kHz) as a function of the delay δt between the beginning of the màsking sound M and the beginning of the test signal (ms). The masking is effected by white noise or by narrow-band noise whose intensity has been adjusted to have the same masking effect in the steady state. Duration of the masking tone given by dark bar M. Transient effects are seen when the 5 kHz test tone is masked by white noise (a), but this overshoot is not present when the same tone is masked by narrow band noise (b) nor when white noise is masked by white noise (c). (From Zwicker 1975)

with M), there also exists a residual masking after M is turned off (*forward masking*) and even another masking such that the audibility threshold of T is worsened if it is present just before M is turned on (*backward masking*). The time course of these masking effects is shown in figure 1.22 in terms of the threshold of a tone T applied before, during, or after the hearing of a masking tone M. It is clear that:

• The threshold increases rapidly during the 10 ms (for low frequencies) or 30 ms (for high frequencies) *before* the beginning of the tone M.

• In contrast, forward masking lasts longer (for about 120 ms) *after* the tone M is turned off.

• Under certain conditions, the beginning of simultaneous masking shows an overshoot when the test is a pure tone (e.g., 5 kHz as in figure 1.22) and M is wide-band noise. In contrast to this, there is no overshoot when the two sounds T and M have similar bandwidths

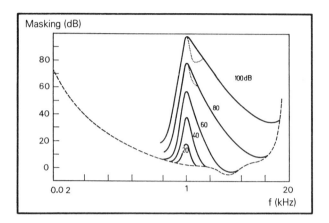

Figure 1.23
Masking of a pure tone by narrow-band noise (bandwidth 90 Hz, centered on 1 kHz) as a function of the pure tone's frequency. Parameter: Masker's intensity level (dB). (From Zwicker 1976)

(both sounds pure tones, or one sound a pure tone and the other narrow band, or both sounds wide band).

MASKING BY NARROW-BAND NOISE: THE CRITICAL BAND AND THE FREQUENCY RESOLUTION OF THE AUDITORY SYSTEM

As long ago as 1940, Fletcher established that when a tone is masked by white noise, only the noise frequencies near that of the test tone play an important part in the masking. (Note that in masking a tone by white noise, no audible beats complicate the issue).

The results of a typical experiment are shown in figure 1.23. In this case, the masking tone consists of a narrow-band noise signal, for example, one that is centered on 1 kHz with a bandwidth of 160 Hz (1000 ± 80). The intensity of the just-perceptible pure tone test signal very clearly shows a maximum value at the central frequency. For frequencies to either side of this maximum, the curves showing the effect of the masking fall very quickly toward the low frequencies; for the higher frequencies, the curves also fall, but with a distinctly lesser slope which depends strongly on the intensity of the masking noise.

Inexorably, the data came to suggest that the minimal bandwidth δf able fully to mask a tone at its particular central frequency f has a physiological correlate in the frequency discrimination of the cochlea itself. This minimal frequency bandwidth thus became defined as the *critical band* δf_c.

A variety of researchers began to exploit diverse ways of estimating the critical band. For example, Zwicker (1975) used narrow-band noise as the test signal T and investigated how it was masked by a combination of two pure tones, one at a higher frequency than T and the other at a lower frequency. When the difference between these two frequencies is diminished to something less than 150 Hz, the test tone's detectability deteriorates, whereas when the frequency separation is greater than 150 Hz, the threshold detectability improves rapidly with increasing frequency separation. The resulting plot of the masking data from experiments such as this allows us to specify the width of a *psychophysical band-pass filter* around each selected frequency.

Some workers criticize this method, however, suggesting that there might be an interaction between the masking and masked tones when they are present simultaneously. Houtgast (1972) made other experiments using nonsimultaneous forward masking. The psychophysical band-pass filters, measured this way, are different from those established by simultaneous masking. First, the pass band is narrower. Second, and more significant, there exist inhibitory zones to either side of the pass band that simultaneous masking does not reveal; this "lateral inhibition" is particularly clear to the high-frequency side.

Whatever might be the details of the matter, the auditory system does seem, from these results, to operate like a system of bandpass filters each having a certain critical bandwidth δf_c. Experiments testing this general concept bring with them the following interesting implications:

The critical bandwidth varies with frequency. Experimentation on this effect carried out by psychophysical techniques in humans and by behavioral techniques in other animals shows much similarity between the shapes of the experimentally established plots of δf_c as a function of f (figure 1.24).

Certain researchers, among them Zwicker (1975; Zwicker & Feldtkeller 1981), have pointed out the probable fundamental importance of a *critical interval*. He used, in this context, a unit larger than the mel but with the same dimensions, called the Bark (1 Bark = 100 mels). The curve of pitch intervals as a function of frequency extends

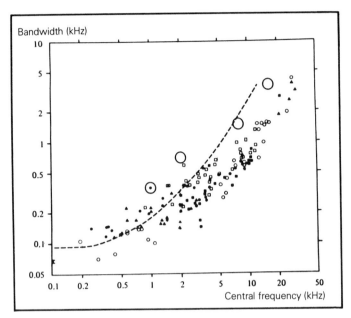

Figure 1.24
Effective bandwidths and critical bandwidths. Comparison of the operating frequencies defined by neurophysiology (effective bandwidth) or by psychophysics (critical band); see text for definitions. The small symbols refer to the effective bandwidth for single nerve fibers as a function of their characteristic frequency for various animals. Each symbol represents one animal (see text). The dashed curve shows the variation of the critical bandwidth as a function of the central frequency. The large circles are critical bandwidths for the cat determined behaviorally. (From Evans 1982b)

over 24 Barks, with a linear section (remember section 3.2) at low frequencies (< 500 Hz) and a log relationship at higher frequencies. This range must be encompassed within the 32 mm of the human cochlea. The interesting fact about the Bark as a unit is that it represents along the whole length of the cochlea the frequency separations corresponding to each critical band (see figures 1.16 and 1.25).

In addition, a comparison of these curves with those showing (in the same system of coordinates) the variation of threshold detectable frequency difference (jnd) as a function of frequency (and of intensity) suggests some striking similarities. At low intensity levels (near 5 dB), the critical bandwidths δf_c vary with frequency just like the jnd δf. This suggests a significant and close relationship between frequency resolution and the critical bandwidth.

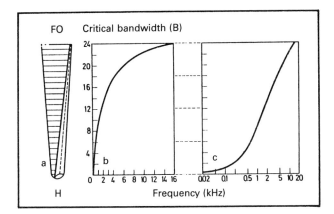

Figure 1.25
Critical bandwidths and distance along the basilar membrane. *a,* Alignment of critical bands along the basilar membrane from the helicotrema (H) to the fenestra ovalis (FO). *b* and *c,* The corresponding disposition of the critical bandwidths in Barks (B) (ordinates, linear scales) as a function of their central frequency. Frequency scale for b is linear and for c is logarithmic). (From Zwicker 1976)

It is also possible to relate the masking power of white noise centered at a particular frequency f to critical bandwidths (Hawkins & Stevens 1950). That is, when the *effective sound level* of the masker (i.e., the noise power within a critical band at f, expressed in decibels above the absolute threshold detectable power level at that frequency) is plotted against its masking effect in decibels, a linear relationship is revealed that is entirely independent of f. Whatever the frequency, the points fall on the same curve (figure 1.26).

Finally, we need to ask whether these entirely external psychophysical stimuli and responses can be assumed to reveal the filtering properties of the basilar membrane itself or an elaboration reached in concert with central mechanisms. The answer to this question is not immediately obvious. Nevertheless, as we shall see in chapter 2, there are corresponding curves that describe the bandpass characteristics of cochlear nerve fibers (e.g., bandwidths defined in essentially analogous ways to those used for specifying critical bands). Experiments show that these bandwidths in general follow the same variations as a function of their central frequency as do the psychophysically determined critical bands, though at any given frequency the nerve bandwidths are rather narrower (see figure 1.24). Evidence in the electrophysiological behavior of nerve fibers also demonstrates

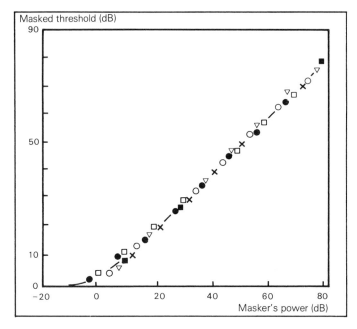

Figure 1.26
Sound power in a critical bandwidth. Relationship between the masking sound power within the critical band corresponding to a certain central frequency f (ratio, in dB, of sound power to threshold detectable power) against the sound intensity of a just perceptible pure tone of the same frequency f applied simultaneously (masked threshold, dB). The relationship is linear and, with this experimental method, is independent of the frequency; open squares, 350 Hz; filled circles, 500 Hz; open circles, 1 kHz; filled squares, 2.8 kHz; crosses, 4 kHz; open triangles, 5.6 kHz. (From Licklider 1951 after Hawkins & Stevens 1950)

flanking inhibitory regions similar to what has been discovered psychophysically by nonsimultaneous masking. Acoustic nerve fiber responses show regions of antagonistic interactions between a centrally placed tone and one situated more laterally to the central regions ("two-tone suppression"). In contrast, two tones existing together in the central regions would be mutually reinforcing.

3.4 TEMPORAL EFFECTS

Below are described, beneath this single heading, data concerned with a wide variety of effects in the psychophysics of hearing. Nevertheless, they all share a common concern with time as the independent variable.

The experimental evidence for forward masking, the masking effect of a sound after it has ceased, involves the measurement of the detectability of a test tone delivered to the subject some time after the end of the "conditioning" tone. In this procedure, the test tone T is turned on immediately after the subject has heard the conditioning (or masking) tone C. The amount of forward masking is measured and the phenomenon is further tested for how the masking changes with respect to three parameters in particular: the intensity level L_c of the masking stimulus, the frequencies of the masking and testing sounds f_c and f_T, respectively, and, finally, the interval τ between the end of C and the emission of T (Garner 1947; Lüscher & Zwislocki 1947; Zwislocki 1978).

The experimental results can be summarized thus:

• For the case $f_c = f_T$, the detectability threshold of T increases above its unadapted value when T is generated less than 200 ms after the end of C. This threshold elevation suggests the existence of an auditory fatigue, or alternatively, demonstrates a loss in sensitivity of the auditory system due to previous exposure to a masking sound (figure 1.27).

• The threshold elevation is greater the greater the intensity L_c of the masking sound. For a fixed delay τ after the end of C, the relationship between the masking effect and L_c is practically linear provided that L_c is greater than some particular value (20 dB in figure 1.28) that depends on the precise conditions.

• In the case $f_T \neq f_c$, the curve $L_T = \Phi\ (L_c)$ depends on the frequency separation, although the form of the curves remains essentially similar.

All the effects just described refer to monaural stimulation. When the same experiments are carried out with C applied to one ear and T to the other, scarcely any loss of detection sensitivity for T is observed. The predominant effect is thus peripheral, not central.

The threshold changes concerned in forward masking should not be confused with other types of phenomena. First, they should be distinguished from a true *auditory fatigue,* which is defined as the modification of hearing sensitivity after prolonged exposure to a

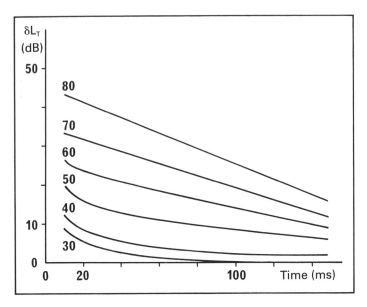

Figure 1.27
Time course of forward masking. The threshold elevations δL_T (dB), measured at times (in ms) soon after the termination of a masking tone pip of duration 400 ms and of the intensity indicated at each curve. Monaural experimentation. (From Licklider 1951 after Lüscher & Zwislocki 1947)

sound. When a sound such as the one described above as "conditioning" (which in the case of masking experiments lasts 1 s at the most) is in fact prolonged for several minutes, then a sensitivity loss is observed that can itself be prolonged and is characterized by (1) a rise in threshold (from 10 to 30 dB for a fatiguing sound of 100 dB); (2) a loss of subjective loudness in a suprathreshold test tone, provided it is 40 to 50 dB less intense than the sound responsible for the fatigue (Botte & Scharf 1980); and (3) a return to normal detection sensitivity that occurs much more slowly in fatigue than in forward masking.

Consider another type of experiment, in which a subject undergoes prolonged exposure to a given tone of constant intensity but this time makes successive estimates of its subjective loudness during that stimulation; this mode of operating is distinct from testing after the end of a stimulus as in the above cases of masking and fatigue. It is then observed that if the sound is feeble (10 dB), the subject experiences a loss of loudness, or what is referred to as a *simple adaptation.* This sort of adaptation is not observed when the constant sound is

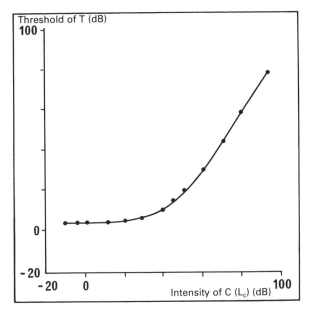

Figure 1.28
Effect of a prior conditioning tone on a test tone. One experimental method is to use conditioning tone C and test tone T that are of different frequencies and to observe the effect *either* of the delay of T after C *or* of the intensity level L_c of C on the threshold for detecting T. In this example, the C–T interval has been fixed at 54 ms and the independent variable is L_c. Notice that the perception threshold increases with increasing L_C demonstrating the conditioning of the system. (From Licklider 1951 after Garner 1947)

more intense (50 dB). However, if the sound is intense (40 dB) and is not constant but is, for instance, modified periodically (say its intensity is increased to 60 dB for 20 s every 15 s) or suffers some other sort of intermittent change, then adaptation is observed once more. This effect is sometimes referred to as *induced adaptation* (Scharf & Buus 1986; Scharf & Houtsma 1986).

ADAPTATION BY MODULATED SOUNDS

A special case of adaptation of the auditory system that is particularly interesting concerns adaptation by sounds modulated in amplitude (AM) or in frequency (FM). Authors have emphasized the importance of using such AM and FM sound stimuli to investigate the auditory system's operation (Kay 1982; see also chapter 3, 1.2).

From a whole range of experiments (which we do not have space to specify in detail), it has been shown that exposure to a given modulated sound (AM or FM) for, say, 10 seconds generates a deterioration in the modulation's threshold detectability for some time immediately after that exposure. The amount of adaptation in modulation detectability is tuned optimally at the adaptor's modulation rate and is less at nearby modulation rates. This adaptation does not occur after exposure to differently modulated or to otherwise dissimilar sounds of comparable intensity. This excludes simple generalized "fatigue" as an explanation of the adaptation. It is a function of the modulation itself. The conclusion is that the auditory system contains a certain number of "channels" dedicated to the detection of AM and FM in sounds that are tuned in modulation rate. These channels might be expected to play a part in detecting the temporal changes of frequency and amplitude that occur in complex sounds. The more familiar experimentation on the auditory system based on click or pure tone detection can only directly correspond with acoustic events that are relatively rarely experienced in day-to-day life by the auditory system. The natural sounds most often encountered are more complex ones than clicks or pure tones, being modulated in amplitude and/or frequency and, particularly importantly in the human case, modulated to generate the speech sounds of the human voice.

INFLUENCE OF STIMULUS DURATION ON THRESHOLD EFFECTS: BRIEF SOUNDS

The threshold effects that we have been concerned with (such as absolute threshold and the differential thresholds of intensity change and frequency change) are independent of time only for stimuli that are present for more than a certain stimulus duration. As we shall see, for lesser stimulus durations, time becomes a limiting factor. The sensitivity of the auditory system depends on how long it can inspect the stimulus.

In audition, as in other sensory modalities, the absolute intensity detectability threshold I of a stimulus (a sound in this case), while it is rather constant for stimulus durations greater than a particular value, increases progressively when the stimulus duration d is shorter than that (Garner 1947).

It has been possible to establish a relationship of the form $L \cdot d = C$ where C is a constant and L is the liminal intensity. This relationship, plotted in log/log coordinates (L in decibels, i.e., log I as a function of log d), yields a straight line of negative slope (log $I = C - \log d$,

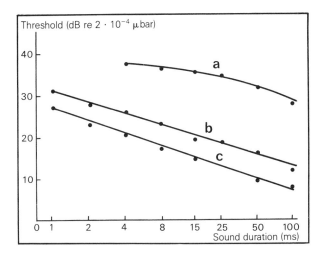

Figure 1.29
Temporal integration of the absolute threshold of sounds. (a) 250 Hz pure tone. (b) Noise. (c) 4 kHz pure tone. (From Licklider 1951 after Garner 1947)

$L_{dB} = C - \log d$). For a variety of sound intensities of pure tones and also of noise signals, these curves are parallel, though separated from one another. But the relationship is only valid for durations less than about 180 ms (figure 1.29).

Another interesting investigation of temporal effects concerns establishing, at a given frequency and sound intensity L, how the duration of an intensity change affects the magnitude of the just perceptible δL (Miller & Garner 1944). Here again there is a duration for which time becomes a limiting factor, in this case at about 400 ms. The curves in figure 1.30 show how $\delta L/L$ increases with decreasing duration of the change δL at different frequencies and sound intensities.

The differential threshold for detecting a frequency change depends equally on its duration (Legouix 1974). It has been established that for tone pips shorter than about 200 ms the threshold δF increases markedly, and consequently, for one given frequency, so does the just-detectable fractional change $\delta f/f$ (figure 1.31).

INFLUENCE OF STIMULUS DURATION ON SUPRATHRESHOLD EFFECTS

The effects of signal duration have been studied for a variety of suprathreshold phenomena, but we shall confine this discussion to three only. We shall see once again that for sounds of less than a given

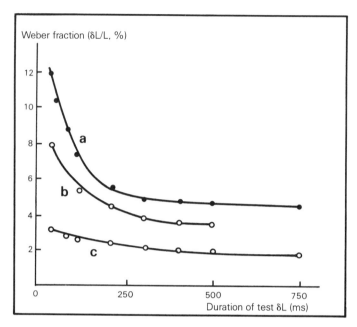

Figure 1.30
Variation of the Weber fraction δL/L. For a sound of frequency f and intensity level
L, the fraction $\delta L/L$ (Weber fraction) for the jnd δL increases the shorter the duration
of the test δL (at <500 ms). (a) 500 Hz, 40 dB; (b) 1 kHz, 40 dB; (c) 500 Hz, 70 dB.
(From Licklider 1951 after Miller & Garner 1944)

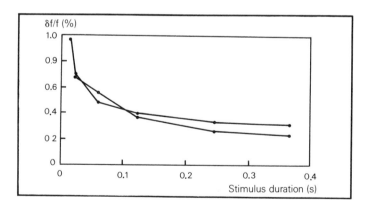

Figure 1.31
**Differential threshold for detecting frequency change as a function of stimulus dura-
tion.** Results for two subjects, 800 Hz pure tone at 40 dB SL. (From Legouix 1974 after
von Békésy 1960)

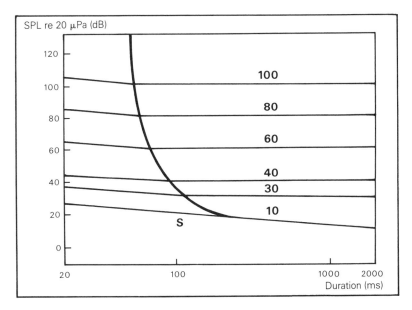

Figure 1.32
Loudness of brief sounds. The intensity SPL (re 20 μPa) of a brief pulse of white noise as a function of its duration (in ms) when it is matched audibly to that of a constant reference of white noise, duration 1 s. Below a certain duration, the subjective impression of intensity decreases; the test sound's true intensity has to be increased to match the reference. The steeply rising curve connects the limiting durations beyond which the sound intensity becomes independent of duration. Parameter: Intensity of the reference tone. (From Licklider 1951 after Miller 1948)

duration, time can become the limiting factor in how suprathreshold signals are perceived, quite apart from its effects on sensory thresholds.

There have been investigations of how the plots of equal loudness for brief sounds vary as a function of their short duration (Miller 1948). In a typical experiment, the subject is asked to match the loudness of a brief white noise signal to that of a long-lasting (1 s) one. This method shows that for signals lasting less than 100 to 200 ms, the subjective loudness diminishes with diminishing duration. This is shown by the plot in figure 1.32, which also makes it clear that the influence of duration is somewhat more marked at increasingly lower sound intensity.

The perceived pitch of brief sounds has also been investigated, covering time durations from about 2 to 500 ms (these might comprise a few sinusoidal waves only). Three separate perceptions have been

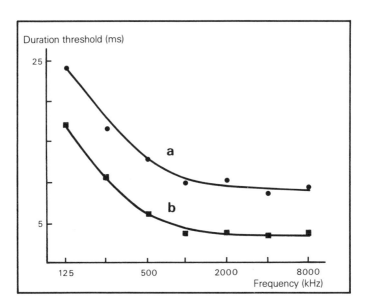

Figure 1.33
The perception of brief sounds. Duration threshold for a sound to be perceived as a click (squares) or as a tone (circles) as a function of frequency. Below 1 kHz it is a minimum number of cycles (2 or 3) that is needed for tonality to be perceived; above 1 kHz this perception needs a particular sound duration. (From Doughty & Garner 1947)

distinguished: First, for very short durations, the sound is perceived as a "click" without tonal quality; at some longer duration, the stimulus is heard as a click but to which is added also some attribute of tonality; an even longer stimulus might be heard as an initial click followed by a tone sensation and then a terminating click.

In a related observation, the minimal duration needed for a single sinusoidal sound to be perceived as possessing a tonal pitch has also been investigated (Doughty & Garner 1947). It has been found that for frequencies higher than 1 kHz a constant *minimal stimulus duration* is needed, whatever its frequency might be, whereas at frequencies below 1 kHz a *minimal number of cycles* of the sound wave must be present. This explains the increases in the curves of figure 1.33 in that lower range of frequencies. As could have been predicted from the findings in the previous paragraph, the curves also show the need for a longer duration of the sound for it to be heard as a tone rather than as a click.

4 BINAURAL EFFECTS

4.1 THE LOCALIZATION OF SOUND SOURCES

This section explores the mechanisms that allow a subject to localize sound sources. In day-to-day life, head movements (and in a variety of animal species movements of the external ear) also can help such localization. Nevertheless, sources can be identified by using purely auditory mechanisms. (Note that under the experimental conditions described, the subject's head will have remained fixed.) These studies tend to concentrate on one or both of two distinct and complementary skills: sound *localization* (in real space) and *lateralization* (distinguishing left from right).

BINAURAL LISTENING

One experimental situation refers to *binaural* conditions in which the subject is asked to listen to a distant source, ideally a point source, either under free-field conditions or in an anechoic room (in either case, ensuring that there should be no echo to interfere with the measurements). Let us consider a source emitting a *pure tone* at a given frequency; the case of transient sound will be considered later.

Localization in the Horizontal Plane
Consider the case of the sound source situated in the same horizontal plane as the ears and more than 1 m away from the subject in an echo-free environment. The subject, under binaural, free-field hearing conditions, is asked to localize the source by specifying its azimuth (the median, vertical, plane being specified as 0° to the front, 180° to the rear, and the vertical plane through the ears as 90° right or left). In these conditions it becomes evident that subject's accuracy in localization is frequency dependent. The maximal errors occur between 2 kHz and 4 kHz (Stevens & Newman 1936a). This nonmonotonic curve of error against frequency provided a logical argument in favor of a *duality theory* of localization mechanisms that has been current since the 1930s. We can easily see that a pure tone emitted by a source placed laterally to the median plane of the head (1) traverses a shorter path to one ear than to the other and (2) encounters the head as an obstruction to its reaching the far ear without hindrance.

The theory predicted (see below) that localization at frequencies less than about 2 kHz would be based on interaural time differences (ITD), whereas above 4 kHz interaural intensity differences (IID)

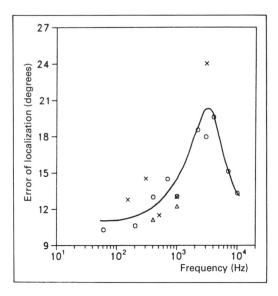

Figure 1.34
Localization in the horizontal plane. The difference in degrees between the reported and actual azimuth of a clickless, filtered, pure tone is plotted as a function of the tone's frequency. Tones at 400 Hz and 4 kHz were at 50 to 60 phons; lower and higher frequencies were at about 30 phons. The subject judged the position of the loudspeaker in steps of 15° at 13 positions from 0° to 180° azimuth. Front/back confusions were not counted as errors. Crosses, earlier measurements; circles, later measurements; triangles, unfiltered tones with broader spectra. The line drawn through the data indicates that the worst localization is in the mid-frequency range, improving below 2 kHz and above 5 kHz. (From Scharf & Houtsma 1986 after Stevens & Newman 1936a)

would be exploited. And it was possible to assume that at frequencies between 2 kHz and 4 kHz neither of these two mechanisms operates near its best efficiency, explaining poorer localization in that intermediate frequency range (figure 1.34).

Localization in the Median Plane

In theory, a source located in the median (sagittal) plane ought to cause complete confusion among sources that are in front of, behind, or above the head, since there are no intensity or phase differences to be expected at the ears. The facts are otherwise, since differences can be found. These are frequency dependent and are concerned with the transfer function of the outer ear (between the open air and the tympanic membrane).

In studying *front-to-back discrimination*, Stevens and Newman

(1936a) showed that confusions were much worse at frequencies below 2.5 kHz (35%) than above, being no more frequent than 10% above 3 kHz. Blauert (1983) has recently added more detail concerning front-to-back differences, showing that a sound to the front is relatively louder than one to the rear for frequencies between 250 and 500 Hz, with the opposite result between 800 and 1800 Hz, returning once more to dominance of the anterior source above 4 kHz (figure 1.35).

Up and down discrimination (for sources between $-13°$ and $+20°$) only seems to be possible at high frequencies.

Localization away from the Median Plane
Away from the median plane, on the other hand, up and down and front-to-back discriminations relative, respectively, to the horizontal and frontal planes passing through the line of the ears are made difficult at low frequencies by the existence of "hyperboloids of confusion" ("cones of confusion"). Sources situated on the surfaces of these generate equivalent interaural disparities.

Precision of Lateral Localization
Mills (1958) set out to determine the accuracy of lateral localization of an effectively point source in terms of the jnd in azimuth $\delta\Theta$ (the minimal angle through which a source needs to be displaced for the subject to perceive a change in position). He was able to show that

• This threshold $\delta\Theta$ is a function of the azimuth, the maximum sensitivity being shown near the median plane for all frequencies.
• Sensitivity decreases with increasing azimuth away from that plane, $\delta\Theta$ becoming very large beyond 60°.
• The magnitude of the threshold is also a function of frequency; near the median plane it is relatively poorer between 1 kHz and 3 kHz, and at very lateral azimuths becomes scarcely measurable in this frequency range (figure 1.36).

DICHOTIC METHODS FOR THE STUDY OF LATERALIZATION AND LOCALIZATION
In current practice, detailed investigations of the mechanisms actually employed in localizing sounds usually exploit *dichotic* stimulation. In this method, each ear receives its own stimulus separately through headphones. The two stimuli can be alike or differ in intensity or in phase or both. During dichotic stimulation a subject perceives a source that can be lateralized (*fused sound image*, or *virtual source*).

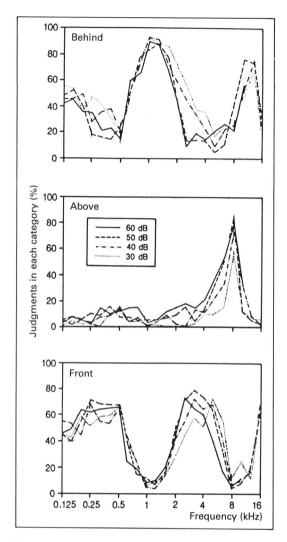

Figure 1.35
Judgments of direction in the median plane. Percentage of judgments that a third-octave-bandwidth signal came from behind, above, or in front plotted as a function of center frequency. Parameter shown for the curves is the signal's sound level in decibels. (Adapted from Blauert 1983 and Scharf & Houtsma 1986)

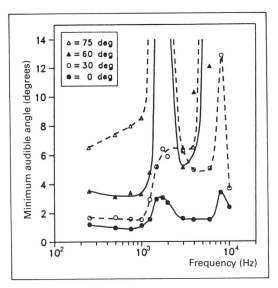

Figure 1.36
Minimum audible angle for pure tones. Source positioned 50 cm in front of the listener's head. On each trial, a 1-s duration, 50-dB SL, tone is first presented from the reference position then moved either to left or right and presented again after a 1-s interval. Subject judges whether source moved to left or to right. Detectable angular change as a function of frequency for four different azimuths. For all azimuths, localization is worst between 1.5 kHz and 2.2 kHz and again deteriorates above about 5 kHz (From Scharf & Houtsma 1986 after Mills 1958)

Although it can be lateralized, it is often perceived as being localized within the head; the sensation of distance is, to an extent, absent under these conditions.

Localization of (Continuous) Pure Tones
Dichotic experiments using pure tones, more than any other method, made it possible to quantify the two mechanisms involved: a *temporal disparity* between the two sounds (which particularly for a sinusoidal signal can also be specified as a *phase* difference)—predominantly at low frequencies (<1.5 kHz) and, at high frequencies (>1.5 kHz) as an *intensity disparity.*

Concerning the *localization of low-frequency sounds,* we have already pointed out that the head is too small compared with the low-frequency sound's wavelength to cast a well-marked sound shadow. Indeed, as long ago as 1896, Rayleigh illustrated this effect with reference to the note C$_4$, 256 Hz. The sound's wavelength is 1.34 m and therefore (the head assumed to be a sphere of 19-cm diameter), diffraction plays a large part; the attenuation of the sound intensity by the head is only about 1%. [Recall that the velocity of sound at normal room temperature of 20°C is 343 m/s. At this temperature, the wavelength (speed/frequency) of audible sinusoidal sounds ranges between 17.1 m at 20 Hz and 1.71 cm at 20 kHz.]

In contrast to the poor directional information from intensity disparity at low frequencies, like C_4, there is no doubt that phase disparity plays an important role.

Physically, one can measure the phase difference in degrees from a point source (ideally) by placing microphones at the position of the ears in a dummy head and using sources of different frequencies placed at different distances from the head. The phase disparity is determined at each frequency as a function of azimuth (Shaw 1974) with the following results: Phase disparity is, as expected, maximal for an azimuth of 90° (sound source on the axis through the ears); and for any one azimuth the phase difference is clearly a function of frequency. [Let Θ be the azimuth of the source with respect to the sagittal plane, l be the interaural distance, and λ be the wavelength, then the following expression serves well enough to estimate the phase difference Φ:

$$\Phi = (2\pi/\lambda) \times l \times \sin\Theta.$$

Using this expression, we find, for example, that for a maximally lateralized source ($\Theta = 90°$), $\Phi = 80°$ at 256 Hz and $\Phi = 980°$ at 3 kHz. This last large value of phase disparity is of little use as a phase-shift reference, for there is an ambiguity; one wavelength involves a phase shift of 360°, but the number of wavelengths in the sound cannot be known to the ears. In contrast, the phase disparity for 256 Hz is clearly unambiguous and very useful for lateralization purposes.]

From such considerations, we can predict that above a particular frequency the phase information becomes ambiguous for the subject. This will start to happen when the half wavelength of the sound becomes about the same as the width of the head (i.e., at about 1.4 kHz for an azimuth of 90°) (figure 1.37).

We also need *physiological* evidence that the phase difference plays a role in the localization of low-frequency sound sources. Mills (1960) first measured the jnd of interaural phase shift as a function of frequency, testing subjects by the *dichotic* method. The characteristics of

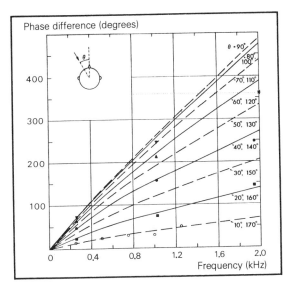

Figure 1.37
Interaural phase difference as a function of frequency. Calculated interaural phase difference for a 8.75-cm radius head, as a function of frequency. Parameter: Azimuth of the source. The symbols are for experimental results from different publications. The star and the dotted line correspond to 360°, the phase angle at and beyond which there is ambiguity (see text). (From Shaw 1974)

this jnd were then compared with the difference of interaural phase that corresponds with the jnd δΘ of a change in azimuth of a *real* source near the median plane (diotic, free-field listening). The strict parallelism of the two as a function of frequency up to 1.5 kHz strongly suggests that phase disparity does indeed play an important part in the localization of low frequency sound (figure 1.38).

Notice that the jnd of phase difference also depends, at a given frequency, on the intensity of the sound (Fedderson et al. 1957). It is optimal for moderate sound intensities and becomes less effective at other, particularly lower, sound levels.

Time intervals corresponding to these phase disparities may be calculated. The smallest perceptible phase difference detectable, 2°, corresponds with a temporal disparity of 4 μs at 100 Hz.

Concerning the *localization of high-frequency sounds* (>1.5 kHz), phase disparities soon become useless as a guide to direction, because as frequency increases the wavelength shortens (with respect to the interaural distance). On the other hand, the shadowing of the sound

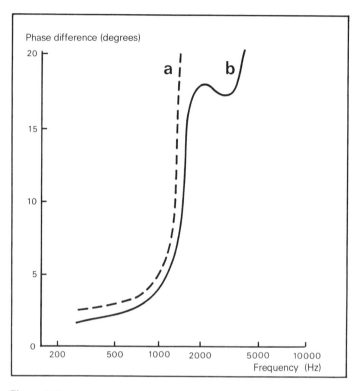

Figure 1.38
Interaural phase differences. (a) Detectability threshold of interaural phase difference, for dichotic listening, as a function of frequency. (b) Phase difference created by a real source moved in the vicinity of the median plane by an angle δΘ the jnd for azimuth change, as a function of frequency. (From Mills 1960)

by the head begins to take on its own importance: The shorter the sound's wavelength, the less diffraction can eliminate the head's sharp shadow. Thus for a wavelength that is half the circumference of the head (i.e., 30 cm, corresponding to 1.2 kHz), the attenuation of sound intensity by the head's shadowing effect is already about 40%.

Purely *physical* studies (like those used to investigate phase disparities) have shown that the interaural intensity disparity from a point source (1) is the greater the closer a source is; (2) is greater the higher the frequency; and (3) plays a larger part the closer the azimuth is to 90° (Fedderson, et al. 1957; see figure 1.39).

Mills (1960), as described above for phase differences, has compared the *dichotic* interaural jnd for intensity difference as a function

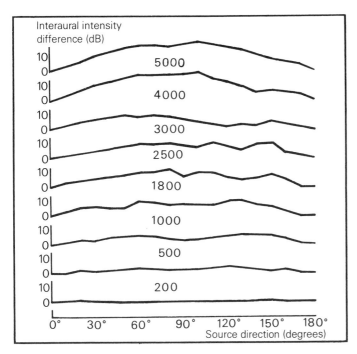

Figure 1.39
Interaural intensity differences as a function of frequency and of source direction (0°
straight ahead, 180° directly behind. Distance of source is effectively constant. (From
Fedderson, Sandel, Teas & Jeffress 1957)

of frequency with the corresponding frequency dependence of the
intensity disparity that is produced by a *real* source moving through
an angle δΘ, the just-perceptible azimuth difference in the vicinity of
the median plane (figure 1.40). The resulting two curves show a strict
parallelism between 1.5 kHz and 5 kHz. Below 1.5 kHz diffraction
around the head is so much in evidence that the interaural intensity
differences are largely subthreshold, in agreement with the discussion above. Nevertheless, there is some disagreement concerning the
validity of the figures arrived at in the above experiment; certain
researchers place the limit of usefulness of intensity differences at a
much higher frequency (nearer 5 kHz). In addition, figure 1.40 shows
that above 6 kHz subjects are only able to discriminate interaural
intensity differences that are much larger, it seems, than the differences that should be available from a point source. Perhaps this difficulty arises from diffraction artifacts in the measurements.

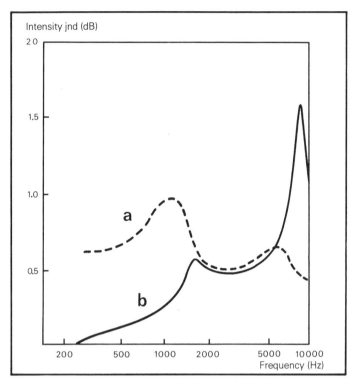

Figure 1.40
Interaural intensity differences. (a) Theoretical jnds of interaural intensity for dichotic listening as a function of frequency. (b) Corresponding intensity differences for a real source moved in the vicinity of the median plane by a jnd of azimuth change as a function of frequency. (From Mills 1960)

Finally, using dichotic techniques it can be shown that, at a given frequency, the differences between the right ear intensity I_R and the left I_L lead to a perceived displacement of the virtual source toward the side with the greater intensity and with a good proportionality between azimuth Θ and the log ratio of the intensities:

$$\Theta = K \log I_R/I_L$$

The above considerations are in reasonable accord with the suggestion that localization errors are maximal around 3 kHz, because at those intermediate frequencies one of the two mechanisms ceases to be useful, while the other is not yet operating optimally.

Note: It has been shown in the case of low-frequency pure tones that a certain phase disparity can be compensated for by an appropriate intensity disparity. This *time-intensity trading* has been studied by both stereophonic loudspeaker binaural methods and by dichotic earphone measurements. A certain phase disparity is first selected that causes a displacement of the virtual source in the sagittal plane. The intensity of the source at the side of most delay in phase is then increased until the subject once more hears the source in its original position. This allows the specification of a trading ratio in μs/dB (David, Guttman & van Bergeijk 1959).

Values published for this trading ratio seem to vary from researcher to researcher, ranging between 1.7 μs/dB and 100 to 150 μs/dB. This time-intensity trading has become a special study in itself and we leave the detail to others (see, e.g., Blauert 1983).

Localization of Other Types of Sound Source
The conditions set up by listening to continuous, long-lasting sounds of well-defined frequency (pure tones in the limit) are clearly not the only possible situation. Rather, this is an exceptional situation compared with normal life when the localization of different and varied sounds is in question. Let us examine certain aspects of the problem.

The first case of interest concerns *brief sounds,* whether they be clicks or preferably tone pips, since these latter transients are characterized by their frequency. Using these signals, it is particularly easy to manipulate independently the two variables δt (the interaural disparity in time of onset) and δI (the interaural intensity disparity) using dichotic listening methods.

When a curve showing the interaural time disparity as a function of azimuth is plotted (Shaw 1974), it is quite clearly at a maximum for 90° and is also independent of the frequency of the stimulus (figure 1.41). The expression giving δt, the time disparity, as a function of azimuth Θ (Shaw 1974) is

$$\delta t = (R/c)(\Theta + \sin\Theta)$$

where R is the radius of the head and c is the sound velocity.

When stimuli of equal intensity are presented simultaneously to the two ears, the subject localizes the transient sound in the median plane "inside the head." When there is a time disparity between the ears of 20 to 40 μs or an intensity difference of 1 to 1.5 dB, subjects still perceive only a single stimulus from a single source that is now

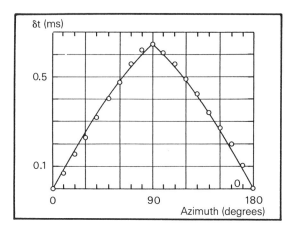

Figure 1.41
Interaural difference in the time of arrival of a sound as a function of azimuth.
Interaural time difference δt calculated for a head of 8.75-cm radius as a function of
source azimuth in degrees (0° straight ahead, 180° directly behind). (From Shaw 1974)

displaced with respect to the mid-line to the side of the first stimulus received or the most intense one.

If δt is increased to 650 or maybe 1000 μs, or δI to 8 or 9 dB, most people perceive the sound as "up against one ear" (the one receiving the first or most intense sound).

When the time disparity becomes even larger (2 to 4 ms), then the two stimuli will be recognized, one to each ear; the first received will seem to be by far the louder and the second much more feeble, even though physically they have equal intensities. This perception of apparent intensity differences carries on until about a 6-ms disparity but soon fades away at greater disparities; all sense of lateralization due to δI disappears and the sounds eventually are clearly heard as two entirely separate stimuli with no influence on each other.

Beyond that time disparity, the *echo threshold* is reached at about 40 to 50 ms. This particular threshold remains about the same for transients, as considered here, or for more complex signals such as the human voice (figure 1.42). We shall return to this topic shortly.

The minimal disparities in t or in I that determine a *jnd* of localization have also been measured (δt_{min} and δI_{min}) with the following results:

• δt_{min} increases very little when δt varies between 0 and 400 μs. In contrast, it decreases with increasing sound intensity, particularly for

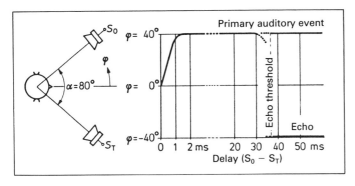

Figure 1.42
Echo threshold. Speech is delivered to left loudspeaker (S_0), followed by same stimulus to right loudspeaker ("echo" S_T). Abscissae, delay (in ms) between left and right (S_0 − S_T). For very short delays localization is close to the midsagittal plane. For longer delays (up to about 35 ms) localization is at the left loudspeaker and the right signal is ignored; for longer delays both stimuli are perceived, the first at the left and the second at the right. Both stimuli, S_0 and S_T, were about 50 dB SPL.

high-frequency transients. Values for δt_{min} range between 10 and 50 μs.

• δI_{min} is relatively independent of I and does not depend much on the frequency content of the transient. In other words, localization determined by interaural intensity asymmetries is much less influenced by the intensity or frequency of the stimulus than that based on interaural time disparities.

Returning to the problem of an echo threshold, if a brief sound is heard from an external loudspeaker and then another click is emitted from a second and differently placed loudspeaker, subjects tend to hear only one sound and to an extent ignore the existence of the second sound and its localization, provided the two sounds are separated by less than 50 ms (namely, below the echo threshold). Being unaware of the echo is the most important part of this phenomenon: It serves well to define the *precedence effect* or, as it is often referred to in acoustics, the *Haas effect*. It has the important consequence (perhaps its main biological function) of allowing the localization of sound sources in spite of the existence of echoes that would otherwise be expected to blur such direction finding (Wallach, Newman & Rosenzweig 1949; Haas 1951). The phenomenon is, thus, far from being a simple curiosity; it is of particular consequence in room acoustics (figure 1.42).

Just as for continuous pure tones, *transients* also enjoy time-intensity trading such that if the sound is referred to one side by a time disparity δt and to the other by an intensity difference δI, it is possible to relocate the sound to the center of the head by appropriate adjustment of the two variables. This compensation can be expressed as before by the ratio $\delta t/\delta I$ (in $\mu s/dB$). This ratio seems to become smaller (smaller δt compensating a given δI) for lower-frequency transients and the opposite for tone pips containing frequencies higher than 1 khz. Essentially, the details of the mechanisms that underpin this compensation are not well known.

Another case is *localization of white noise*. Remarkably, subjects are perfectly able to localize white noise during dichotic listening, apparently on the basis of phase difference because experimentally the two ears receive the same stimulus with simply a time disparity introduced between one ear and the other; the instantaneous noise fluctuations remain the same and are only displaced in time.

Finally, an effect of current interest is the localization of transients encountered in the general environment, particularly speech. The latter contains many high frequencies, and we might therefore postulate intensity differences as the main mode of localization. But in fact, it is the *envelope* of the speech sounds that is used, namely, a succession of short-lasting variations, not the individual frequency components. For these variations in the envelope, the temporal disparity is the more definitive cue.

We have sketched the results of tackling certain sound localization problems by dichotic experimentation, a method that is admittedly very artificial. Many other factors are likely to intervene in more natural situations and it would be wrong not to mention them also:

1. So far we have not properly considered how sound is mapped and attains such spatial dimensions as are, for example, experienced in stereophony. In principle, this technique assumes that stereo recordings should be made using two or more microphones that are differently placed with respect to the sound source and that each separate recording should eventually energize a separate loudspeaker. The auditory physiologist, however, finds enormous problems in stereophony. These cannot be discussed in detail here, but they concern the fact that the auditory system is constantly receiving a variety of sounds with different intensities and temporal disparities, and at the same time coping with the complications of reverberations and echoes. The mechanisms described above, though certainly im-

portant, appear to us only to resolve a part of this problem and do not in themselves allow a full explanation of the creation of a spatial sound field and its perception.

Even in its purely technical and practical aspects, stereophony poses serious problems. It is particularly necessary to distinguish between true stereophony and "pseudostereophony" (see, e.g., Condamines 1978; Blauert 1983).

A true impression of an external sound space is attained by using two receivers (microphones) placed at two locations in the sound field from which the two sound signals are eventually applied to two separate loudspeakers. One problem is faithfully to maintain the differences between these two signals throughout the whole process of transmission. At present in radio transmission, it is usual to exploit a modulation of the radiofrequency carrier wave that permits a simultaneous transmission of the two signals. Similarly, for stored signals (discs, cassettes, and the like), stereophony is preserved by using a variety of processes that allow the independent reproduction of the two signals (even when, as on a disc, the two signals are cut in the same groove).

The many tricks used in pseudostereophony are quite different. The general principle is to apply to two loudspeakers, two signals that derive from an originally *single* recording. The two signals are technologically made to differ from each other (e.g., by mutual phase-shifts) by manipulating the original mono information. Listening to this sort of output can, to some extent, create the impression of an artificial sound space.

2. Sound localization with head movements eliminated scarcely corresponds to any natural situation except perhaps the case of a transient sound arriving unexpectedly with no chance for subsequent exploratory movements. In more commonplace occurrences, the subject has time to carry out head movements that help localize the source not only with respect to the median plane but also within that plane (up/down) and to make front/back judgments with equal precision. Subjects who suffer quite large inequalities in sensitivity between the two ears are nevertheless able to achieve a reasonably good spatial localization, no doubt thanks to the extra information available from head movements.

3. It is also important to remember continually, as did the very earliest researchers in the field, the important role played by the external ear, with its complex folds, in localizing sounds. People who

suffer a profound unilateral deafness need to exploit the directional characteristics of the external ear to the full (Shaw 1974). Even in the normal subject, front/back and up/down discriminations owe a great deal to the transmission characteristic of the external ear as a function of the direction of arrival of a sound.

4. There is also the question of sorting out different sounds. A subject who is surrounded by many and varied ambient sounds can in fact usually distinguish one source from another, localize them separately, and, for example, concentrate on one conversation while disregarding others (the classic "cocktail party effect"). This case, however, introduces extra aspects that belong to mechanisms of attention as well as to purely auditory difficulties. We do not have the space here to discuss this effect in the necessary detail.

4.2 OTHER BINAURAL EFFECTS

Let us examine, quite briefly, some other problems concerned with binaural hearing that have been addressed by using dichotic stimulation.

BINAURAL SUMMATION AND ABSOLUTE THRESHOLDS

For several years, researchers have studied whether the absolute threshold, measured with simultaneous input to the two ears, is lower than the same threshold obtained monaurally. The earliest results were often quite equivocal because of uncertainties about the precise characteristics of the stimuli presented. Technical advances have allowed the use of well-controlled stimuli in experiments that suggest the following conclusions:

• The binaural threshold of a sound's detectability—specified in terms of the minimal pressure at the eardrum—is, as a general rule, smaller than its monaural value.

• In principle, if each ear had an identical monaural threshold and if at some level in the central nervous system there were a perfect summation of the effects, the binaural threshold ought to be 50% of the monaural (i.e., smaller by 3 dB). It has been possible to demonstrate this in a rather limited number of cases (i.e., when both ears have the same absolute threshold and also in cases in which slight differences in sensitivity have been compensated for exactly in the sound input.)

• Most often the monaural thresholds of the two ears are appreciably different, sometimes by as much as 6 dB; the difference between the binaural threshold and the monaural threshold of the more sensitive ear then becomes about 1 dB. That difference also corresponds in this case to perfect summation of the sound power applied to each ear (Colburn & Durlach 1978).

DIFFERENTIAL INTENSITY THRESHOLD

In essence, the differential binaural intensity threshold is a little lower than the monaural, but the reasons for this are still a matter of discussion. Peripheral factors have been proposed as well as central influences. The argument proceeds as follows: Experiments show that the energy transfer in each canal varies continuously, the best efficiency of transmission being shown sometimes on the right, sometimes on the left. The mechanism for these variations is not certain, but it could at least engender some central nervous system effect that continually selects the most favorable input for further processing.

BINAURAL INTENSITY SUMMATION (SUPRATHRESHOLD)

Researchers agree in general, differing only in detail, that a sound applied to two ears appears to be louder than when it is applied to one. After a systematic study using sounds of different frequencies but the same intensity levels and applying one to one ear, the other to the other, von Békésy (1960) was able to show that the two sounds do summate and do so the more effectively the closer their individual frequencies (f and f') are. Maximal summation (figure 1.43) occurs when $\delta f = |f - f'| = 0$.

INTERAURAL SUMMATION AND INHIBITION DURING MASKING

The next important question, since it is the most commonly encountered situation in practice, is whether the discrimination of a sound being masked by noise is better achieved in binaural or in monaural listening.

It has been shown that when subjects are exposed to rather weak masking noise signals, binaural listening is more effective than monaural. The binaural threshold for detecting the masked signal is lower than the monaural. But the opposite is true when the masking noise is intense. This *interaural inhibition* (Hirsh 1948) is particularly severe at low frequencies (figure 1.44).

Other studies have considered in more detail the effects of the way the sounds and masking noise are presented to the subject. It has

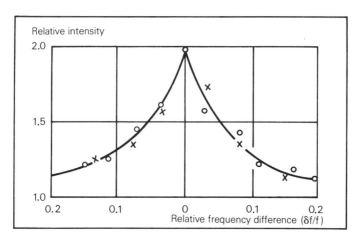

Figure 1.43
Binaural summation of sound intensity. Two sounds of equal physical intensity (40 dB) but differing slightly in frequency (relative frequency difference $\delta f/f$) are presented simultaneously, one to each ear. The subject is asked to equalize the sound intensity perceived to that when only one of the sounds is presented monaurally. The relative intensity for the combined tones is shown. Notice that summation is maximal for δf = 0. The same curve fits data for 500 Hz (circles) and 2 kHz (crosses). (From Licklider 1951 after von Békésy 1929; see von Békésy 1960)

been shown, for instance, that for a sound of 500 Hz masked by noise the threshold for detection of the sound is about 9 dB *higher* binaurally if the two signals, sound and noise, are each applied *similarly* to the separate ears, that is, either with each applied in phase-opposition or with each applied in-phase (when, in silence, without masking, the binaural threshold is 3 dB lower than the monaural). In contrast, when the sound and the masking noise are presented *in different ways* to the two ears—sound in phase and noise in antiphase, or vice versa—the binaural threshold for detecting the sound is in this case *lowered* by 15 dB compared with the monaural. One refers to this as a *masking level difference* or a *binaural unmasking* (Colburn & Durlach 1978). It has also been demonstrated that this effect in binaural masking, which depends on the interaural phases, depends also on the frequency of the masked sound, being most evident around 500 Hz and virtually absent near 1.5 kHz. The underlying mechanisms of the phenomenon have been the object of some theoretical speculation and even of some model-building, but they are still not very well understood.

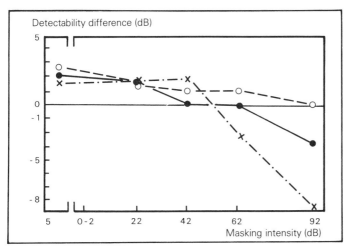

Figure 1.44
Binaural summation and inhibition. A binaural masking noise causes a difference between the detectability of a tone supplied monaurally and the same tone applied binaurally. The section above the horizontal line (+) indicates binaural summation, binaural threshold is smaller; and that below (−) indicates an inhibitory interaction, binaural threshold is larger than monaural. For 250 Hz (crosses), 1 kHz (filled circles), 4 kHz (open circles). Note that when the masking noise is intense, the binaural threshold for the low-frequency sound is the most increased. (From Licklider 1951 after Hirsh 1948)

DIPLACUSIS: INTERAURAL DIFFERENCES IN PITCH

Otologists are very familiar with *diplacusis,* the perception of different pitch levels when sounds of the same frequency are applied to one or the other ear. The effect can be studied quantitatively by measuring the difference in frequency of the two sounds needed to give the same pitch sensation in each ear. Note that the disparity between "normal" ears is a function of frequency and it decreases with increasing sound intensity (Stevens & Egan 1941) (figure 1.45).

It is particularly clear-cut in normal subjects after exposure of one ear to high sound intensity of a given frequency. After such an exposure for several minutes at 130 to 150 dB, even a disparity of one octave has been observed.

5 TONAL SENSATIONS, MUSICAL SOUNDS, AND MUSICAL SCALES

In this section, we shall discuss (very incompletely, owing to space limitations) a whole range of problems concerned with musical acous-

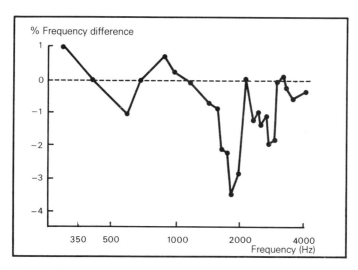

Figure 1.45
Diplacusis for a normal subject. The frequency of a tone supplied to the left ear is adjusted to the same pitch as a reference frequency earlier supplied to the right ear. The % frequency difference is shown for different frequencies. (From Licklider 1951 after Stevens & Egan 1941)

tics, a study that since von Helmholtz (1863), Rayleigh (1945, 1896), Brillouin (1958), Bouasse (1926), and many others has existed as a multidisciplinary interface between studies of the physical nature of sound and of the physiological properties of the auditory receptors. As we shall soon see, it is not always easy to disentangle what is a property of one domain and what of the other.

5.1 SPECIFICATION OF MUSICAL INTERVALS BETWEEN PURE TONES

A subject asked to listen to two tones simultaneously will describe them as either a consonance (agreeable in some way) or a dissonance (disagreeable). (These characterizations hold for those accustomed to Western classico-romantic music and may not pertain for subjects from different cultures or for those familiar with very modern Western works.) The physical counterparts of these subjective judgments have been continuously developed and elaborated since the introduction of the notion of *frequency* in the seventeenth century. Until then, the concept of an *interval* (ratio) was the basis of all discussion, an idea already familiar to the Greeks, who knew that, given two strings under equal tension but of different lengths l_1 and l_2, the quality of their combination depends on the ratio of their lengths l_1/l_2 (Bouasse 1926; Wood 1944; Danielou 1959).

An impression of unison, or perfect consonance, is attained when the two frequencies are in the ratio $2:1$, comprising the *octave*. Earlier civilizations had realized that consonance is obtained when there are *simple ratios* between the lengths of their musical strings (e.g., $5:4$, $4:3$, $3:2$), whereas more complex ratios (e.g., $30:29$, $16:15$) result in dissonance. Thus the specification of the relationships between musical tones had from the earliest times been based on *ratios* l_1/l_2 between the lengths of strings. [Remember that for a length of vibrating string, $f = p \cdot 1/2l \cdot \sqrt{(P/\mu)}$, where f is the frequency of the sound, l is the length of the string, P is the stretching force exerted on the string, μ is the mass per unit length of the string, and p is an integer greater than 1 specifying the order of the partial produced. This implies also that the relationships between musical tones depend on frequency *ratios* f_1/f_2, not on frequency *differences*.]

Such considerations resulted in the introduction of a logarithmic scale to specify the intervals I between sounds in terms of these ratios. The musical interval between two sounds of frequency f_1 and f_2 is given by

$$I = k \log f_1/f_2,$$

where k is a constant that determines the size of the chosen unit of interval. It is worth bearing in mind that the unison to its octave interval ($f_1/f_2 = 2$) is given by $I = k \log 2$, or, put in another way, $k \times 0.301$.

In practice, two units for intervals are currently adopted: One (the most frequently used in France) is based on $k = 1000$ and defines intervals in *savarts* (σ). For this choice of unit:

$$I(\sigma) = 1000 \log_{10} f_1/f_2,$$

and the octave interval $= 300\ \sigma$.

A second unit, originally considered by Helmholtz, consisted in regarding the equal-tempered semitone (see below), one twelfth the octave interval, as base. This interval divided into 100 parts gives the widely used interval unit the *cent*. Thus an equal-tempered semitone $= 100$ cents and an octave $= 1200$ cents; in these units the interval f_1/f_2 is given by:

$$I \text{(cents)} = \{1200/\log_{10} 2\} \{\log_{10} f_1/f_2\} \approx 4000 \log_{10} (f_1/f_2)$$

(An interval specified in cents is thus about 4 times its value in savarts; an equal-tempered semitone is about 25 savarts.)

The use of logarithmic scales for musical intervals has the clear advantage of allowing intervals to be added—instead of using ratios—while at the same time conforming very well with the nature of the auditory mechanisms and arrangements upon which pitch interval perception is based.

It is of interest here to specify the just-perceptible interval of frequency in these units. For frequencies above 1 kHz where, as we have seen earlier, $\delta f/f$ is independent of f, the minimal detectable interval is given by $\delta f/f = 0.002$, or about 4 cents (1 savart). At lower frequencies ($f < 1$ kHz) where δf is relatively constant, the interval $\delta f/f$ depends on the frequency. It varies between about 50 cents (13 σ) at 60 Hz to the 4 cents (1 σ) of 1 kHz.

In musical practice, the minimum perceptible interval is conventionally considered to be the *comma*; this corresponds with $f_1/f_2 = 81/80$, $\delta f/f = 0.012$, a value approaching 20 cents (5 σ). (Refer to section 5.4 below and to tables 1.17 and 1.18 for information on musical scales and musical intervals with their various schemes of nomenclature in France and elsewhere.)

5.2 PERCEPTION OF REAL SOUNDS

ATTRIBUTES OF PURE TONES

We have already mentioned (in the section on pitch scale), that the concept of tonality and consonance of octaves is accepted as an attribute of a sound, although it is not the same as pitch level. Whereas the pitch level distinction "low-high" represents a *monotonic* variation along the entire audible range of frequencies, the idea of tonality and octave consonances constitutes a *cyclic* relationship between frequencies, such that two pure tones an octave apart share a pitch similarity even though they have no spectral coincidence. Nevertheless, the nature of octave perception has been widely argued (e.g., by Burns & Ward 1982) and two points should be mentioned: (1) The perception of musical intervals and tonality applies in only part of the whole range of pitch levels; its existence extends at the most between 60 Hz and 5 kHz. (2) The relative importance of what is inborn (i.e., an authentic purely sensory process) and of what is acquired (as a consequence of cultural influences, Western in particular) constitutes an ongoing debate.

Intensity (dB)

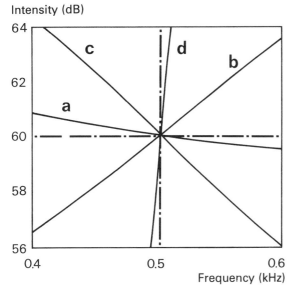

Frequency (kHz)

Figure 1.46
Isophonic frequency/intensity contours for four attributes of sounds. The reference sound, represented at the center of the diagram, has a frequency of 500 Hz and an intensity of 60 dB. (a) Locus of frequencies and intensities that have the same loudness. (b) Curve representing the intensity of sounds at different frequencies that give the same impression of volume (equal volume curve). (c) Equal density curve. (d) Equal pitch curve (see text). (From Boring 1942 after Stevens 1934)

In addition to loudness and pitch, pure tones present a whole series of other subjective dimensions whose quantitative specification is difficult and even controversial, no doubt in part because of their subjective nature. Thus the list of psychophysical and psychoacoustic studies includes three other attributes (Boring 1942):

- Clarity (a "bright" sound, a "dark" sound)
- Volume (an "expansive" sound, a "pinched" sound)
- Density (a "massive and dense" sound, a "delicate and diffuse" sound)

We can recognize, for example, that a not very intense low-frequency sound gives the same impression of volume as a high-pitched tone of greater intensity. As for curves of equal density, they do not parallel those of volume but, on the contrary, seem to be of opposite slope; as frequency increases the volume decreases but the density increases (figure 1.46).

Another subjective quality perceived with pure tones is *roughness*. This is experienced, for example, when a pure tone, say 1 kHz, is amplitude-modulated at a much lower frequency, say 50 Hz. A variety of psychoacoustic studies has been devoted to this phenomenon (based on quantitative estimates using methods such as Stevens employed; see Buser & Imbert 1982). Here are some results:

• For a given modulation frequency, the subjective impression of roughness (r) is proportional to the square of the modulation index m ($m = \delta p/p$; see "Intensity Differential Threshold," above). Thus

$$r = k \cdot m^2.$$

• The intensity of the modulated sound does not seem to play an important role.
• For a sound of a given frequency, the roughness varies with the modulation frequency, beginning around 20 Hz, then increasing rapidly with f_{mod}, and eventually decreasing rapidly at a higher modulation rate (Zwicker 1976). The maximal roughness occurs at an f_{mod} that depends on the frequency of the sound that is modulated: 40 Hz for 120 Hz, 50 Hz for 250 Hz, 70 Hz for 1 kHz, and 90 Hz for frequencies above 2 kHz.
• At least in the lower range of frequencies ($\leq$ 1 kHz), the highest modulation frequency at which roughness begins to disappear is about equal to the critical bandwidth (the lowest frequency being always near 20 Hz). When the modulation rate exceeds the critical bandwidth, it no longer directly interferes with the perceived quality of the modulated tone. The tone does not then appear to be roughened (figure 1.47).

HEARING TWO PURE TONES SIMULTANEOUSLY

We also need to examine the wide variety of subjective perceptions elicited when two sinusoidal pure tones are presented simultaneously whose intensities are about equal and whose different frequencies, f_1 and f_2, bear certain relationships to each other. When the difference between the frequencies f_1 and f_2 is about 2 to 3 Hz, a single tone is heard whose intensity varies periodically. The sound is perceived to beat in a rhythm equal to $\delta f = f_1 - f_2$. These *beats* are best heard for δf values that vary with the pitch of f; these values also vary between subjects. Thus a wide range of values of effective δf has been reported. According to some researchers, beats cease for δf

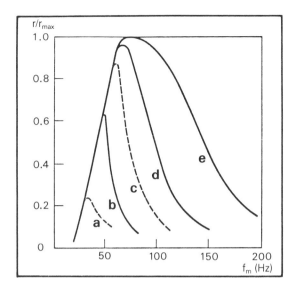

Figure 1.47
Roughness in a sound. Relative roughness r/r_{max} as a function of modulation frequency f_m of amplitude-modulated pure tones at different modulation frequencies: (a) 120 Hz, (b) 250 Hz, (c) 500 Hz, (d) 1 kHz, (e) >2 kHz. (From Zwicker 1975)

$\geq$ 6 Hz at mid-range audiofrequencies. This is equivalent to an interval of 8 to 12 cents (2 to 3 σ) at 1 kHz; others report beats for intervals up to 60 cents (15 σ), which at 1 kHz corresponds to δf = 35 Hz (von Helmholtz 1863; Bouasse 1926; Roederer 1979).

Whatever the precise conditions needed for beats, when the difference δf (or the relative disparity $\delta f/f$) increases any further the sound acquires a roughness (which we have already discussed), with its "maximal unpleasantness" being attained at a δf that depends upon f and lies between 60 and 120 cents (15 and 30 σ). Not surprisingly, the boundary between perceiving tonal beats, on the one hand, and hardness or roughness in a tone, on the other, is quite variable from subject to subject and, according to the experimenters, the two perceptions can very easily overlap near the boundary. (In these intermediate conditions, sounds specified as "voix celeste" or "vibrato" in certain instruments, e.g., the organ, are generated by just the sort of superpositions of separate tones discussed here.)

At much higher frequency separations the two individual sounds are heard simultaneously and are judged to be consonant or

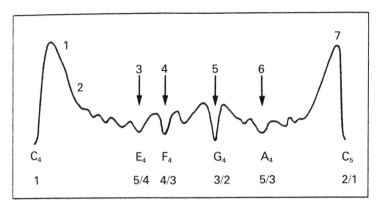

Figure 1.48
Hardness of a complex sound as a function of frequency ratios. The note C_4 is played continuously on one violin and a second violin sound is added that traverses the octave range to C_5, passing via E_4, F_4, G_4, A_4. Note the transitions through (1) a strong discord to (2) a roughness, then through consonances at the intervals of the third (3), fourth (4), fifth (5), and sixth (6), then before reaching the octave, a further zone of roughness (7) and once more an obvious dissonance. (From Wood 1944 after Helmholtz 1883)

dissonant depending on the ratio of their frequencies, the closest consonance being realized when, as we have seen above, $f_1/f_2 = 2$. Consonance is also experienced when the frequency ratios are 5/4 (major third), 4/3 (fourth), and 3/2 (fifth). There are some subtle variations in these ratios, as we shall see below, that depend on the precise musical scale in question. Between these special ratios, the subject hears a mixture of the two sounds that is more or less consonant or dissonant. This applies to pure tones but also to real instruments that do not generate pure tones, such as the violin (figure 1.48).

PURE TONES AND NONLINEARITIES

Other phenomena only affect the perception of pure tones when they have reached a particular sound intensity. In fact, at high sound levels distortions are produced that are universally attributed to nonlinearities in the auditory system; this applies to several distinctly different phenomena.

When a subject is exposed to an isolated single pure tone, free from any physical harmonic distortion, then beyond a certain intensity the subject hears harmonics. When such harmonics are not present in the sound itself and are clearly subjective, they are often referred to

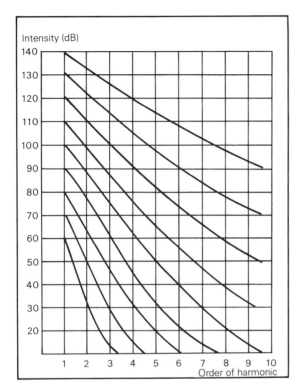

Figure 1.49
Aural harmonics. Chart of the relative intensities of subjective aural harmonics. Each curve cuts the vertical at $x = 1$ at the intensity of the fundamental (pure tone) and the successive aural harmonic amplitudes are at the intersections with 2, 3, etc. (From Wood 1944 after Stevens 1938)

as *overtones* or *aural harmonics* (Stevens & Newman 1936b). [These effects, created by the ear, must be distinguished from objective, physical harmonic distortion in the sound reproducer such as can be registered and measured by linear physical receivers independently of any observer.]

As mentioned at the beginning of this section, the perception of these harmonics exposes a nonlinearity in the ear: It distorts the signal, transforming the original purely sinusoidal vibration into a more complicated periodic wave that can be defined by Fourier analysis as consisting of a certain number of harmonics, multiples of the original stimulus' frequency. This original frequency has now become merely the fundamental component of this more complex wave (figure 1.49).

When a pure tone of frequency f_1 is sounded and then there is added to this another pure tone of frequency f_2 of about the same intensity, the perceived loudness of f_1 can become less than normal as the intensity of f_2 is increased. This might be described as a mutual inhibition (or antagonism) between the two sounds. A sound of 7 kHz, for example, is influenced in this way by tones between 5 and 12 kHz.

In other conditions, when listening to two simultaneously presented tones, not only the primary sounds f_1 and f_2 are heard but also some of a whole series of other *combination tones* with frequencies of the sort $mf_1 \pm nf_2$. The sounds $mf_1 - nf_2$ are called *difference tones* and the others, $mf_1 + nf_2$, are *summation tones*. [Generally speaking, these tones can be the more easily identified by using an exploratory tone, particularly when the combination tone is rather weak. After the addition of another tone of frequency f', which is very near to the combination tone's frequency f, the subject will appreciate its presence the more clearly by hearing beats at a rate $f - f'$. An alternative method is by cancellation. A third tone is applied and is adjusted in frequency, intensity, and then phase until it cancels the perception of the combination tone.]

In general, difference tones are much more evident than summation tones, as witnessed by the latter usually being detected after the difference tones have first become clearly present—it is sometimes very hard to be sure that summation tones are there at all. Two combination tones are particularly notable: One is the *simple difference tone* $f_2 - f_1$ (for $f_2 > f_1$) and the other is the *cubic difference tone*, given by $2f_1 - f_2$.

These effects were discovered by Sorge in 1744 and by Romieu in 1753. But it was Tartini (1754) who claimed to have observed them as early as 1714—an old-time scientific controversy! Tartini being the more influential publicist, they became known as "Tartini tones." They were soon well recognized by organ builders; for example, by using two organ pipes, one of 16 ft sounding C_1 ($f = 32$ Hz) and another of 10 ft 8 in. sounding G_1 ($f = 48$ Hz), the (difference) combination tone resulting from sounding them together is C_0 ($f = 16$ Hz), which can otherwise only be obtained from a much larger, 32-ft single pipe (figure 1.50).

It was noticed that the success of such combinations of organ stops depends on the accuracy of their intonation. If in the above example the two pipes were slightly out of tune, the difference tone would

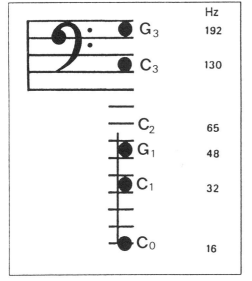

	Hz
G₃	192
C₃	130
C₂	65
G₁	48
C₁	32
C₀	16

Figure 1.50
Combination tones. A combination tone of pitch C_0 (16 Hz) is heard when G_1 (48 Hz) and C_1 (32 Hz) are sounded simultaneously. The bass clef, with G_3 and C_3 marked, is in the diagram to identify the tones musically.

disappear and a chord of the fifth would be heard instead. The transformation between the two sensations is abrupt: The difference tone and the chord are not heard simultaneously. We seem in this case to be dealing with two sensations that are invoked in entirely different ways.

Still more complex interactions are observed when subjects listen to a sound comprising several frequencies, each of which is effectively a harmonic of a fundamental frequency that is not itself actually present in the mixture of sounds; for example, playing 700, 800, 900, and 1000 Hz simultaneously. Under these conditions, subjects hear either a difference tone that is the common fundamental of the separate components (the *missing fundamental,* 100 Hz in this case) or a summation tone with a frequency that is a common multiple of the separate components; this latter situation is very rare.

Helmholtz (1863) was the first to propose an explanation for these phenomena that attributed both aural harmonics and combination tones to nonlinearity of the auditory system (but without specifying what part of the system). He proposed this when authors before him had postulated different interpretations based on a complicated set of rules for linear interactions that generated a variety of different beats. However, given a whole range of conditions, those hypothesized interactions were only able to explain difference tones and could not at the same time cope with summation tones. It was these latter that Helmholtz specifically discovered.

Helmholtz' theory ran, in principle, as follows: Given a sound $a\cos\omega t$, the resulting vibration of the mechanical system (in this case, the auditory detectors) might be a linear function of the sound, thus $X = a\cos\omega t$.

The hypothesis is to suggest that if a becomes too large, the relationship beween X and the sound is no longer linear but can be expressed in the form:

$$X = a_1 \cos\omega t + a_2 \cos^2\omega t + \ldots + a_n \cos^n \omega t,$$

the number of terms brought into play depending, of course, on the incident intensity. In addition the powers of $\cos\omega t$, $\cos^n \omega t$ reduce to $\cos n\omega t + k$. In other words, frequencies appear that are multiples 2, 3, . . . , n of the originally single incident frequency.

If two incident frequencies are simultaneously present initially, we may write that within the limits of linearity

$$X = a\cos\omega_1 t + b\cos\omega_2 t.$$

When the system ceases to respond linearly, the rules for transforming the powers of the original linear vibrations and of their summed actions generate terms representing diverse combinations of vibrations of the type $\cos(m\omega_1 \pm n\omega_2)$, from which arise difference and summated combination tones.

In chapter 2 we will examine how the evidence for cochlear function, both mechanical and electrical, emphasizes the presence of nonlinearities and, in appropriate cases, can even quantify the mechanisms that lead to it. However, even at the level of acoustic psychophysics alone, some recent researches on combination tones cast considerable doubt on Helmholtz' (polynomial) hypothesis.

Given sounds of two frequencies f_1 and f_2 simultaneously present, with $f_1 < f_2$, one can list the following effects (Goldstein 1967):

1. *The simple difference tone* ($f_2 - f_1$). Since this is not in fact perceived except for high intensities of the two sounds presented (>100 dB), the sort of situation postulated by Helmholtz holds, where nonlinearity is a result of the intense sound exciting the receptors beyond their linear range.

2. *The cubic difference tone* ($2f_1 - f_2$). Here the situation is much more complicated. It now seems certain that its existence is not limited to

the presentation of intense tones; it can be generated even by relatively weak sounds (30 dB). It has been shown in this context that when two stimuli f_1 and f_2 ($f_1 < f_2$) with moderate and equal intensities (50 dB) are presented, then the cubic difference tone can be as much as 10 dB when $f_2/f_1 = 1.1$. In contrast, with constant and equal intensities, as the ratio f_2/f_1 increases (i.e., the disparity between the two frequencies becomes greater), the intensity of the cubic difference tone diminishes linearly with the increase in f_2/f_1. It becomes scarcely observable except for $1.1 < (f_2/f_1) < 1.5$.

The existence of the cubic difference tone is confirmed by the fact that, first, its perception as a frequency ($2f_1 - f_2$) can be suppressed by simultaneously playing a third, real, external tone of frequency ($2f_1 - f_2$) whose phase and amplitude have been adjusted appropriately; second, playing a third tone at the same time as f_1 and f_2 of a frequency near ($2f_1 - f_2$) generates beats; and third, the perception of ($2f_1 - f_2$) can be masked by narrow band noise centered on ($2f_1 - f_2$) (figure 1.51).

[To explain the salience of the cubic difference tone, we might assume that one effect of distortion is to introduce a combination tone of the type $(\cos 2f_1 + \cos 2f_2)^3$. Remembering that $f_1 < f_2$, the resulting distortion should introduce the following frequencies: f_1, $3f_1$, $3f_2$, f_2, $2f_1 + f_2$, $2f_1 - f_2$, $2f_2 - f_1$, among others. For all these possible combination tones, only $2f_1 - f_2$ is quite certainly less than f_1 and f_2 and consequently, considering other effects and particularly masking, it will be the most audible.]

3. There are much less prominent combination tones of the type $(n + 1)f_1 - nf_2$ where $n > 1$. The only ones that can be perceived are $3f_1 - 2f_2$ and, to the slightest degree, $4f_1 - 3f_2$.

From purely psychophysical evidence, then, an essential nonlinearity appears to exist in the auditory system that is connected with frequency selectivity and its characteristics but not necessarily (as Helmholtz suggested) needing an overload imposed on the system by excessive stimulation. In chapter 2, we shall consider whether this essential nonlinearity is in the basilar membrane, or in the transducing hair cells, or both.

PERCEPTION OF COMPLEX SOUNDS

One of the most exciting but difficult problems in psychoacoustics is the perception of complex sounds that comprise either mixtures of pure tones or consist in a fundamental and its harmonics.

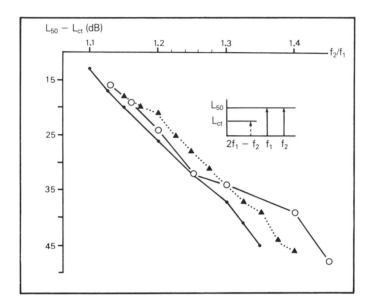

Figure 1.51
Amplitude of the cubic difference tone $2f_1 - f_2$. The intensity of the cubic difference
tone (L_{ct}) as a function of f_2/f_1 is shown for two subjects. L_{ct} is measured by asking
subjects to cancel the perception of the difference tone by adjusting the intensity of
another, external, sound of frequency $2f_1 - f_2$ that is out of phase with the combination
tone. The two tones f_1 and f_2 each have an intensity of 50 dB (L_{50} in the inset) and the
difference, $L_{50} - L_{ct}$, is plotted. The experiments were monaural, using an earphone.
Results for the two subjects are shown as dots and open circles. The second subject also
participated in a different measurement of the difference tone (triangles). Free-field
experimentation was used. The subject heard either the sound when (f_1 and f_2) are
fed to a loudspeaker or the sound from an externally generated ($2f_1 - f_2$) applied to
the loudspeaker. The intensity of the latter was adjusted by the subject, step by step,
until it matched the intensity of the perceived difference tone from the addition of f_1
and f_2. Note that the two methods (open circles and triangles) agree quite well but the
second method is much more time consuming. (From Goldstein 1967)

It has long been known that, given a little training, the human
auditory system can recognize a certain number of pure tones that
are the components of a complex sound, each by its own pitch, up
to the fifth harmonic of the fundamental periodicity of the sound. As
described by Helmholtz, this is an analytical skill in hearing, in contrast to the often synthetic hearing of everyday life, as, for instance,
the recognition of a complex melody by the global periodicity of its
envelope rather than by concern with the details of its spectral
composition.

But to return to the analytical properties of hearing; this was elevated to the status of a law by Georg Simon Ohm (1843). It was he

who established a firm link between the components of a complex sound recognized subjectively and the harmonic components revealed in Fourier analysis. His work was made possible by the introduction (in Germany) of the siren, an apparatus developed by Cagnard de la Tour which for the first time allowed the production of sounds whose frequency could be well controlled and varied.

This and subsequent work of the same kind was the basis, confirmed later by a great variety of masking experiments, upon which to found the idea that the auditory system can be regarded—at least in its early stages—as a bank of band-pass filters in parallel.

This having been said, analytic hearing also implies, apart from the indispensible first peripheral analysis, a well-targeted process of selective attention that is a matter of purely central processing and thus is not part of our present considerations.

In the enthusiastic pursuit of these ideas, other observations stimulated controversies that would have remained of historic interest only if it were not for the fact that they bear upon certain ways of regarding cochlear mechanics.

Seebeck (1841) opened the debate. He used a siren that by the arrangement of its holes could supply two different tones, each provided with its own series of harmonics. The surprising result was that the loudness of the dominant sound was not that predicted by Fourier analysis. The lowest tone heard was much louder than would be predicted by the amplitude of that harmonic. Seebeck concluded that a Fourier series did not allow one to predict subjective loudnesses.

Helmholtz, discussing the definite hearing of an absent or feeble fundamental, attributed it to an essential nonlinearity in the operation of the cochlea which created difference combination tones including the tone $f_1 - f_2$. These tones, having the frequency of the fundamental, can reinforce it, or even create it when it is absent.

Much later, Schouten (1940) upset Helmholtz' theory in considering the same question of the missing fundamental. Although the simultaneous provision of sounds of 1000 Hz, 1200 Hz, and 1400 Hz certainly evoked the perception of an absent sound of 200 Hz, he showed that supplying 1040 Hz with 1240 Hz and 1440 Hz (i.e., raising every component by the same small frequency change of 40 Hz), which should equally have allowed 200 Hz to be heard did not do so. In fact the second series (notice it is *enharmonic*) generated the perception of a pitch equivalent to 205 Hz. This weakened Helmholtz' hypothesis that the lower pitch relied on difference tones.

What is more, it was possible to show that the tone perceived as 200 Hz (in the first case) did not beat when another external tone was supplied at a nearby frequency (202 Hz). Neither was the 200 Hz perception masked by noise centered at 200 Hz, although it was well masked by noise spanning the original harmonic complex. From such experiments, Schouten proposed the hypothesis that low-frequency harmonics in a series enjoy the rather good frequency reso-lution of the low-frequency cochlear filters and each is well defined in pitch; in contrast, the higher harmonic frequencies do not enjoy an equally good frequency resolution. They constitute a tonal "resi-due" that the ear cannot analyze as precisely as lower harmonic com-ponents but to which hearing will still allocate a pitch that is not part of the original sounds. Thus, once more there arises a perception like that of a "missing fundamental" but not necessarily precisely where expected.

Schouten's ideas have in their turn been debated by more recent researchers. These later observations have generally concluded that central processes contribute to the assignation of a pitch to complex sounds; studies in this area include, among others, those of Houtsma and Goldstein 1972; Gerson and Goldstein 1978 (theory of optimal central processors); Wightman 1973 (central pattern transformations); and Terhardt 1979 (virtual pitch), to which we should now add the two-channel central model of van Noorden (1982). A full discussion of these recent theories, ranking their merits or indeed defects, can-not be undertaken here.

A complex sound is also perceived with a certain *timbre*. The defi-nition of timbre recommended by the American Standards Associa-tion is about as broad as possible, being the subjective impression that allows one to distinguish between two sounds of the same fun-damental loudness and pitch, presented in the same way.

Quite clearly, timbre is a multidimensional attribute, and psycho-acoustics researchers have worked to discover what factors are impor-tant. One well-known factor is the number of harmonics contained in the total sound (we return to this in the next section when dis-cussing the timbre of musical instruments). One problem is to find out what other characteristics of the components determine timbre. It is clear that timbre depends on the amplitude of the components present in the sound, particularly harmonic components. We shall see that these assist the identification of different musical instru-ments. The precise influence of the *phase* of the components is more difficult to ascertain (Plomp 1970).

It is clear from the outset that when two waves are superimposed their phase relationships affect the resulting waveform: In this respect the phases can be regarded as definitive. But, in a wider context, it has emerged experimentally that phase plays a more important part the lower the audiofrequency and the closer together the frequencies of the two components are,—in particular, when they share the same critical band (see Zwicker & Feldtkeller 1981).

Let us now consider consonance and dissonance for complex sounds that are characterized by possessing a considerable number of harmonics of considerable magnitude. These can be high or low in pitch, or both.

Helmholtz supplied many data on this subject. According to him

• Consonance between two sounds is more marked the greater the number of shared coincident or close harmonics.

• Dissonance results from beats existing between certain harmonics.

• This dissonance is increasingly disagreeable the lower the order of the beating harmonics.

• Certain intervals give a greater impression of dissonance than others; the worst interval (to a Western ear) is around 100 to 120 cents, which is near a semitone in all musical scales.

Another attribute of a complex tone is its *sharpness* or *harshness.* This seems to be closely related to its density, as discussed above with respect to pure tones (and investigated by Stevens in depth). Using subjective methods of evaluation, it seems that the sharpness of a noise signal or a complex tone with multiple harmonics depends on how far its upper frequencies extend. Essentially, the impression of sharpness is doubled when the upper frequency cut-off is tripled. For narrow-band noise, the sharpness, clearly, can only depend on its central frequency.

5.3 GENERAL STRUCTURE OF THE SOUNDS OF MUSICAL INSTRUMENTS

Our intention in this section is to move on from the tonal impressions given by simple sounds to consider those more complex tones that are common in everyday life, and in particular, to study the case of musical instruments. As a general rule, an instruments is enabled by its construction to generate many notes, with frequencies $f_1, f_2, \ldots ,$ f_i, called *partials* (Bouasse 1923; Wood 1944).

Musical instruments are divided (by other criteria) into two sorts:

• Those that generate a set of nonsustained oscillations, i.e., oscillations resulting from a single impulsive force (percussion, plucked string, struck string). Physically, the system is in free oscillation. [Mathematically this means that the second term in the differential equation of movement is in the limit a Dirac impulse.] Under these conditions the instrument can emit the many frequencies of its partials that *do not necessarily comprise a harmonic series.*

• Those that generate sustained oscillations (i.e., that are forced into an oscillation), which to a rough first approximation might be like a sinusoid. [Here the differential equation of movement would have a sinusoidal second term. *This is just an approximation, since in most cases the driving force is not sinusoidal but a relaxation oscillation.*] This sort of oscillation is generated, for example, in the bowed strings of the violin family and by the embouchure of wind instruments (e.g., flute, horn) and the excitation of reed pipes (e.g., organ, oboe). In these cases, the sound, although periodic, is almost invariably complex, having a fundamental component but also harmonics of this fundamental. The frequency of each of these will either coincide with or be very close to one of the partials of the instrument.

Without going into the technical details of instrumental design, we can see that each will generate its own particular spectral content according to its shape and mode of attack (violin bow, hammers of the piano, quills of the harpsichord). It is the precise timbre that each instrument creates that allows its identification; this implies that for the same fundamental each must also generate its own particular series of harmonics, the amplitudes of which will vary greatly from instrument to instrument. Figure 1.52 shows some detailed examples. [Some instrumental sounds are also frequency modulated, as, for instance, when a violin is played with vibrato (e.g., at A_4, a frequency modulation of $\delta f = 10$ Hz has been observed at a modulation rate of $3/s$; the sound's frequency spectrum therefore spans approximately $(440 - 10 - 3)$ Hz to $(440 + 10 + 3)$ Hz (Zwicker & Feldtkeller 1981).]

Table 1.8 summarizes the essentials of a simple classification of the different ways musical instruments generate their sounds, and figure 1.53 illustrates the frequency ranges of a variety of instruments.

Two additional classes of instrument should be kept in mind:

• In some cases, instruments have partials that are very different from the harmonics of the fundamental. Here, only one frequency, the fundamental, will be strongly reinforced; thus it seems sensible to regard these instruments as *resonators* (e.g., hollowed out spheres, "Helmholtz resonators").

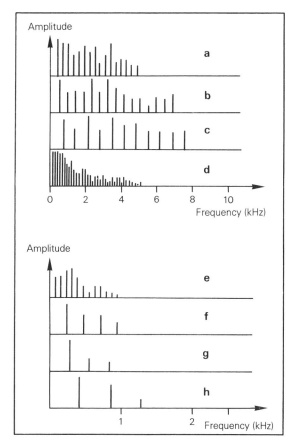

Figure 1.52
Line spectra of different instrumental sounds. (a) Violin D string, D_4 = 288 Hz. (b) Violin A string, A_4 = 426 Hz. (c) Violin E string, E_5 = 640 Hz. (d) Viola C string, C_3 = 128 Hz. (e) Horn, E_2 = 80 Hz. (f) Horn, B_3 = 240 Hz. (g) Horn, D_4 = 288 Hz. (h) Horn, A_4 = 426 Hz. The frequencies are in the natural scale for which A_4 is at 426 Hz (see table 1.18).

Table 1.8. Classification of (Western) Musical Instruments

Stringed Instruments	*Wind Instruments*
1. Plucked strings	1. With flute embouchure
a. With fingerboard: guitar, lute mandolin	a. Multiple pipes: Pan pipes
b. Without fingerboard: lyre, zither, harp	b. Single pipe:
c. Keyboard: spinet, virginal, harpsichord	i. With mouthpiece: recorder (conical tube)
2. Struck strings	ii. No mouthpiece: flute (cylindrical tube)
a. No keyboard: cimbalom	2. Reed pipes[a]
b. Keyboard: pianoforte (antecedent, square piano)	a. Single beating reed[b]: clarinet, basset horn (cylindrical tubes), saxophone (conical tube)
3. Bowed strings	b. Double reed: krummhorn (medieval), oboe (cylindrical tube), cor anglais, bassoon, contrabassoon, bagpipes (conical tubes)
a. Straight bow: viols, violin, viola, cello, double bass	
b. Rotating bow: hurdy-gurdy	c. Free reed[c]: harmonica, harmonium, accordian
Percussion Instruments	3. Horn embouchure (lips as reed): trumpet, trombone (cylindrical tubes), horn, cornet, tuba, serpent bugle, saxhorn (conical tubes)
1. Of definite pitch	
a. No keyboard: timpani, bells, xylophone	
b. Keyboard: celesta, glockenspiel	4. Organ: ranks of reed pipes (with beating reeds) and diapasons (flutelike)
2. Of indefinite pitch	
a. Struck skin: tambour, sidedrum bass drum	*Electronic Instruments*
b. Struck metal: triangle, gong (tam-tam), cymbals, rattle	1. Ondes Martenot (heterodyne)
c. Struck wood: castanets	2. Organs and synthesizers

[a]Reed: blade or blades maintained in vibration by an air current. These together determine the rate of alternating release and cutoff of the air.
[b]Beating reed and [c]free reed: single vibrating tongues which do and do not entirely cut off the air flow, respectively.

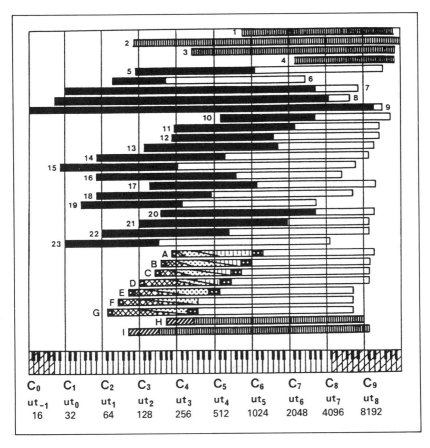

Figure 1.53
Frequency ranges of a few noises, instrumental sounds, and the various registers of human voices. The octaves are designated by what at present appears to be the convention most commonly used internationally, together with the Latin nomenclature, starting at ut^{-1}, and the corresponding ut^{-1} frequencies in the natural scale (see table 1.17). 1, jangling keys; 2, handclaps; 3, cymbals; 4, triangle; 5, xylophone; 6, bass drum; 7, harp; 8, piano; 9, organ; 10, piccolo; 11, flute; 12, oboe; 13, clarinet; 14, bassoon; 15, contrabassoon; 16, horn; 17, trumpet; 18, trombone; 19, tuba; 20, violin; 21, viola; 22, cello; 23, double bass. *Human singing voices*: A, soprano; B, mezzo-soprano; C, alto; D, contralto; E, tenor; F, baritone; G, bass. *Speaking voices*: H, female; I, male. *Symbols for instrumental sounds*: black, zone of fundamentals; white, zone of harmonics; barred, zone of indeterminate frequencies (noise). *For the singing voice*: cross-hatched, chest voice; dotted, middle register; barred, head voice. *For the speaking voice (H and I)*: hatched, zone for words; barred, zone of indeterminate frequencies. (Modified from Dunker 1972)

• Other instruments, such as bells, are almost invariably asymmetrical with respect to their geometric axis and can generate many systems of partials. According to where they are struck they can produce one particular tone (together with its harmonics), or a different tone (with its own individual harmonics), or, most often, excite both sounds simultaneously, allowing the existence of many complex systems of beating between the many different components.

5.4 REMARKS CONCERNING THE SUBDIVISIONS OF THE OCTAVE

At this stage, let us introduce a brief study of the ways in which musicians have come to define the different intervals in the octave, the only interval that has been uniformly accepted as being completely consonant at all times and in all latitudes (see above, "Specification of Musical Intervals Between Pure Tones"). The information in this section has been culled from many different publications, particularly the following: von Helmholtz 1863; Bouasse 1926; Wood 1944; Brillouin 1958; Danielou 1959; de Candé 1961; Philippot 1968a,b; Barraud 1968).

A musical scale is a sequence of selected notes within the octave. Let us consider the intervals between these notes, such as are specified in a scale of Western music, without for the moment closely defining the exact frequency intervals. A working definition might be "according to the white keys of the piano" starting on C. The interval between the first two successive keys is the *second*, between the first three keys the *third*, the *fourth* and *fifth* being the intervals to the fourth and fifth keys, respectively, with the *sixth* and *seventh* following the same rule.

The next step, anticipating a little, is to consider the idea of a *tone* (T), *semitone* (t), and *quarter tone* ($t/2$). The real magnitudes of the intervals so defined have varied with the passage of time; essentially, their magnitudes have not been far from 200 cents, 100 cents, and 50 cents, respectively.

These considerations enable us to distinguish between different types of scales according to the precise intervals they employ from the tone, semitone, and quarter tone selection. The *diatonic scale* uses tones and semitones, the *enharmonic scale* uses all three possibilities, while the *chromatic scale* only exploits semitones. In the diatonic and enharmonic scales, where all the intervals are not identical, one can also specify different *modes* by the different sequences of intervals they use. These modes have varied from age to age in the history of music.

Table 1.9. Ancient Greek scales and modes

	Type of scale		
Mode	Diatonic	Enharmonic	Chromatic
Dorian	t, T, T	$t/2, t/2, 2T$	$t, t, T + t$
Phrygian	T, t, T	$2T, t/2, t/2$	$T + t, t, t$
Lydian	T, T, t	$t/2, 2T, t/2$	$t, T + t, t$

From musical history, one might infer that our Western scales and modes originate in the ancient Greek's "tetrachord" which, limited by the number of strings in the lyre, long used a system of four adjacent notes that spanned a short scale of a fourth, i.e., $2T + t$. [In that age it was customary to specify a scale in descending pitch: So specified, this scale would be A–E on the white notes of the piano. Nowadays we normally specify scales as ascending, so E–A in this case.] The total interval, less than one octave, could itself be divided in three particular types of scale, *diatonic* of the type containing $2T + t$, *enharmonic* of the sort $2T + t/2$, and *chromatic* $1\frac{1}{2}T + 2t$. Upon this basic scheme three principal modes were adopted, called *Dorian*, *Phrygian*, and *Lydian*. Table 1.9 draws up the nine possible arrangements. (*Note*: There is considerable doubt about the exact authenticity of the precise arrangements supposed to have been used in ancient times.)

Next, a second tetrachord was introduced. Toward 700 B.C. two tetrachords were used with a common central string, giving a "heptachord." That was at the culmination of the Greek classical age and it was not until later, under Pythagoras' influence (530 B.C.) that an eight-string lyre was constructed, introducing a whole tone T ("disjunctive") between the two tetrachords to allow the realization of note sequences that could now cover a whole octave ($2T + t, T, 2T + t$). Under this new arrangement, many combinations become possible, including different types of scales and modes. For example, table 1.10 shows the possibilities using scales of the diatonic type.

The Greek modes provided the musical basis of worship in the primitive Christian Church, but thereafter they were simplified little by little. A certain number of them survived and were incorporated in the plainsong of the twelfth century. With the introduction of polyphony and, more important, of harmony, the choices became more restricted, and effectively the only present-day survivors in Western music are the major mode (the Lydian diatonic) beginning on C and a certain number of minor modes.

Table 1.10. Modes and Pythagorean scales

Dorian	*t*	*T*	*T*	*T*	*t*	*T*	*T*
Phrygian	*T*	*t*	*T*	*T*	*T*	*t*	*T*
Lydian	*T*	*T*	*t*	*T*	*T*	*T*	*t*

Table 1.11. Scale based on intervals of the fifth

F_1	C_2	G_2	D_3	A_3	E_4	B_4
2/3	1	3/2	$(3/2)^2$	$(3/2)^3$	$(3/2)^4$	$(3/2)^5$
2/3	1	3/2	9/4	27/8	81/16	243/32

Remember that we have only been discussing Western music. In fact, many other scales and modes have been developed (the pentatonic scales of Chinese, Native American, and Celtic music; and the complex scales of Indian, Iranian, and Arabian music). We clearly cannot treat them in adequate detail here.

The theoretical approach of Pythagoras was quite fundamental in other ways. He was the first to emphasize the need for an arithmetical basis: He saw the need for simple relationships between frequencies. Using musical strings of different lengths, he established that the particular character of the octave—when two different sounds become as alike as possible—resulted from a length ratio of 2. He then introduced as a fundamental interval the ratio 3/2 (which is a fifth in our modern scale) to be the optimal ratio for his system. A series of notes separated from one another by a fifth could then be arranged that result (using present-day nomenclature) in a sequence of the sort in table 1.11. In this system, every time a note is raised by a fifth, its frequency is multiplied by 3/2; when it is lowered by a fifth, its frequency is multiplied by 2/3.

By gathering together all the notes of table 1.10 into the same octave, one can construct the *Pythagorean scale*. This is shown in table 1.12 with the notes arranged in succession and with their relative frequencies and their corresponding frequency intervals indicated. In this way one arrives, via a "cycle of fifths" (a system also known to the Chinese), at a scale constructed by *TTtTTTt*, with the Pythagorean major tone interval being 240 cents and the Pythagorean semitone, the "limma," being an interval of 90 cents. The difficulties that arise in using this scale are that merely by the arithmetical rules Pythagorean fifths impose a ratio of 3/2, and certain other chords sound, to expert ears, "hard" and not properly consonant (e.g., the third C–E of 408 cents and the sixth C–A of 906 cents).

Table 1.12. Pythagorean Scale

Scales and ratios							
C_2	D_2	E_2	F_2	G_2	A_2	B_2	C_3
1	9/8	81/64	4/3	3/2	27/16	243/128	2
Intervals: ratios and cents							
9/8	9/8	256/243	9/8	9/8	9/8	256/243	
204	204	90	204	204	204	90	

Table 1.13. Natural harmonic scale and ratios with frequencies f, $2f$, $3f$, etc.

C_2	C_3	G_3	C_4	E_4	G_4	B_4	C_5
1	1/2	1/3	1/4	1/5	1/6	1/7	1/8

Table 1.14. Arithmetic scale and ratios with corresponding frequencies f, $6f/5$, $3f/2$, etc.

C_2	E_2	G_2	C_3	G_3	G_4
6/6	5/6	4/6	3/6	2/6	1/6

Other schools, opponents of the Pythagoreans, then saw the light of day, among them those of Aristoxenus (300 B.C.) and Didymus (63 B.C.), followed later by others who expounded the virtues of dividing the scale according to *harmonic* ratios. Two ways of specifying the notes became predominant:

• The series formed by *natural harmonics*, corresponding to frequencies f, $2f$, $3f$, $4f$, etc. as shown in table 1.13.
• A series known as the *arithmetic*, with the gamut arranged in six equal parts with frequencies corresponding to f, $6f/5$, $3f/2$, $2f$, $3f$, $6f$, etc., as in table 1.14.

These two arrangements, harmonic and arithmetic, had each its own advantages: The first contained the perfect major chord (C–E–G) and the second the perfect minor chord (C–E^b–G). However, each also contained mistuned "sharp" intervals, the third in the first and the sixth in the second case. These two types of scale appeared to be entirely incompatible; however, compromise solutions to the problem were proposed.

In the sixteenth century, one solution was developed by and attributed to Zarlino. This new dividing of the scale became known as "the physicist's scale" and "natural" or "just" temperament ("because it is particularly pleasing and agreeable," said Helmholtz). In fact, more detailed historical research seems to show that this just temperament scale, also known as the "mean-tone" scale, was arrived at not only by Zarlino's efforts in 1560 but also with the less well-known participation of Salinas in 1577 (von Helmholtz 1863). The principle was to consider only those intervals that can be expressed as simple fractions. Zarlino chose the seven "natural" sounds of the scale of C major (table 1.15), selecting for each of the five other sounds (the black piano keys) a particular interval, sharped and flatted, respectively, between the adjacent notes. As a consequence of these arrangements, harmonies were excellent in C major or A minor. But in other keys, since slightly different divisions between the two sorts of tones and the two sorts of semitones are demanded for the scale to remain "natural," the intervals sound increasingly false the more sharps or flats there are in the key signature (i.e., the further the key is away from C major).

The scale has advantages: It contains three perfect chords F–A–C, G–B–D, and C–E–G, with the ratio of their extreme notes equal to 3/2 (the Pythagorean fifth); it also contains a harmonic third 5/4. As for the intervals A–C and E–G, they are in the ratio 6/5 of the arithmetic scale.

But there are problems, too, that are to some extent the result of the complex nature of the scale. It comprises three types of intervals: a major tone (9/8; 204 cents); a minor tone (10/9; 184 cents), and a semitone (16/15; 112 cents). The extra intervals introduced are the minor semitone, or diesis (25/24), and the limma (135/128). Note that the difference between the major and minor tones is precisely 1 comma (81/80; 20 cents).

There are other difficulties associated with this scale, particularly in key transpositions. Thus the fifth D–A is not an interval of 3/2 but of 3/2 × 80/81, i.e., the fifth reduced by a comma (680 instead of 704 cents, a so-called weak fifth or flat fifth). In the same way, the fourth F–B is an interval 45/32 = 592 cents, whereas the interval in the descending fourth C–G = 500 cents but in the ascending fourth A–D = 520 cents (strong fourth, sharp fourth), and so on.

Another attempt to reconcile the irreconcilable—namely, to try to square the existence of just fifths (iteration of the ratio 3/2) with the existence of octaves (multiples of 2)—gave rise to the compromise proposed by Weckmeister (1645–1706) called the *equal-tempered* scale. [The equal-tempered scale, presaged by Weckmeister, was not in fact widely accepted until much later. German organ builders used it in the eighteenth century, whereas in the United Kingdom piano manufacturers did not introduce it until 1850, nor the organ builders

Table 1.15. Natural Scale

Scale and ratios

C_2	D_2	E_2	F_2	G_2	A_2	B_2	C_3
1	9/8	5/4	4/3	3/2	5/3	15/8	2

Intervals: ratios and cents

9/8	10/9	16/15	9/8	10/9	9/8	16/15
204	184	112	204	184	204	112

Table 1.16. Equal-tempered scale

Scale, ratios, and cents

	D^b		$D^\#$	F^b	$E^\#$	G^b		A^b		$A^\#$	C^b	
C	$C^\#$	D	E^b	E	F	$F^\#$	G	$G^\#$	A	B^b	B	C
1	$2^{1/12}$	$2^{1/6}$	$2^{1/4}$	$2^{1/3}$	$2^{5/12}$	$2^{1/2}$	$2^{7/12}$	$2^{2/3}$	$2^{3/4}$	$2^{5/6}$	$2^{11/12}$	2
0	100	200	300	400	500	600	700	800	900	1000	1100	1200

Intervals: ratios, cents, and tones

$2^{1/12}$	$2^{1/12}$	$2^{1/12}$	$2^{1/12}$	$2^{1/12}$	etc.
100	100	100	100	100	etc.
	T		T	t		T		T		T	t

before 1860, there being a general reluctance to part with the "natural" temperament.]

The principle is to divide the octave into twelve equal intervals, with the frequency ratios of adjacent notes being $\sqrt[12]{2}$. This interval equals, by definition, 100 cents and is the equal-tempered semitone. The equal-tempered tone interval is thus 200 cents and the octave comprises 1200 cents. The equal-tempered scale is shown in table 1.16.

The advantage of the equal-tempered scale is that it allows all possible transpositions; in particular, it is possible to write for a piano so tuned in all 24 musical keys, major and minor. Bach demonstrated this virtue to great effect (twice! once in 1722 and again in 1744) in his "Well-Tempered Clavier," lovingly referred to as "The Forty-Eight." [The scale also almost reconciles the irreconcilable, at least once. There are, very nearly, 12 fifths in 7 octaves.]

It is inconvenient to have to recognize that, compared with the natural scale, all the intervals apart from the octave are slightly mistuned. Thus the fourth and fifth deviate from the ideal by 2 cents, and the major and minor thirds and the sixth are all mistuned by about 15 cents (but these errors are a small fraction of each total interval).

This fundamental series of notes can be used for two types of musical scales:

- The *chromatic*, comprising all twelve notes of the equal-tempered scale.
- The *diatonic*, in which a musical composition uses a subassembly of the series, usually according to two different modes: the *major mode*, in which the basic structure is *TTtTTTt*; and the *minor modes*, characterized by beginning (*T* + *t*). The possible combinations in this sort of scale are many and the sequences are different in ascending and descending; for example, *TtTTtT* + *tt* (ascending) with *TTtTTtT* (descending).

The diatonic semitone of the musician (passing from one note to the next adjacent) and the chromatic semitone (flatting or sharping a note without changing its name) are identical in the equal-tempered scale (e.g., $C^{\#} = D^{b}$), but they are not so in other scales, in particular in the natural scale. This identity of note actually qualifies it as being enharmonic, one that has a far from simple ratio with a note of the same name.

If we want to be very literal about what would be the ideal musical mathematics, the transposition of the *tonic*, the first note of the scale in use, to a different tonic should, in principle, have no effect of any sort on the melody or harmony. In practice, skilled musicians recognize that each key has its own tonal *color*. This no doubt arises from the "mistuning" of intervals within the scale that results from making all semitones equal.

The equal-tempered chromatic scale of twelve notes is, of course, not the only possible one. In fact, a variety of other temperaments have been thought up, such as dividing the octave into 53 ninth-tones ($\sqrt[53]{2}$), or 31 fifth-tones ($\sqrt[31]{2}$), or 24 quarter-tones ($\sqrt[24]{2}$). Debussy liked to limit himself to 6 tones ($\sqrt[6]{2}$). Some contemporary musicians, such as Stockhausen, have chosen at one stage to abandon the elementary interval $\sqrt[12]{2}$ and instead to divide the interval between a fundamental tone and its fifth harmonic into 28 equal parts ($\sqrt[28]{5}$). The road is clearly free for other excursions. . . .

A final point of some importance concerns recognizing the successive octaves and knowing their frequencies and, incidentally but necessarily, how they are designated.

Beginning with this latter topic, we cannot fail to notice the virtual anarchy that seems to reign over the naming of octaves. In table 1.17 we have used the Latin nomenclature ut_{-1}, ut_0, ut_1, . . . , ut_7, even

Table 1.17. Nomenclature of notes and scales

Frequency[a]	Latin	Standard	Helmholtz	Other	Organ[b]
16	ut_{-1}	C_0	C_2	C_2	32 ft
32	ut_0	C_1	C_1	C_1	16 ft
64	ut_1	C_2	C	C	8 ft
128	ut_2	C_3	c	c^1	4 ft
256	ut_3	C_4	c'	c^2	2 ft
516	ut_4	C_5	c''	c^3	1 ft
1024	ut_5	C_6	c'''	c^4	6 in.
2048	ut_6	C_7	c''''	c^5	3 in.
4096	ut_7	C_8	c'''''	c^6	1.5 in.

[a]Frequency of each C in the succession of octaves of the natural scale.
[b]Corresponding length of open organ pipes.
Note that the German nomenclature is like the Anglo-Saxon (standard) except that H is used for B and B is used for B^b.

though the French nomenclature does not always use ut_0 and starts therefore at ut_{-2} (recognizing also that the Latin nomenclature "ut" is now often and quite happily replaced by "do"). The designations used in non-Latin countries have been specially diverse. They include the method that we have finally selected in this book (which seems to be the standard choice at present), but other older and more recent nomenclatures are still current. For example, there is the list that Helmholtz particularly favored that runs C_1, C, c, c', c'', c''', c'''', etc., and yet others (C_1, C, C^1, C^2, etc.).

Even more important has been the choice of a reference frequency. Once this is fixed, all the other notes can be specified according to the rule selected for dividing the octaves, the actual choices being, in practice, between the natural and the equal-tempered scales.

The "physicist's reference" selects not one note but specifies all the C's as increasing in frequency by powers of 2 successively (16, 32, 64, etc.). The values in this scale are usually coupled with the lengths of the open organ pipes that generate them (in feet or inches; see table 1.17). Given these C frequencies, the octaves can be divided either into natural scale steps or into equal-tempered frequency steps, as shown in table 1.18.

But through the history of music the selection of reference frequencies has not proceeded exactly in that way. The note A_4 within the octave C_4–C_5 (ut_3–ut_4) has been chosen as the single specified reference standard with all the other frequencies being calculated from

Table 1.18. Frequency of the notes C to B in the octave C_4–B_4

Standard	C_4	D_4	E_4	F_4	G_4	A_4	B_4	C_5
Helmholtz	c'	d'	e'	f'	g'	a'	b'	c''
Latin	ut_3	re_3	mi_3	fa_3	sol_3	la_3	si_3	ut_4
Natural scale frequencies[a]	256	288	320	342	384	426.5	480	512
Equal-tempered scale frequencies[a]	256	287.4	322.5	341.7	383.5	430.5	483.2	512
Natural scale[b]	264	297	330	352	396	440	495	528
Equal-tempered scale[b]	261.6	293.6	329.6	349.2	392	440	493	523.2

[a]Scale based on the choice of powers of 2 for the frequency of successive C's. Here C_4 = 256 Hz.
[b]Scale based on the reference A_4 = 440 Hz.

Table 1.19. Comparison of the octave divisions in the Pythagorean (P), Zarlino's or ▶ natural (Z), and Werckmeister's or equal-tempered (W) scales

To the left, intervals from the lower C are indicated in cents (first column) and in savarts, σ (second column); for definitions see section 5.1. For each scale, P, W, and Z, five columns show respectively from left to right (1) name of the interval; (2) interval from lower C in savarts, σ; (3) frequency ratio to lower C (frequency f_0); (4) standard non-Latin nomenclature of the notes; (5) intervals within each scale (tones T, halftones t): Augm, augmented; m, minor; M, major. Standard flat and sharp symbols.
(Compiled from a variety of sources: von Helmholtz 1863; Bouasse 1926; Wood 1944; De Candé 1961; Roederer 1979).

that basis, once more with different values that depend on whether the natural or equal-tempered scale is used.

In addition, the reference frequency chosen for A_4 has changed considerably through the centuries, and even sometimes from year to year. In 1885 A_4 was fixed at 435 Hz, then in 1939 the standard was raised to 440 Hz. For that reason alone, the equal-tempered C_4 changed from 258.65 Hz (based on 435) to 261.63 Hz (based on 440).

Finally, using the present standard of 440 for A_4, the frequencies of all the other notes once more depend on the type of scale chosen. This is illustrated in table 1.18 for sequences in the natural scale and the equal-tempered scale in the octave C_4–C_5. These themselves differ from the values appropriate for C_4 = 256 of the "physicist's scale." The three main ways of dividing the octave into musical scales are shown in table 1.19.

cents	σ	Pythagorean (P) σ	f/f₀	note	interval	Natural (Z) interval	note	σ	f/f₀	Tempered (W) interval	σ	f/f₀	note
1200	300	300	2.000	C₁	Octave	Octave	C₁ / B# / G♭	300 / 290 / 283	2.000	Octave	300	2.000	C₁
1100	275	278 / 255	1.898	B / A#	M Seventh *(Limma)*	M Seventh / m Seventh	B / B♭	273 / 255	1.875 / 1.800 *(t_M)*	M Seventh	275	1.887	B *(t)*
1000	250	250	—	B♭	m Seventh *(T_M)*	m Seventh	A# / B♭♭	245 / 232	*(T_M)*	m Seventh	250	1.781	A#B♭ *(T)*
900	225	227 / 204	1.687	A / G#	M Sixth	M Sixth	A	222	1.667	M Sixth	225	1.681	A
800	200	198	1.580	A♭	m Sixth *(T_M)*	m Sixth	A♭	204	1.600	m Sixth	200	1.587	G#A♭ *(T)*
						m Sixth	G# / A♭♭	194 / 186	*(T_M)*				
700	175	176	1.500	G	Fifth	Fifth	G / G low	176 / 170	1.500	Fifth	175	1.498	G
600	150	153	—	F#	Augm Fourth	Triton	G♭	153	1.422	Triton	150	1.414	F#G♭ *(T)*
		147 / 130	—	G♭ / E#	Triton *(T_M)*		F#	148	1.406 *(T_M)*				
500	125	125	1.333	F	Fourth *(Halftone & Limma 256/243 = 23σ)*	Fourth	F	125	1.333	Fourth	125	1.334	F
						M Halftone	F / E# / F♭	125 / 114 / 107	*(M Halftone t_M = 16/15 = 28σ)*				*(Halftone t 2^(1/12) = 25σ)*
400	100	102 / 96 / 79	1.266	E / F♭ / D#	M Third	M Third	E	97	1.250	M Third	100	1.260	E *(T)*
300	75	73	1.184	E♭	m Third *(T_M)*	m Third	E♭	79	1.200 *(m Tone)*	m Third	75	1.189	D#E♭
200	50	51	1.125	D	Second *(Tone T_M 9/8 = 51σ)*	Second	D♯ / E♭♭	68 / 61	1.125 *(T_m = 10/9 = 46σ)*	M Second	50	1.122	D
						m Tone	D / D low	51 / 46	1.111 *(M Tone)*				
100	25	28 / 23	—	C# / D♭	Apotome / Limma	M Halftone	D♭ / C#	28 / 17	1.066 / 1.041 *(T_M 9/8 = 51σ)*	m Second	25	1.059	C#D♭ *(Tone 2^(1/6) = 50σ)*
						m Halftone / Quartertone Z Comma	C	10 / 5.4	*(51σ)*				
0	0	5.8 / 0	—	C	P Comma					W Comma	5	—	C

The Auditory Receptor System

First of all we shall consider the general gross anatomy of the mammalian peripheral organ of hearing, then, in more detail, the morphology of the receptor region itself (figure 2.1).

1 THE OUTER EAR

From an anatomical point of view the outer ear comprises the ear canal, or external auditory meatus; the concha, which links the auditory canal to the exterior; the pinna, which often takes the form of an "ear trumpet" to collect the sound. In animals (but not in humans) it can be oriented toward the source of a particular sound by the use of muscles located within the pinna itself (17 of them in the horse!).

The human pinna, with its characteristic folding, is essentially constructed of cartilage covered with skin. This cartilaginous region extends into the concha, which forms the outer third of the auditory canal. The wall of the innermost two thirds of the canal is defined by bony structures. Sebaceous and ceruminous glands are present in the cartilaginous portion.

2 THE MIDDLE EAR

The middle ear, or tympanic cavity (figure 2.2), situated between the outer and inner ear communicates with the nasopharynx via the eustachian tube. Normally this is closed, but it opens briefly during swallowing.

At the inner end of the ear canal is the *tympanic membrane* (eardrum), which has a flared, conical shape. The central tip of the cone (*umbo*) penetrates a little into the middle ear cavity. The tympanum is made of three layers; an external, squamous epithelium that joins with that of the external auditory meatus; a middle layer of fibrous tissue, comprising both radial and circular arrangements of fibers that maintain a certain tension; and an inner layer of mucous tissue that is continuous with the lining of the middle ear cavity.

The middle ear cavity, comprising the tympanic cavity proper and

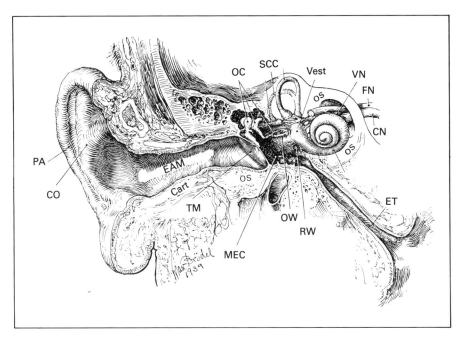

Figure 2.1
Longitudinal section of the human auditory apparatus. PA, pinna; CO, concha; EAM,
external auditory meatus; Cart, cartilage; TM, tympanic membrane; OC, (middle ear)
ossicular chain; SCC, semicircular canals; OW, oval window; RW, round window;
MEC, middle ear cavity; Vest, vestibule; VN, vestibular nerve; FN, facial nerve; CN,
cochlear nerve; ET, eustachian tube. (From Wever & Lawrence 1954 after *Brödel's Anatomy of the Human Ear*, 1946, Saunders)

an upper portion extending above the tympanum (epitympanic recess, or attic), communicates with the inner ear at the oval and round windows.

The *tympanum* and the *oval window* are connected via the *ossicular chain*. In practically all mammals, the ossicles comprise three bony structures: the malleus (hammer), the incus (anvil), and the stapes (stirrup).

The *malleus* has two distinctive parts, the *head* (*capitulum*) and its *handle* (*manubium*), the latter being attached to the tympanum along a radius reaching up to the umbo. By the forces that the malleus transmits it maintains the shape of the cone of the tympanic membrane, concave toward the interior of the tympanic cavity.

The *incus* consists of a short process, whose articulatory surface contacts the head of the hammer, and a long process, which articu-

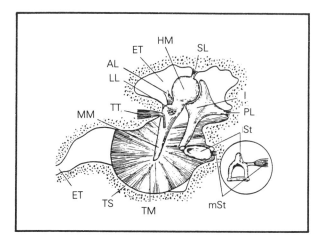

Figure 2.2
Diagram of the middle ear as viewed internally from near the oval window. TM,
tympanic membrane; TS, tympanic sulcus; MM, manubrium of malleus (handle of
the hammer); ET, eustachian tube; TT, muscle fibers of tensor tympani; AL, anterior
ligament; LL, lateral ligament; SL, superior ligament; PL, posterior ligament; HM, head
of malleus; I, incus (anvil); ET, epitympanic recess; mSt, stapedius muscle; St, stapes
(stirrup). *Inset*, View of the stapes and the stapedius muscle from another angle. (From
Møller 1974a)

lates with the head of the *stapes*. The other extremity of the *stapes* has
a *footplate* that is attached to the margins of the oval window.

The *tympanic cavity* proper contains the manubrium of the malleus,
the long process of the incus, and the stapes; the head of the malleus
and the body of the incus are situated in the *epitympanic recess*.

The malleus is suspended by four ligaments: anterior, posterior,
lateral, and superior (the latter being smaller than the others). The
incus itself possesses a posterior ligament. The malleus-incus connection is rigid in most species and in humans it only allows very limited
movement, except perhaps in the very young child. In contrast, the
incus-stapes connection appears to be much more flexible, thus
allowing the stapes more freedom of movement.

Finally, there are two muscles, the tensor tympani and the stapedius, that control the mobility of the system. The *tensor tympani muscle*
inserts in a canal adjacent to the eustachian tube; its tendon crosses
the tympanic cavity and is inserted into the medial surface of the
manubrium near its neck. It is innervated by a motor branch of the
trigeminal nerve and its contraction exerts tension on the tympanum,
directed toward the interior of the middle ear cavity. The *stapedius*

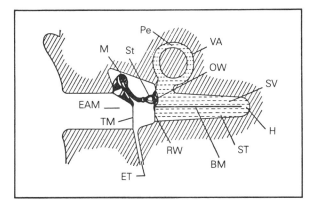

Figure 2.3
Schematic diagram of the human ear in a longitudinal section with the cochlea represented as "unrolled." EAM, external auditory meatus; TM, tympanic membrane; M,
malleus; ET, eustachian tube; St, stapes; RW, round window; Pe, perilymph; VA,
vestibular apparatus; OW, oval window; SV, scala vestibuli; H, helicotrema; ST, scala
tympani; BM, basilar membrane. (From von Békésy & Rosenblith 1951).

muscle, the tendon of which issues from a tiny bony "pyramid," inserts into the neck of the stapes. The nerve to the stapedius branches
from the facial nerve near the pyramid. Contraction of the stapedius
tilts the stapes in such a way as to increase the rigidity of the incus-
stapes articulation.

The middle ear muscles are notable for their rich motor innervation;
the number of muscle fibers per motor unit is generally small, about
7 for the tensor tympani and 14 to 20 for the stapedius and is thus
not unlike the motor innervation of the oculomotor muscles.

We shall see below that the whole ossicular chain acts like a lever
and that the two muscles, contracting in synergy, underpin the rather
impressive mechanical rigidity of the system.

3 THE INNER EAR

The inner ear, encased in the temporal bone (figures 2.1, 2.2, 2.3), is
made up of a series of intercommunicating cavities: the *cochlea,* the
vestibule, and the *semicircular canals.* Together these constitute the *bony
labyrinth* (see also Buser & Imbert 1982, chapter 3).

3.1 GENERAL STRUCTURE

At the level of the cochlea, the bony labyrinth connects with the
middle ear via the oval window and its membrane, to which the
footplate of the stapes is attached, and also by the round window,

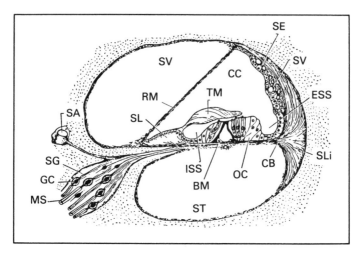

Figure 2.4
Diagrammatic, generalized cross section of the cochlea. SV, scala vestibuli; ST, scala tympani; TM, tectorial membrane; RM, Reissner's membrane; StV, stria vascularis; CC, cochlear canal (scala media); SLi, spiral ligament; BM, basilar membrane; SL, spiral limbus; SG, spiral ganglion; OC, organ of Corti; SA, spiral artery; GC, ganglion cell of SG; MS, myelin sheath of a cochlear nerve fiber; SE, secretory epithelium; ESS, ISS, external, internal spiral sulcus; CB, crista basilaris. (From Davis 1951)

which is closed by its own membrane. The bony cochlea, shaped like a snail shell, is a few-turn spiral, with two and a half turns in humans (see figure 2.1).

In transverse section, the cochlea is seen to be divided into two spiralling parts; the upper *scala vestibuli* connects with the vestibule, and the lower *scala tympani* terminates in the round window. These two divisions are themselves interconnected at the apex of the spiral, the *helicotrema* (figures 2.3, 2.4, 2.5).

The scala vestibuli and scala tympani both belong to the *perilymphatic space*. Between them, near the axis of the cochlea, is the *cochlear canal (scala media)*, which is separated from the scala tympani by the basilar membrane and from the scala vestibuli by Reissner's membrane. The cochlear canal, or *membranous labyrinth,* belongs to the *endolymphatic space.*

Reissner's membrane is formed from two layers of cells. The one facing the cochlear canal has an ectodermal origin, while that on the perilymphatic side is mesodermal. The two layers are separated by a thin fibrous layer. Reissner's membrane is not impermeable: it seems that certain exchanges can take place between perilymph and endolymph (see below).

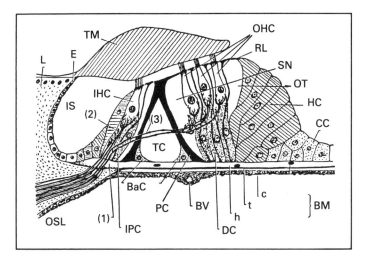

Figure 2.5
Transverse section of the cochlea. The inner edge of the spiral is to the left. IHC, inner hair cell; OHC, outer hair cells; PC, pillar of Corti; BaC, basal cells; TM, tectorial membrane; RL, reticular lamina; TC, tunnel of Corti; BM, basilar membrane with components: c, connective tissue, t, transverse fibers, h, homogeneous layer; BV, blood vessel; HC, Hensen's cells; CC, Claudius' cells; OSL, osseous spiral lamina; L, spiral limbus; DC, Deiter's cells (outer supporting cells); E, epithelium of internal sulcus; IS, internal sulcus; SN, space of Nuel; OT, outer tunnel; IPC, inner pharyngeal cells; (1), nerve fibers entering via the habenula perforata; (2), inner spiral fibers; (3), tunnel fibers. (The relationship of the cilia of IHC and OHC to the TM remain under discussion; see text). (From Davis 1951)

The *basilar membrane* extends between the outer spiral ligament and the inner osseous spiral lamina (the *modiolus,* near the axis of the cochlear spiral) (figure 2.6). In transverse section it is seen to possess two distinct parts; the inner region, from the modiolus to the outer pillar of Corti is called the *pars* (or *zona*) *tecta* or *pars arcuata;* the outer part from the outer pillar of Corti to the spiral ligament is the *pars pectinata.* The two parts are made up of similar cellular layers but are different in the number of layers of elastic fibers: one layer only in the pars tecta and two superposed but distinct layers in the pars pectinata.

The *organ of Corti* rests on this membrane within the cochlear canal. It comprises the receptor cells, various supporting and accessory cells and specialized pillar cells known as the *pillars* or *rods of Corti*. These latter delimit a particular space called the *tunnel of Corti,* which is filled with *cortilymph*. The composition of this fluid and its detailed

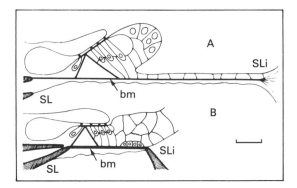

Figure 2.6
Morphological variation of the organ of Corti along the cochlea. Note that the basilar membrane (bm) is wide at the apex (A) and narrow at the base (B). SL, spiral lamina; Sli, spiral ligament; scale bar: ~ 50 μm. (From Spoendlin 1979)

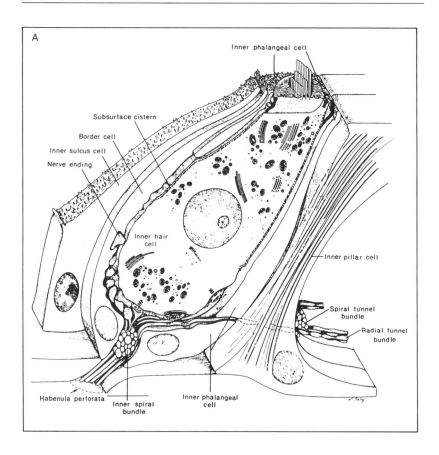

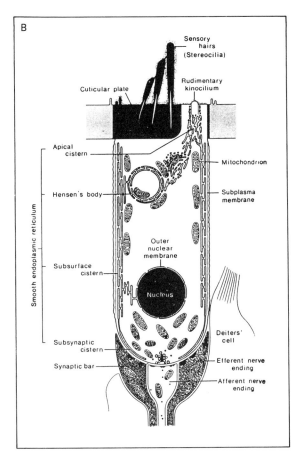

◀ Figure 2.7
Artist's conception of inner hair cell (A) showing organization of cell organelles that is distinct from that of outer hair cells and (B) schematic diagram of outer hair cell showing various cell organelles. Note interconnecting cisternal structures such as apical cistern, Hensen's body, subsurface cistern, subsynaptic cisternae. (Drawings by Nancy Sally in Lim 1986)

morphological siting suggest it to be part of the perilymphatic space. We will discuss this further.

3.2 THE RECEPTOR CELLS

There are two separate populations of ciliated receptor cells (figures 2.7, 2.8), the *outer hair cells* (OHC) and *inner hair cells* (IHC). In humans, there are three to five rows of OHC ranged along the cochlear tunnel; they number between 12,000 and 19,000. They do not rest on

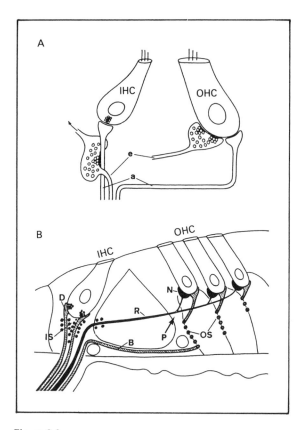

Figure 2.8
Afferent and efferent innervation of hair cells. *A* shows how efferent fibers (e) form axodendritic contacts with the afferents (a) to the inner hair cell system (IHC) while efferents to the outer hair cells (OHC) form axosomatic contacts. *B,* Routes of afferent (hatched) and efferent (black) fibers to the inner (left) and outer hair cells (right). D, afferent dendrites on IHC (inner radial fibers); the inner spiral fibers (IS) are the efferents forming axodendritic contacts (as in *A*). Afferents to OHC first cross the tunnel of Corti as basal tunnel fibers (B) and then form the outer spiral fibers (OS) around accessory cells to reach the OHC. Efferents to OHC cross the tunnel as upper radial fibers (R) to contact the hair cells (at N). P, pillar of Corti. (From Spoendlin 1979)

the basilar membrane itself but on the supporting cells called *Deiter's cells*. The IHC form only one rank along the tunnel and number about 3,500 cells. They are surrounded by different supporting cells (*inner supporting cells*) but the IHC themselves rest directly in contact with the basilar membrane.

Deiter's supporting cells, and also the cells of the inner and outer pillars of Corti, contain large numbers of tonofibrils that confer on them a certain rigidity; in addition, the pillar cells are firmly fixed to the basilar membrane by some sort of cement.

Lateral to the OHC and to the Deiter's cells there exists a border of cells called *Hensen's* and *Claudius' cells*. Cells other than receptor cells are also situated at the inner border of the cochlear tunnel (see figure 2.5).

The *tectorial membrane* extends over the receptor cells. It is a fibrous and gelatinous structure formed from a principal body of essentially radial fibers wrapped in an amorphous substance. It extends from the spiral lamina, where it inserts medially, to the level of Hensen's cells, where it forms a *marginal band* which in turn is attached to the reticular lamina by another marginal band. Below this band there is a structure called the *median band of Hensen* and another called the *amorphous band of Kimura* (see figure 2.5; Lim 1986).

At the outer wall of the cochlear tunnel there exists a specialized region called the *stria vascularis*, which plays an essential role in maintaining the peculiar composition of endolymph, as we shall see below. The blood vessels that irrigate this region come from the modiolus and cross the scala vestibuli. The stria is formed of three populations of cells, *marginal* at the endolymphatic side, *intermediate*, and *basal* at the perilymphatic side (Kuijpers 1969).

Finally, the cochlea spirals around a hollow bony axis, the *columella*, which accommodates the entry of the fibers of the cochlear nerve. The cell bodies of these primary fibers are situated within a canal in the osseous spiral lamina, where they form the *spiral ganglion*.

Table 2.1 lists some numerical data concerning the morphology of the peripheral organ of hearing in the human, cat, dog, and guinea pig.

3.3 FINE STRUCTURE OF THE RECEPTOR CELLS

There are essential structural differences between the inner and outer hair cells.

Table 2.1. Quantitative morphological data

	Human	Cat	Dog	Guinea pig
Meatus				
Cross section	0.3–0.5 cm^2			
Diameter	0.7 cm			
Length	2.7 cm			
Volume	1.04 ml			
Tympanum				
Area	50–90 mm^2	32–48 mm^2		23–28 mm^2
Thickness	0.1 mm	0.03 mm		
Malleus				
Weight	23 mg	10–11 mg		
Length	5.5–6.0 mm			
Incus				
Weight	25 mg	3–4 mg		
Stapes				
Weight	2–4 mg	0.2–0.9 mg		
Area	2.6–3.7 mm^2	1.1–1.3 mm^2		0.8–0.9 mm^2
Windows				
Oval (area)	2.0–3.7 mm^2	1.1–1.3 mm^2		1.4 mm^2
Round (area)	2 mm^2	2.8–3.3 mm^2		1.0 mm^2
Cochlea				
Number of turns	2.2–2.9	3	3.2	4.9
Basilar membrane				
Length	25–35 mm	19–25 mm	14–16 mm	18.8 mm
Thickness	<0.003 mm			0.007 mm
Breadth (base)	0.04 mm			
Breadth (apex)	0.36 mm			
Hair cells				
IHC (number)	3500	2600	1600	
OHC (number)	20,000	9900	6100	
Ganglion cells				
Number	30,000	50,000		

INNER HAIR CELLS

These have an ovoid, piriform cell body (35 μm long and 10 μm diameter in the chinchilla). Their upper surface comprises a cuticular thickening (1 to 2 μm) into which two or three ranks of cilia, called *stereocilia*, are implanted by their "roots." Each cell carries 60 to 100 cilia in all. A very small part of the upper surface of the cell has no cuticular covering. Here there is found a basal corpuscle and a centriole (in the rat and guinea pig, though not in the cat). By all appearances, this seems to indicate the vestiges of a kinocilium, which is known to exist in the vestibular cells of the adult (Buser & Imbert 1982) but which disappears toward the end of embryonic life in the auditory cells. The cilia do not all have the same length. The longest (6 to 7 μm) are near the basal corpuscle and the pillars of Corti; the shorter hairs are closer to the modiolus. The stereocilia are grouped together in a widely open V shape (almost in a straight line). The open end of the V faces inward, with the basal corpuscle situated toward the outside and consequently near the pillars of Corti. The IHC nucleus is central. Endoplasmic reticulum is found below the cuticle, and the cytoplasmic region above the nucleus contains Golgi complex and lysosomes. Ribosomes and mitochondria are found in the infranuclear region. Note that the IHC typically form only a single rank along the whole length of the tunnel of Corti.

OUTER HAIR CELLS

The OHC are cylindrical (25 to 45 μm long, depending on their location, and 6 to 7 μm in diameter). They also have a cuticular surface and stereocilia. The cilia are arranged in three or four ranks and grouped in a rather clear V or W shape, opening out inward. At the point of the V there is again a noncuticular zone and a basal corpuscle representing what remains of kinocilium. Sometimes, a vestigial kinocilium can be seen (figure 2.9). Here again, the longest stereocilia are outermost.

The OHC nucleus is basal, and mitochondria are present under the cuticle as well as below the nucleus. Endoplasmic reticulum and glycogen can be seen along with clear indications of a highly energetic metabolism. This observation accords well with other data revealing the existence of contractile proteins in the OHC (discussed later).

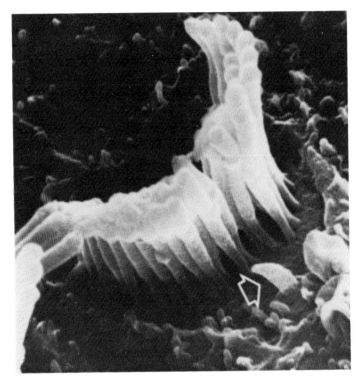

Figure 2.9
Arrangement of cilia in macaque OHC; scanning EM view. Note the clear V arrangement, with its open end facing internally (toward the upper left in this view), formed
by the several rows of stereocilia. In this animal, which was at least 3 to 4 months old,
there were clearly signs of a vestigial kinocilium (arrow) at the outer tip of the V (i.e.,
downward to the right) in a large number of OHC. This is not normally the case in
primates (see text). Microvilli of the supporting cells can also be clearly seen. (From
Ades & Engstrom 1974)

ARRANGEMENT OF THE RECEPTOR CELLS

Consideration of further structural details concerning the arrangement of the hair cell system is essential for understanding the relevant operating mechanisms (see Hudspeth 1985).

The upper, cuticular surfaces of the hair cells (both inner and outer)
are, for the whole population, bounded by a common *reticular lamina.*
This layer allows only the stereocilia to penetrate it and forms an
impermeable barrier between the hair cells and the cortilymph, on
the one hand, and the endolymph proper, on the other. Thus only
the stereocilia, which pass through the layer, are bathed in endo-

lymph. Electron micrograph sections also show that, between the hair cells, there are microvilli showing contact with supporting cells (particularly Deiter's cells for the OHC). In this way, the mammalian scala media forms a morphologically enclosed space, an endolymphatic space into which the cilia of the hair cells can extend, while the rest of the receptor cell occupies perilymphatic space. We shall consider the functional importance of this fact below (Anniko & Wroblewski 1986).

Both the OHC and the IHC show arrangements of their cilia that are precisely and identically spatially organized with respect to their relative orientation to the tunnel of Corti and to the axis of the cochlear spiral. If we justify the use of such morphological data as a basis for making close comparisons between systems, then such an analogy with the vestibular cells leads one immediately to consider the possibility of linking the functional depolarization of the cochlear receptors with reference to the arrangement of their cilia. (*Note:* The mechanical analogies with the vestibular receptors must not, however, be pushed too far. The cupular and macular hairs are in fact much longer than the cochlear, whereas the otolith and cupular membranes are much less rigid than the tectorial membrane.)

Investigations aimed at specifying the contractile proteins found in the cells show the presence of actin filaments oriented parallel to the long axis of the cilia. These pass through the reticular lamina and penetrate the apical plate of the receptor cell into a region where there also exists a truly three-dimensional actin filament network, which is itself surrounded by an annulus of actin filaments. Lower in the cell body, a network of fibers once more running parallel to the major axis of the cell is seen in the cytoplasm (reviewed by Zenner 1986). Other contractile proteins, in particular myosin and tropomyosin, also appear to be present. The existence of these proteins has profoundly modified our ways of viewing possible cochlear mechanisms; they contribute a modifiable stiffness to certain hair cell structures and also mediate actual cellular contractions, as we shall discuss below.

Another problem that has arisen in cochlear mechanics, the solution of which will no doubt also be based on morphological data, concerns the precise relationships between the cilia and the tectorial membrane (TM), particularly in the mammal. A view that has already become outdated was that all the cilia, whether IHC or OHC, made firm connections with the TM at their extremities. Studies with scanning electron microscopy after cryofracture have profoundly altered that view. While it is almost certain that the OHC cilia (particularly the longest, i.e., the outermost, hairs) are solidly anchored into the TM at the level of the amorphous membrane of Kimura, the question is not so well resolved for IHC. At their locations, the TM presents a feature called the *band of Hensen* on its internal face, and any coupling between that with the IHC cilia remains doubtful. The electron microscopic evidence in this region is far from clear-cut. In essence, the present prevailing thought is that the IHC cilia are free from attachment (Lim 1986).

Finally, other morphological studies have recently shown the presence of fine filaments that make transverse couplings between adjacent cilia in each bundle in such a way that the longer cilia will pull along all the others with them.

Phylogeny of the Auditory Apparatus

In a whole range of vertebrates, the labyrinth comprises a practically identical architecture, with a utricle, saccule, and semicircular canals (Buser & Imbert 1982, Vol. II). In contrast, it is clear that the auditory organ shows quite remarkable modifications from the fish to the mammals. Since material from nonmammalian vertebrates is much used to explore the detailed properties of ciliated cells, we need to be aware of these evolutionary aspects of their morphology.

Any *outer ear* structure is usually negligible in nonmammalian vertebrates. The tympanum is superficial in fish and amphibians; in reptiles and birds it occurs in a depression called the *auditory meatus.*

The *middle ear* shows a more interesting evolution. In fish there is a whole series of very different organizations. In certain groups (teleosts, including salmon, perch families, and many marine species), the mechanical vibrations in the water are simply transmitted across the soft tissues of the animal to the inner ear without any special intermediates. In other groups (teleosts, including the herring family) the swim bladder serves as an amplifying transformer of pressure thanks to the bubble of gas it encloses. This bladder has effectively developed diverticula that make contact with the inner ear, increasing its intensity sensitivity and extending its useful frequency range. In yet other groups (Ostariophysi, including the carp and catfish families) there is a remarkable specialization in which there has arisen, between the swim bladder and the inner ear, a chain of *ossicles of Weber,* which in fact are part of the four first vertebrae. These notably extend the range of audible frequencies. Finally, certain species exploit a diverticulum situated at the level of the gills which acts as an air bubble amplifier (freshwater fish of Africa, Anabantidae).

All terrestrial vertebrates—amphibians, reptiles (apart from the urodela and ophidia), and birds—possess a middle ear, an air-filled cavity that communicates with the pharynx and contains a rigid structure (*colu-*

mella) which connects the tympanum to the inner ear and which serves as an acoustic impedance transformer as in mammals. The columella is the embryological homologue of the mammalian stapes. It consists of a cartilaginous part proximally (near the tympanum) and a distal bony portion. In certain groups, these two parts are even anatomically distinct and form the *extra columella* and the *columella proper*, respectively. In the Urodela, a group close to aquatic life, the columella is enclosed in soft tissue; in snakes there is neither a tympanum nor a middle ear cavity, the columella extending between a cranial bone and the inner ear.

The *inner ear* is first represented in fish and amphibians as a simple diverticulum of the saccule of the labyrinth, the *lagena*. This contains a small platform of ciliated cells that comprise the macula of the lagena. In amphibians, the lagena is a little more developed, and it contains not only a macular neuroepithelium but also, very close to that, a formation of ciliated cells called the *basal papilla*.

In reptiles and birds this basal papilla acquires an increasing importance. It extends along the whole length of the lagena, which in its turn is perceptibly lengthened to become an independent cochlear canal connected to the saccule by a simple tube. The papilla becomes associated with a basilar membrane upon which stand both ciliated cells and supporting cells. The macular lagena, in contrast, ceases to be predominant.

In all cases it seems that the cilia of the receptor cells are free standing in fluid without any accessory structure playing a part, in contrast to the mammalian OHC with their cilia fixed to the tectorial membrane (figure 2.10).

3.4 INNERVATION OF THE RECEPTOR CELLS

The mammalian cochlea is innervated by tens of thousands of sensory neurons (afferents), by about 50,000 in cat (in which species diameters are <7 µm) and by about 30,000 in humans. In addition, there is a limited number of efferent fibers (500 to 2,000); see Spoendlin 1970, 1979 and figure 2.8).

AFFERENT FIBERS

The afferent fibers cell bodies reside in the spiral ganglion that is sited in the modiolus on the internal surface of the spiral lamina. The cell body is generally bipolar, with its peripheral branch penetrating the cochlear canal by a system of apertures in the spiral lamina called *habenulae perforatae*. At these apertures all the myelinated afferents shed their myelin sheaths.

The pattern of afferent innervation is complicated. The IHC enjoy about 95% of the innervation by afferent fibers; each fiber connects with only one cell, but each cell is innervated by about 20 separate afferent fibers. This establishes a clearly divergent arrangement be-

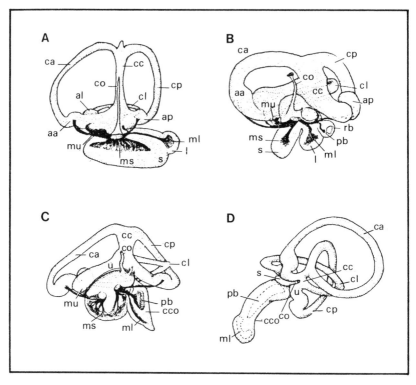

Figure 2.10
Evolution of the inner ear (vestibuloauditory apparatus). *A*, Teleost (perch). *B*, Amphibian (toad). *C*, Reptile (turtle). *D*, Bird (passerine). ca, cp, cc, cl: semicircular canals, respectively vertical anterior, vertical posterior, part common to both vertical canals, lateral ("horizontal") canal. aa, ap, al, anterior, posterior, and lateral ampullae; co, otic canal; u, utricle; s, saccule; l, lagena; cco, cochlear canal; mu, ms, ml maculae of the utricle, saccule, and lagena; pb, basilar papilla and basilar membrane; rb, basilar recess. (From Baird 1974)

tween the receptors and the central nervous system (3,000 IHC supplying 20,000 afferent output fibers).

The connection between each afferent and its hair cell receptor shows a particular fine structure: The swollen terminal bouton is poorly granulated, while at the cell surface opposite there exists a structure with a greater optical density that is surrounded by vesicles. This suggests that the synapse functions in the direction receptor toward fiber and that we are dealing with a truly afferent termination, therefore with an afferent dendrite. These afferent terminals are distributed over much of the cell body. The trajectory of the fibers innervating the IHC occurs radially, that is, toward the modiolus, for which they are named the *inner radial fibers* (Spoendlin 1979).

The OHC receive an innervation notably different from that to the IHC. Here only 5% (2,000 to 3,000) of the sensory fibers serve the population of around 20,000 OHC; thus each separate afferent innervates about 10 OHC. Each cell receives afferents from about 4 separate fibers. Thus, unlike the IHC, the afferent innervation to the OHC is largely convergent. Its fibers enter the cochlea, cross the tunnel of Corti near the basilar membrane (as *basal tunnel fibers*), then, when they reach the vicinity of the OHC, take on a spiral trajectory such that each travels along the cochlea by 0.6 to 0.7 mm (as *external spiral fibers*) before innervating the OHC (see figure 2.8). The terminals of the afferents to the OHC are essentially similar to those to the IHC except that they tend to be more concentrated toward the base of the ciliated OHC.

There is a present day tendency to emphasize a difference that might exist between the afferent innervation of the IHC and of the OHC, even though the facts remain controversial. In the spiral ganglion it is clear that 95% of the cells are bipolar and have a myelinated centrally projecting fiber. These cells, called type I, extensively innervate IHC. What is more, there appear to be three categories of type I fiber with large, medium and small fiber diameters. Each IHC might receive a fiber of every type, a thick fiber's terminal tending to make contact at the outer side of the cell and medium and thin fibers distributed to the modiolar side. In contrast, type II fibers from the remaining 5% of the ganglion cells innervate OHC. According to some publications, these cells do not have a central projection and should thus be classified as monopolar. Other researchers consider that central projections do exist but are unmyelinated and thus simply are difficult to identify properly in their trajectory toward the cochlear nucleus (Liberman & Oliver 1984). The former hypothesis is to some extent reinforced by the fact that exploration of the fibers of the cochlear nerve (downstream from the spiral ganglion in consequence) has not so far shown the bimodal nature of the afferents that would be expected if there really were two types of afferents in the projection to the brainstem. However, given the possibility that some of the afferents are very thin and difficult to trace, the question remains unresolved; the possible presence of monopolar neurons without central projections does not appear to be tenable with any certainty.

Neurochemical Data

The search for neurotransmitters at the afferent synapses is now directed toward excitatory amino acids. Autoradiography (Eybalin, Calas & Pujol 1983) and immunohistochemistry (Fex & Altschuler 1986) have in fact demonstrated the involvement of glutamic acid in the IHC lateral system (type I fibers). The characterization of neurotransmission at the OHC (type II fibers) remains a matter for discussion.

EFFERENT FIBERS

Electron microscopy shows that, apart from the connections with afferent dendrites, there are other terminals in the immediate vicinity of the receptor cells that have the characteristics of efferent influences. These terminals are, for example, rich in granules and vesicles, suggesting centrifugal synaptic interactions.

These efferent connections arise from the olivocochlear bundle, a tract whose organization and origin (in the superior olive) we shall describe later in detail. It contains fibers that are relatively thick and myelinated but also others that are thin and unmyelinated.

The number of large myelinated fibers reported varies with species (and the research worker) but is always a minority. A present estimate of the total number of fibers is 1350 for the cat and guinea pig (Warr 1975).

The thin *fibers innervating the IHC* occupy only two tracts. Some originate in the contralateral superior olive but most arrive, uncrossed, from the ipsilateral olive (dorsolateral and lateral periolivary nuclei). They take a spiral trajectory, that is, they follow the contours of the cochlea for a certain distance (inner spiral fibers) and make axodendritic connections with individual afferent fibers. These fibers constitute about 58% of the total efferents and form the *lateral efferent system* (figures 2.7, 2.8, 2.11).

The *fibers innervating the OHC* are thicker and a little fewer in number (42%). They cross the tunnel of Corti in its upper regions (*upper radial tunnel fibers*) and innervate the OHC, axosomatically in this case (i.e., terminating on the receptor cell body itself). Earlier in their tract they have generated branches, with the result that 800 fibers can innervate the whole population of 20,000 OHC. They achieve their final connections by an incident radial trajectory (*outer radial fibers*). These fibers innervating the OHC constitute the *medial efferent system.* As we shall see below, they originate in the nuclei of the medial trapezoid body and in the dorsomedial periolivary nuclei. They make

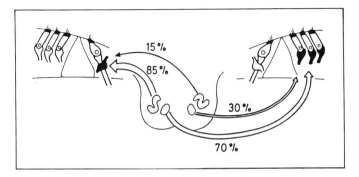

Figure 2.11
Schematic diagram of the origin and distribution of the efferent olivocochlear bundle fibers that innervate the inner and outer hair cells. Efferents to OHC arise from large neurons in the periolivary nuclei close to the trapezoid body. The great majority of them (70%) cross the midline (medial efferent bundle). Efferents to IHC arise from smaller cells in the medial superior olive. Most of these fibers remain ipsilateral (lateral efferent bundle). (From Spoendlin 1979)

---

some ipsilateral connections but are predominantly crossed from the contralateral side.

Note that the terminations on the OHC do not seem to be identical at all parts of the cochlea. The efferent innervation influences all the cells in the basal turn, but farther along the cochlea it fails to reach the third rank of OHC and farther still fails to reach the second rank also. Only the first rank of OHC seems to be innervated right up to the apex.

The ways in which the efferent fibers make their connections with OHC are probably even more complicated than the account above suggests: Apart from their axodendritic connections on the thin (spiral) afferent terminals, they probably equally make contact (en passant) with radial fibers and perhaps also make axosomatic contacts with some IHC.

Neurochemical Data
Recent studies (Eyberlin & Pujol 1984a,b, Fex & Altschuler 1986), have specified some of the transmitter actions between the efferents and the hair cells. Their data may be summarized thus:

• The presence of choline acetyltransferase (ChAT) in the fibers belonging to the lateral and medial systems, both in their cells of origin and in their terminals, suggests that most of the efferent innervation is cholinergic.

• A limited number of fibers in both systems demonstrate immunore-activity to glutamic decarboxylase (GAD) and to gamma-amino-butyric acid (GABA). Thus the possibility of a system of cotransmit-ters (acetylcholine and GABA) has not been eliminated.

• The existence, this time in the lateral system only, of opioid pep-tides (notably of enkephalin) suggests the possibility that they might cooperate with acetylcholine in the axodendritic synaptic actions on the sensory afferents of the IHC.

Finally, it has also been reported that there are thin noradrenergic fibers in the eighth nerve. It seems that they probably do not enter the cochlea, and at present their function is unknown (Eybalin, Calas & Pujol 1983).

II. PHYSIOLOGY OF THE RECEPTOR ORGAN

The sound stimulus first enters via the external and middle ear that together ensure an efficient transmission of the acoustic energy to the inner ear, where the receptor mechanisms act. We shall consider in turn the two main operations, first the transmission of the sound, then its reception and coding into afferent signals. (All the data dis-cussed below, with the exception of the section on cochlear transduc-tion, will be concerned with mammalian audition.)

IIA Sound Transmission

4 THE OUTER EAR

In question here is the function of the complex geometry of the outer ear in the reception of sounds. Two aspects are customarily discussed separately: to what extent the outer ear generates a gain in sound pressure, and to what extent it contributes to the localization of sounds.

4.1 PRESSURE GAIN

Essentially, the *ear canal* contributes most to pressure gain. This is demonstrated by the difference between the sound pressure level immediately adjacent to the tympanum and the incident free-field sound pressure level measured at the entry to the ear canal. Indepen-dent variables to consider are, on the one hand, the frequency of the sound and, on the other, the direction of arrival of the sound relative to the axis of the ear canal. In practice, very few measurements have been made for all azimuths. The most precise data that we will discuss here concern the horizontal plane, the angle Θ being measured with respect to the sagittal plane, with the axis of the ear canal being specified as 90°. In these measurements the outer ear receptor system is assumed to be fixed with no intervention from musculature that might alter its directional sensitivity.

The results essentially establish a relative pressure increase at the tympanum compared with the free-field sound pressure between 1.5 and 7.0 kHz, with some sort of plateau between 2.5 and 5.0 kHz. The gain can be as much as 20 dB. It arises from a resonance linked to the various reflections that occur within the ear canal. This effect is little modified by change of azimuth.

[The resonance can be predicted theoretically from a model consisting of a closed pipe energized by a sound field, though, admittedly, resonance would be much sharper for a tube with rigid walls than it is for the auditory canal.

This boundary problem relates also to estimating an acoustic impedance for the outer ear. Precise calculations of this are difficult. Theory predicts that for a tube of diameter d the acoustic impedance is increased by a factor $1/d$. For a tube of diameter $d = 0.4$ cm, the impedance, which is about 42 cgs in a free-air field should become (with this sort of estimate) about 104 cgs in the external auditory meatus.]

Shaw (1974) estimated the relative contributions of the auditory canal proper and of the concha to this resonance. The central peak at 2.5 kHz is probably essentially due to the canal but with a certain influence from the concha. The concha itself plays a more definite role at higher frequencies (5 kHz). Measurements of this sort in the cat have led to similar conclusions (figure 2.12).

4.2 SOUND LOCALIZATION

It is hard to conceive that the pinna plays no role in the localization of a sound source, particularly concerning up/down and back/front discriminations for which, as we have seen, intensity and phase disparities each give ambiguous information. This extra help in localization is likely to be particularly effective when the pinna is fully mobile thanks to muscle activity . Nevertheless, the treatment of this is quite complex, and most often the necessary data are not available. However, we may certainly predict that the higher frequencies are most likely to be involved (having short wavelengths with respect to the size of the pinna). The effect is particularly well marked in echo-

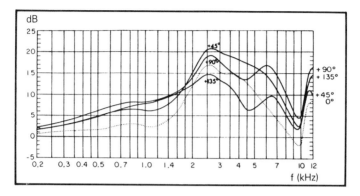

Figure 2.12
Sound transmission in the outer ear. Mean increase in sound pressure at the tympanum in decibels (dB) over the SPL at a source in the external free field in the horizontal plane, as a function of frequency f (kHz) and for different values of azimuth in that horizontal plane (0°, +45°, +90°, +135°). The pressure is measured with respect to what it would be (in the absence of a subject) at the point occupied by the center of the head. Zero azimuth is straight ahead in the sagittal plane and 90° azimuth in the plane perpendicular to that, in line with the ears and at the ipsilateral side. (From Shaw 1974)

locating bats, and for them we know that directional sensitivity depends on the emission and reception of sounds of frequency up to 100 kHz in some species. The relatively large size and mobility of both the pinna and tragus of the outer ear of several members of Chiroptera (the horseshoe bat, Rhinolophidae, for example) are clearly relevant to their direction-finding skills.

5 THE MIDDLE EAR

The acoustic vibrations in the air set the tympanum into vibration. This movement is transmitted via the malleus, incus, and stapes, the latter being firmly attached to the oval window. Thus the sound energy is transferred to the organ of Corti. The arrangements in the ossicular chain play an essential role in the effective transfer of the vibrations, and many, often complex, studies have contributed to its elucidation. We examine certain aspects of these below.

There have been a variety of ways of attacking this problem. The independent variable may be a given sound pressure at the tympanum or the frequency; measurements may be concerned with the displacement of the stapes or with the velocity of its displacement, with the pressure at the oval window, or with the pressure at the level of the basal turn of the cochlea. The success of these diverse

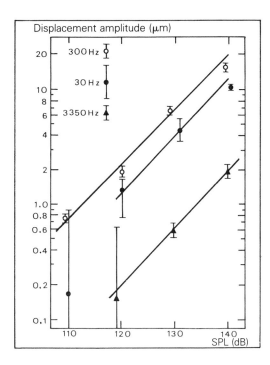

Figure 2.13
Stapes displacements. Amplitude of displacement of the stapes as a function of sound pressure (SPL) at the tympanum, for three frequencies (30 Hz, 300 Hz, and 350 Hz). Each point is the average of five to ten measurements. (From Guinan & Peake 1967)

investigations has proved to be strongly dependent on improvements in the design of the various detectors (of pressures or of movements) and to some extent because of this the results cannot be regarded as final.

5.1 OVERALL TRANSFER FUNCTION OF THE MIDDLE EAR

Let us first of all consider the overall transfer function of the middle ear with the stapes movement as the dependent variable.

Several researchers (Guinan, Møller, and Wilson, among others) have examined the movement of the stapes effected by a given pressure at the tympanum.

For a given frequency, the transmission obeys a linear law; more precisely, the log of the displacement of the stapes increases linearly with the sound intensity. This linearity is, however, normally only observed below 70 dB, because the acoustic reflex due to the middle ear muscles comes into play at higher intensities. If the reflex is prevented, linearity is seen up to 120 dB (figure 2.13).

For a given constant sound pressure applied to the tympanum the amplitude of vibration of the stapes behaves as follows as a function of sound frequency (for cat and guinea pig): the curve is practically

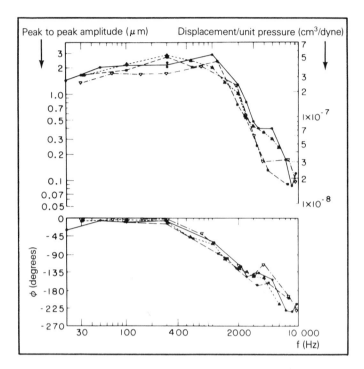

Figure 2.14
Transfer functions of the cat middle ear (4 animals). *Above,* Peak-to-peak amplitude
(μm) of stapes movement and displacement/unit sound pressure (for 120 dB SPL).
Below, Phase shift in degrees (φ). (From Guinan & Peake 1967)

horizontal up to 0.4 kHz, then falls by 12 dB/octave to 2 kHz and
more rapidly (20 dB/octave) beyond that (figure 2.14). Stapes vibration is in phase with tympanic vibration below 0.3 kHz, then phase
differences develop, up to $-150°$ at 3 kHz and $-225°$ at 10 kHz.

5.2 MECHANICAL FACTORS IN THE TRANSMISSION PROCESS

THE TYMPANUM

Helmholtz had recognized that the tympanum is a cone, whose shape
is determined by the equilibrium state of the arrangement of its radial
and circumferential elastic fibers. von Békésy was able to show from
his studies of cadavers that the tympanum is not normally under
tension and that it has a uniform elasticity at all places ($12.0 \cdot 10^{-4}$
dynes $\cdot$ cm^{-2}).

von Békésy also studied the tympanic modes of vibration using a
sensitive capacitative detector. The measurements established that

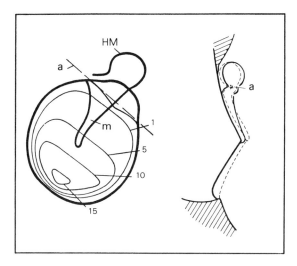

Figure 2.15
Movements of the tympanum. *Left,* Vibrations of the human tympanum for a frequency of 2 kHz; equal amplitude contours of (relative) movements. At this frequency the tympanum behaves as a rigid body turning around an axis of rotation. HM, head of the manubrium (m). *Right,* The same seen in profile; note the effect of the axis of rotation (a) of the manubrium on the movement of the tympanum (dotted line). (From von Békésy 1951)

up to 2.4 kHz all the central part of the tympanum, including the malleus (with which it firmly connects), vibrates as one. However, this vibration does not, as might be imagined, simply occur along the axis perpendicular to its surface but effectively is a rotation around an axis situated near the upper regions of the membrane, parallel with its plane and passing through the head of the malleus. For a given stimulus, it is possible, with this sort of measurement, to trace contours of equal amplitude of vibration and to show that the maximal vibration occurs in the lower part of the drum at the opposite slope of the cone to where the manubrium is situated (figure 2.15). In humans, for a tympanic surface area of 85 mm^2, the central area of effective vibration at frequencies below 2.4 kHz extends over 55 mm^2. Above 2.4 kHz, the tympanum ceases to vibrate as a unit but shows several nodes; these diminish the effective vibrating area. In the main, these rather old observations are still accepted as correct (Khanna & Tonndorf 1972).

Both theoretical arguments and experimental studies have been made on the transfer of vibratory forces from the tympanum to the manubrium. Helmholtz' initial hypothesis was that, since the tympanum appears to be a slightly incurved cone, the effect of sound pressures would be to modify the radius of curvature between the peak of the cone and its peripheral attachments and thus to generate a vibratory component normal to the plane of the tympanum. This normal force would act on the manubrium in such a way that the system would constitute a *pressure amplifier.* However, more recent work does not appear to confirm this idea. The suggested power amplification assumed that the displacement of the tympanic membrane was considerably greater than the corresponding movement of the manubrium; thus the leverage can be effective. Measurement contradicts this hypothesis of Helmholtz. Experiments show that the displacements of the tympanum are of a similar magnitude as those affecting the manubrium. Other considerations that also refute the "lever effect" are concerned with the effects of changing the air pressure in the neighborhood of the tympanum either by increasing (positive pressure) or decreasing (negative pressure) the pressure in the middle ear. Helmholtz' hypothesis would predict that during negative pressure conditions the gain would increase, and conversely it would decrease under the influence of positive pressure. But recent observations have shown that hearing always deteriorates when the middle ear pressure is changed from its normal value, whether increased or decreased.

These studies were carried out in humans by changing the intraaural pressure either by an oral injection of air or by exploiting the Valsalva maneuver. (The latter consists of a forced expiration against closed lips and nostrils, creating a positive pressure in the middle ear via the eustachian tube. Conversely, a deep inspiratory movement in the same conditions will produce a pressure drop in the middle ear.) Animal experiments have used direct injection or extraction of air from the middle ear via a tube introduced from the opened bulla. In humans, the dependent variable measured is the perception of a sound (its threshold in particular); in animals, the magnitude of the cochlear microphonic is used.

To summarize the results:

• In humans, the threshold deteriorates when the pressure is changed, whether positively or negatively. The deterioration increases (by as much as 20 dB) the greater the pressure change.
• The effect is most clearly seen at lower frequencies (<2 kHz).
• In animals, the effects of increasing or reducing the pressure are

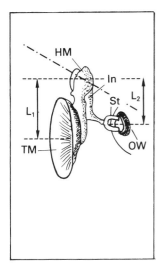

Figure 2.16
Lateral view of the middle ear components. TM, tympanic membrane; the handle of the manubrium is attached to this membrane and the head of the manubrium (HM) abuts against the incus (In), which in turn moves the stapes (St), the footplate of which is connected with the oval window (OW). The line of dashes and dots represents the axis of rotation of the ossicular chain passing through the head of the manubrium, drawn in perspective. It is parallel to the plane of the tympanic membrane. L_1, L_2, lengths of the handle of manubrium and the arm of incus, respectively. Note that $L_1 > L_2$ (see text). (Modified from Pickles 1982)

very similar; the ensuing reduction in sensitivity to sound signals affects low frequencies more than high.

• The reduction in transmission by pressure change is very much less if the ossicular chain is interrupted, showing that it is at the tympanum (and not the oval window) that pressure change exerts its effects.

• Bone conduction of sound (transmission of sound to the inner ear but not from airborne sound) is similarly affected but by a quite different mechanism (see section 2.6 below).

THE OSSICLES

In its turn, the functioning of the ossicular chain has also been the object of various investigations. One of the first aspects to be explored was the mode of vibration of these interconnected bony structures (figure 2.16). It is agreed that the tympanic vibrations move the manubrium conjointly, generating a rotation of the ossicular chain around an anterior/posterior axis passing from the anterior ligament of malleus across the small process of incus and its posterior ligament, the mass of the ossicles being in this way equally distributed about this axis. Note that section of these ligaments only affects the vibration of the stapes at low frequencies.

Since von Békésy there has also been much interest in the movements of the stapes. He had concluded, from work on cadavers, that there is a rotatory movement around an axis passing through one end of the footplate (figure 2.17a). More recent work demonstrates,

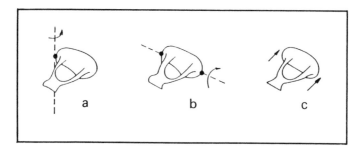

Figure 2.17
Modes of vibration in stapes. The dashed lines show the axes of rotation. *a*, Rotation around an axis passing through the posterior portion of the footplate; this is the vibratory mode that von Békésy observed in the human cadaver with very low frequency stimuli of moderate intensity. *b*, Rotation around the major axis of the footplate, same conditions *c*, Piston movements seen in the cat for stimuli < 140 dB, reported by Guinan & Peake. (From Guinan & Peake 1967)

in contrast, a translational movement along the stapes axis of symmetry: a pistonlike movement (Guinan & Peake 1967; figure 2.17c). Only at very high intensities is rotation observed around an axis in the plane of the footplate, whether it be anterior/posterior and coinciding with the footplate's major axis (figure 2.17b) or perpendicular to that.

We have already seen that at a given frequency the ossicular transmission shows an excellent linearity (e.g., it does not distort an applied sinusoidal stimulus); in contrast, the gain and phase shift of the system vary in a more complicated way with frequency. This divergence poses a problem for the reason that, since the phase shift exceeds 180°, there is no question of trying to fit the mechanics of the middle ear to a classic second-order model (i.e., to a system composed of simple frictional, elastic, and inertial components).

Such considerations have led to (1) regarding the transmission chain as a formal second-order system below 2.5 to 3.0 kHz and as at least third order at higher frequencies; (2) describing the complex high-frequency behavior as arising from the existence of a finite elasticity at the incus/stapes junction. On examination of the movements of the ossicles, the following facts have been established:

• To a first approximation, the malleus/incus articulation appears to be rigid (in the adult), although there is still some discussion on this matter.
• In contrast, the malleus/stapes junction seems to possess a certain elasticity.

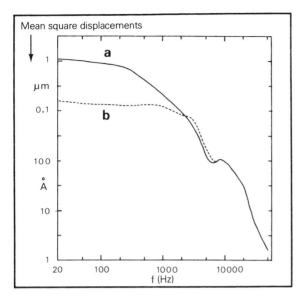

Figure 2.18
Displacements of the long process of the incus. Averaged and smoothed displacements of the long process of the incus, immediately adjacent to the stapes, as a function of frequency for a constant sound pressure of 100 dB SPL at the tympanum, in guinea pig. *a*, Tympanic bulla open. *b*, Bulla closed. The real curves include irregularities that have been ignored here. (From Wilson & Johnstone 1975)

• This elasticity is influential at high frequencies (> 2.5 kHz), in which frequency range the gain of the system (at least that estimated as the pressure gain) becomes relatively poor.

Differences are also noticed according to whether the experiments are conducted under "open bulla" or "closed bulla" conditions. The former was the case in most direct investigations of the cochlea (particularly the older ones), whereas the latter experiments usually derived their results from observing the afferent nerve activity. It seems that opening the bulla is accompanied by a relative (artificial) increase in displacement amplitudes at very low frequencies, < 0.4 kHz (Wilson & Johnstone 1975; figure 2.18).

These measurements, interesting as they are, in fact become more so if the velocity rather than the displacement of the stapes is considered. We shall see that the adequate cochlear stimulus at the oval window is a pressure that is proportional to the velocity of displacement da/dt, not to the displacement amplitude a. Therefore, considerations of impedance will very usefully complement other data.

5.3 IMPEDANCE MEASUREMENTS

Remember that acoustic impedance is given by the ratio between the pressure applied to a medium and the velocity of displacement of the medium. This impedance is purely resistive when only frictional components are involved and becomes reactive according to the extent to which the system contains elements that can store mechanical energy, whether they are related to inertial mass (representing the mechanical equivalent of electrical inductance) or to elastic elements (compliance, the mechanical equivalent of electrical capacitance).

A variety of devices has been used to measure the impedance of the acoustic system at the level of the tympanum. These measurements (see Zwislocki 1985) were variously used for such aims as optimizing the design of earphones or supplying a differential diagnosis for middle ear troubles. (We will briefly return to these tympanometric applications later in Appendix A.) But for the present, let us concentrate on the fundamental aspects of the problem (Møller 1963, 1974).

We shall not go into the details of the methods, which are simple in principle but harder to negotiate in practice. Basically, an output device is inserted into the ear canal in the vicinity of the tympanum so that it is effectively sealed from the exterior. The instrument is supplied with two tubes connected in parallel to separate external condenser microphones, one serving as a sound source (with frequency and intensity variable and well controlled) and the other acting as a probe to measure the reflected vibrations. In the calculations, the space delimited by the plane of the output device and the tympanum is assumed to be a lossless transmission line.

Consider first the absolute values of impedance in terms of resistance and reactance (see chapter 1, 1.2). We already know how each of these components varies with frequency in a variety of species. Figure 2.19 illustrates such data in cgs units for the human, cat, and rabbit. Notice the constancy of the resistive component (except at high frequencies), which contrasts with the rapid increase of reactance. We can say that between 1 kHz and 3 kHz the impedance is essentially resistive. But above 3 kHz, certain irregularities show up.

However, it is more informative to consider how the modulus $|Z|$ of the impedance and its phase vary together as a function of frequency *for a constant sound pressure acting on the tympanum*. In this

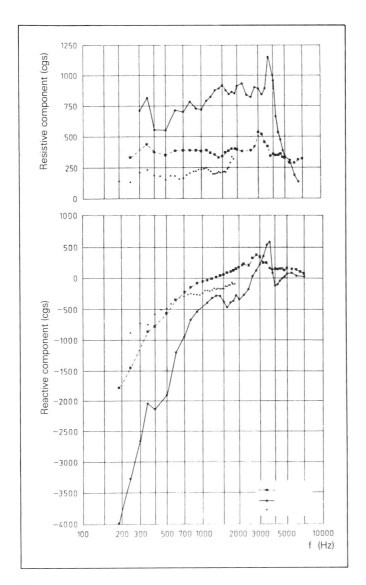

Figure 2.19
Acoustic impedance of the ear in the human (triangles), cat (squares), and rabbit
(**continuous line**). *Above*, Resistive components. *Below*, Reactive components, as a
function of frequency f. (From Møller 1974)

representation $|Z|$ is expressed as its ratio (in decibels) to 100 cgs units. Under these conditions we obtain curves of the sort in figure 2.20, which are data for the cat. Note therefore that $|Z|$ decreases up to 1 khz (at about 12 dB/octave) thereafter to become constant between 1 khz and 3 khz, and then shows irregularities that include a peculiar peak near 4 khz. Note in passing that in SI units the impedance magnitude at the tympanum has been estimated as 1680 $N \cdot s \cdot m^{-3}$ for the cat.

To summarize, the impedance is minimal and essentially resistive in a range 1 to 20 khz (at least in the cat and guinea pig). At lower frequencies it becomes greater because of the relative rigidity of the structures (tympanum, ligaments) at low frequencies. At frequencies higher than the zone of minimal resistive impedance, the massive inertial component begins to dominate and, what is more, at the same time the useful vibrating area of the tympanum begins to decrease, deteriorating the sound transfer.

Another essential question is the following: to what extent does the *impedance* correspond, following its very definition, with the quotient *pressure* exerted on the tympanic membrane divided by *velocity* of movement of the manubrium, which we have seen is firmly connected to that membrane? Is there anything like a constant correspondence between them? Actual measurements made on the velocity of the manubrium for a constant tympanic pressure do in fact reveal an excellent correspondence (see the two curves in figure 2.20). The impedance varies, as it should, effectively in the same way as the inverse of the velocity of vibration of the manubrium, at least in the band 0.2 to 2.5 khz. Therefore, in this frequency range the malleus acts as a rigid system, converting the sound into vibration of the manubrium. Above 2.5 khz the results are somewhat at variance, this being particularly due (as we have seen above) to the tympanum ceasing to vibrate as a single unit.

The same sort of experiment can be carried out but using the *amplitude* of the cochlear microphonic as an indicator. As we shall see below, this electrical wave is proportional to the velocity of the cochlear fluid, which is itself proportional to the velocity of vibration of malleus. Here again, the correspondence between the impedance and the power transfer is clearly shown between 0.5 and 3 khz. At lower frequencies a certain discrepancy shows up which might be due to an attenuation of the cochlear microphonic in the region of the round window. Above 4 khz it is thought, once more, that the

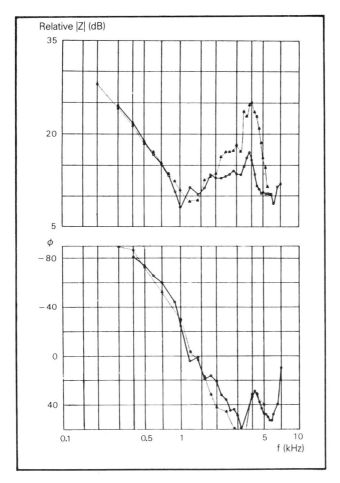

Figure 2.20
Frequency variation of the acoustic impedance at the tympanum and of the reciprocal
of velocity of manubrium movement, for a constant sound pressure at the tympanum.
Above, Frequency variation of the modulus $|Z|$ (ratios in dB) (solid line) and of the
reciprocal of the velocity (v^{-1}) of manubrium, in this case to an arbitrary reference
(broken line). *Below,* Phase angles ϕ of the same two variables. (From Møller 1975)

behavior of the tympanum itself comes into play. It no longer acts like a piston. At higher frequencies the transmission is probably also affected by the finite elasticity of the incus/stapes junction. Quite a series of different measurements have thus been used to distinguish the separate factors that determine the overall impedance measured in the vicinity of the tympanum. The impedance is certainly determined by the combined contributions of the tympanum itself, of the elements of the middle ear, and of the cochlea. From this arises the interest in making diverse estimates of the separate effects.

In particular, the experiment described above measuring the manubrium's velocity has been repeated but using not the velocity of the malleus but of the long process of the stapes instead. These results again agree, confirming that the malleus/stapes articulation is rigid, at least below 2.5 kHz.

One might also ask to what extent the system stapes/oval window (i.e., finally the cochlea itself) contributes to the total impedance. To this end, comparisons have been made between normal impedance curves and those obtained after interruption of the incus/stapes junction. The results show that although the reactive component is little affected, the resistive component is considerably diminished, particularly around 4 kHz, emphasizing the particular influence that the system stapes/oval window/cochlea normally exerts in this frequency range.

Earlier workers suggested the acoustic impedance of sea water (1.5 $\cdot 10^6$ N $\cdot$ s $\cdot$ m^{-3}) to be an appropriate value for the cochlear impedance, to a first approximation. In fact, more recent theoretical and experimental treatments (Khanna & Tonndorf 1971) conclude that smaller values are appropriate, around 2 $\cdot 10^5$ N $\cdot$ s $\cdot$ m^{-3} at 1 kHz, for the cat. The impedance value for the cochlea itself depends little on frequency since it is essentially resistive. The cochlear impedance being notably greater than that of the middle ear (1680 N $\cdot$ s $\cdot$ m^{-3}), we can, without too much error, suggest that if the gain G of the transfer function of the middle ear is the ratio P_s/P_t, where P_s is the pressure at the stapes and P_t is the pressure at the tympanum and if Z_c is the cochlear impedance, then:

$$G = P_s/P_t,$$

where $P_s = Z_c \times V_s$ and V_s, the velocity of the stapes, can also be written $d(a)/dt$ where $a(t)$ is the excursion of the stapes. Thus

$$V_s = d(a)/dt = P_t \times (G/Z_c)$$

and

$$Z_c = \{G \times P_t\} \div \{d(a)/dt\}.$$

This expression allows us to predict that at a constant tympanic pressure P_t the impedance is practically proportional to the inverse of the stapes velocity (and of the malleus' velocity also).

5.4 THE MIDDLE EAR AS AN IMPEDANCE TRANSFORMER

One of the problems concerning the transformation of an airborne vibration into a cochlear vibration is precisely that of matching the two impedances. We have seen above (chapter 1, 1.2) that expressions for the transmission and reflection of mechanical vibrations at a boundary between two media emphasize the role of their respective impedances. It is agreed that if the airborne vibrations were to act directly on the oval window, at least 98% of the sound energy would be reflected, and thus the efficiency of the auditory apparatus would be greatly diminished. It is thanks to the tympanum/ossicles/oval window system's action as an *impedance transformer* that the coefficient of transmission is so much improved.

In general, the impedance transformation is governed by three factors (Khanna & Tonndorf 1971, 1972; Møller 1965):

1. The most important concerns the differences in surface area between the tympanum on the one hand and the stapes footplate on the other. The pressure increases inversely with the surface area.
2. A second factor is the lever action of the ossicular chain. The handle of malleus and the long process of incus (see 5.2 above) have different lengths (L_1 and L_2 in figure 2.16); because of this the force exerted by the stapes is increased and its speed is reduced, compared with those elements at the tympanum.
3. A last consideration is related to the modes of vibration of the tympanum itself, which suffers changes in its curvature under the impact of sound pressures. Such changes could cause the handle of the malleus to be displaced less than the tympanum, which also could give rise to a diminution of the velocity but an augmentation of the force exerted by the ossicular system. (This mechanism was initially proposed by Helmholtz and is in fact not universally accepted

and seems to be partially denied by more modern work, as discussed above already.)

It is quite clear that the quantitative evaluation of these factors relies on the exploration of the movements of each of the diverse elements of the system and that this in turn relies on suitably refining the methods of investigation used to this end. No doubt this latter consideration explains the often very different values in the work published at different times, by different researchers, on different species.

In humans the effective tympanic area (55 mm^2) and stapes area (3.2 mm^2) gives factor (1) above a value of 17. For the cat the corresponding figures 42 mm^2 and 0.2 mm^2 give a higher value of 35.

As for factor (2), concerned with the different lengths of the handle of malleus and the long process of incus, it can be estimated thus: If the length difference increases the force by a factor r it also reduces the velocity by the factor $1/r$. Thus the impedance, being the ratio of the pressure to the velocity, is increased by r^2. For humans, older measurements give factor (2) a value of 1.3 at moderate frequencies; more recent work for the cat gives $(1.15)^2 = 1.32$. Guinan (1967) publishes a value of 2.

Finally, factor (3), less well known and usually neglected, might change the impedance by $2^2 = 4$ in the cat (force doubled, velocity halved; figure 2.21).

Overall, then, the transformation ratio has been given as around 18 for humans, probably as no more than a guess, and the more recent estimates for the cat give $35 \times 1.32 \times 4 = 185$.

We need also to note the general values given for impedances: 430 N · s · m^{-3}) for air, about 1700 N · s · m^{-3}) at the tympanum, and finally $2 · 20^5$ N · s · m^{-3}) for the cochlea, all at approximately 1 kHz. Calculation from the values of impedance transformation shows that the ultimate power absorbed is about 67% of the incident airborne sound power, an excellent state of affairs compared with the 2% that would be absorbed in the case of a direct transfer of airborne sound to the cochlea fluids. (Essentially these estimates relate to mid frequencies, around 1 kHz in humans, and from 1 to 20 kHz in the cat and guinea pig.)

5.5 EFFICIENCY OF POWER TRANSMISSION BY THE MIDDLE EAR

Having now some measures of the impedance, it is equally necessary to get a more exact idea of how well the ear transmits tympanic

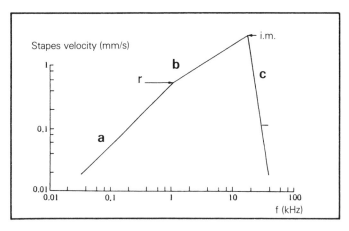

Figure 2.21
Frequency response of the middle ear of the cat estimated from the stapes velocity for a constant tympanic sound pressure. The curve for a constant sound pressure 100 dB SPL comprises a first segment (a) rising at 6 dB/octave, an inflection (at r) followed by a second section (b) at 4 dB/octave and then an abrupt reversal of the slope, section (c), to −36 dB/octave. The inflection at r involves a change in stiffness; the reversal (at im) is concerned with the inertial mass. (From Evans 1982a).

stimuli throughout the whole audible frequency range. In fact, remembering that the adequate stimulus is not the stapes displacement but its velocity, it is important to find how that quantity varies with frequency at a constant tympanic sound pressure. The curve suggested for this variation (Evans 1982a) for the cat shows an increase at 6 dB/octave, then 4 dB/octave up to 20 kHz, therefter falling at −36 dB/octave, resulting in an optimal response between 1 and 10 khz (figure 2.21).

We might also plot a corresponding curve of the threshold for vibrations in the middle ear as a function of frequency. It can then be affirmed that this threshold (in decibels SPL) decreases, passes through a minimum, and then increases rapidly with frequency increase (see also figure 2.33, below).

5.6 FUNCTION OF THE MIDDLE EAR MUSCLES

M. STAPEDIUS AND M. TENSOR TYMPANI

The contractions of the middle ear muscles can be followed by electromyographic recording. The movement of the tensor tympani can also be followed by measuring the displacement of the tympanum that this contraction produces. The tympanum is effectively moved toward the interior of the middle ear cavity under these conditions; in contrast, the stapedius only generates a very small movement, since it pulls in a direction practically perpendicular to the direction of the pistonlike movement of stapes (i.e., it moves parallel to the plane of the footplate). In addition, contractions of these muscles change the magnitude of the cochlear microphonic, change the acoustic imped-ance of the ear, and also, as psychophysics shows, affect the thresh-old of hearing.

The stimulus adequate to initiate reflex contraction of these muscles is a sound input. With a unilateral stimulus, contractions affect both pairs of muscles, stapedius and tensor tympani, on each side. In humans the stapedius seems to be the more activated by sound.

A study of the latency of the reflex leads to some interesting conclu-sions. Its magnitude is some 14 ms for the stapedius and 18 ms for the tensor tympani in the cat for intense contralateral sound stimula-tion. In humans, indirect methods have suggested values of 150 ms at threshold and 25 to 35 ms at greater stimulus intensities.

Combined neuroanatomical and neurophysiological studies enable us to outline the neuronal pathways comprising the reflex arcs of the two muscles (figure 2.22). Let us first recall that motoneurons to the stapedius are localized in the medial division of the ipsilateral nucleus of the facial nerve (VII) and that those to the tensor tympani are in the ventrolateral division of the ipsilateral trigeminal (V) nucleus.

Three or four neurons are concerned in the stapedial reflex: (1) the afferent auditory neuron, (2) a neuron from the ventral cochlear nucleus terminating in (3) the ipsilateral nucleus of stapedius (nu-cleus of VII) and passing through the trapezoid body. Another possi-ble complementary pathway is more complex, with a neuron issuing from the cochlear nucleus to the medial nucleus of the superior olive and from there a third neuron traveling to the ipsilateral and contra-lateral nucleus of VII.

As for the tensor tympani reflex, given the absence in this case of direct connections from the cochlear nucleus to the nucleus of V, an indirect pathway (in particular via the olive) is indicated.

It should be noticed that these muscles can equally be activated by nonacoustic stimuli such as body movements, closing the eyes, a jet of air playing on the orbit, vocalization, or cutaneous stimulation of the outer ear and around the auditory canal (or by electrical stimula-tion of the latter).

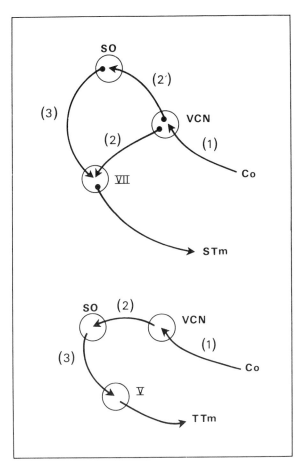

Figure 2.22
Highly simplified diagram of the reflex pathways for activating the middle ear muscle reflexes. *Above,* Audiostapedius reflex pathway: (1) from the cochlea (Co) to the ventral cochlear nucleus (VCN); (2) short route from VCN to nucleus of facial nerve (VII) innervating the stapedius muscle (STm); (2') less direct route from VCN through superior olive (SO) to the seventh nerve nucleus (3). *Below,* Audiotensor tympani reflex pathway: (1) from Co to VCN, then (2) from VCN to SO, then (3) from SO to the fifth nerve nucleus (V) innervating the tensor tympani muscle (TTm).

Leaving aside a variety of older observations, the most precise present data on the effects of these muscles are furnished by measurement of changes in middle ear impedance when they contract. In particular, it has been shown that such impedance variations are proportional to the magnitude of the integrated electromyogram of the stapedius. Therefore, measuring this impedance can be exploited to evaluate the strength of the audiomuscular reflex as a function of the intensity and frequency of sounds and to explore the effectiveness of middle ear transmission when these muscles contract. These experiments have mostly been made on the awake rabbit and, also as far as is possible, on humans.

Impedance and the Audiomuscular Reflexes
First of all, let us consider how measuring impedance allows us to trace the generation of the audiomuscular reflexes. (Borg 1972a,b; Møller 1974a,b). The impedance measurement is made (in humans and rabbits) using a tone of 800 Hz which, as we have seen, is in the frequency range where impedance is at a minimum and where small (unwanted) changes in the volume of the ear canal have little effect, whereas contraction of the muscles produces clearly measurable variations. These are evaluated by a null method, using a detector placed close to the tympanum. The sound probe used to measure the impedance must be at an intensity that does not itself trigger the reflex (<75 dB).

The *reflex response* is elicited by an intense stimulus—ipsilaterally, contralaterally, or bilaterally—sufficiently loud to cause an impedance change, the characteristics of which are essentially as follows:

• The threshold for the reflex, defined as the stimulus needed to generate a response that is 10% of the maximal, has been measured as a function of frequency. The threshold is high at 500 Hz (100 dB) and decreases at 12 dB/octave up to 4 kHz, where it is 80 dB. The threshold for the stapedius is about 10 dB lower than that for the tensor tympani (see figure 2.25; see Borg 1972a,b).

• At a given frequency, the size of the reflex response is a function of the intensity of the auditory stimulus. In the rabbit, the response increases according to a generally sigmoid function (with intensity in decibels, i.e., a scale of log pressure) to attain a plateau near 100 dB (figure 2.23).

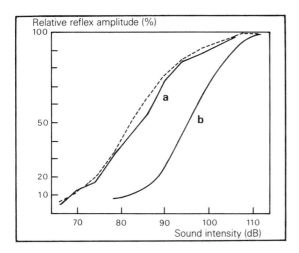

Figure 2.23
Stimulus/response characteristics for the complete ipsilateral audiomuscular reflex and also after tenotomy of one of the middle ear muscles (tensor tympani or stapedius). The dashed curve shows the usual normal response with intact musculature. Curve (a) was determined three months after section of tensor tympani: little effect. Curve (b) is from another experiment two months after stapedius had been sectioned. Stimulus: 2 kHz, 0.5 s. (From Borg 1972b)

• The response threshold is a little less for the muscles of the ipsilateral ear compared with the contralateral. Figure 2.24 shows the reflex amplitude/stimulus intensity function for ipsilateral and contralateral stimulation in humans.
• When a wide-band signal (i.e., noise) is used to elicit the reflex, the reflex threshold is lower than for a pure tone.

Having once established the amplitude/intensity characteristics of the reflex, animal experiments have been conducted to study the contribution of the individual muscles. By tenotomizing or denervating either tensor tympani or stapedius and remeasuring the amplitude/intensity characteristic, it was found that elimination of the tensor tympani has hardly any effect on these curves, whereas elimination of the stapedius' effects displaces the curve in such a way that for a given stimulus intensity the reflex becomes much more feeble, particularly for lower-frequency stimulation.

Effect of the Reflex on Middle Ear Sound Transmission
For these (animal) experiments the experimental set-up is more complicated. The stimulus is applied to one ear and impedance changes

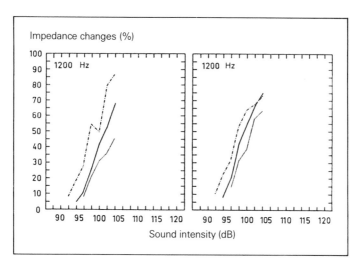

Figure 2.24
Acoustic impedance and the middle ear muscle acoustic reflex. Relative change, in the human, of acoustic impedance as a function of stimulus intensity for 500 ms stimulation at 1.2 kHz. *Left,* Left ear stimulation. *Right,* Right ear stimulation. Solid line, impedance change in stimulated ear; thin line, response to contralateral stimulation; dotted and dashed line, response to binaural stimulation. (From Møller 1974a).

are measured in the contralateral ear, thus testing the effect of the crossed audiomuscular reflex from the stimulated ear. This is followed by a block of the stapedius, or tensor tympani, or both, in the *stimulated ear,* which affects the transmission of sound to its cochlea. According to the quality of the sound transmission in that ear, the sound will initiate a correspondingly greater or lesser contralateral response, Thus, measuring the amount of any impedance change in the test ear can determine what effects on the stimulated ear's middle ear transmission have resulted from experimental modifications to its integrity. Measurements of the amplitude/response characteristics first before, then after blocking one of the two muscles in the stimulated ear reveal that the curve is displaced along the abscissa; this shift demonstrates that the presence of the two inner ear muscles introduces a certain *attenuation.* For a given sound stimulus, more sound reaches the stimulated ear's cochlea in the absence of the muscles. As an indication of the order of magnitude of this effect, increasing the stimulating sound's intensity by 1.0 dB at the level of the tympanum only augments the sound level at the cochlea by 0.3 dB

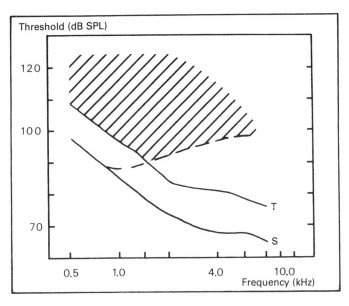

Figure 2.25
Properties of the acoustic reflexes, variation with frequency, and their role in middle ear sound transmission. Solid lines indicate mean thresholds for eliciting the stapedius reflex (S) and tensor tympani reflex (T) (at 10% the maximal responses) in the unanes-thetized rabbit for *ipsilateral* stimulation by pure tones. The hatched area is the zone in which either muscle makes a noticeable change in the middle ear transmission (determined as described in the text). The thresholds for changing impedance and for modifying transmission are effectively the same at low frequencies, whereas above 0.8 kHz the muscles can contract without affecting the transmission characteristics. (Modified from Borg 1972a)

when the muscles are contracting, indicating an effective attenuation by their reflex activity of 0.7 dB/dB.

This attenuation is a function of frequency. In general, it is present at lower frequencies for all values of sound intensity beyond that at which the reflex contractions of the stapedius and tensor tympani first occur. At higher frequencies (>1 kHz), however, the attenuation seems to affect only intensities that are notably higher than those that initiate the muscular contractions (30 dB at 4 kHz) (figure 2.25).

Finally, let us emphasize once more that, except at lower frequencies, these actions are almost entirely due to the stapedius. [This modification of middle ear transmission is related to the fact that the muscular contraction increases the stiffness component of the impedance which, as we have seen, is exactly what diminishes transmission at lower frequencies.]

A certain number of experiments, similarly using impedances as a measure, have been carried out in humans, particularly patients with a temporary unilateral paralysis of the stapedius (e.g., Bell's palsy). In essence, the results, inevitably sketchy, agree with the indications from animal work fairly closely, except that the threshold for reflex contraction of the stapedius seems to be somewhat higher in humans (86 to 102 dB) than in the rabbit.

FUNCTION OF THE MIDDLE EAR MUSCLES' CONTRACTIONS

The above experiments show how the middle ear behaves in the presence and absence of its muscles' activity. We might conclude that their contraction constitutes an adjustment to the presence of relatively high stimulus intensities by a closed-loop negative feedback that acts on middle ear transmission of the incident sound to the cochlea. The paralysis of these muscles would therefore effectively open the loop.

The possibility that other, more precise functions are also controlled by the stapedius, and to a lesser extent the tensor tympani, has been explored, and three effects of their contractions have been proposed:

• *Augmentation of the dynamic range of the cochlea.* In fact, in the absence of these reflex attenuations the high stimulus intensities would exceed the upper operating limit of the inner ear. The attenuation of these stimuli increases the operating range by avoiding receptor saturation (see section 7.3, below).
• *Preferential attenuation of low frequencies.* We have seen that lower-frequency sound is relatively more affected than higher frequency by the middle ear reflexes. Again, we know (chapter 1, 1.3.3) that low frequencies can powerfully mask high frequencies. A preferential attenuation of lower frequency (i.e., like inserting a high-pass filter) would therefore have the effect of relatively favoring the hearing of higher frequencies. A particular example of this is the reception of speech, the intelligibility of which might in this way be to some extent safeguarded.
• *Cause an effective adaptation to continuous high-intensity sounds.* This is the action that has most often been adduced. From all the evidence, the contraction cannot protect the auditory system at a sudden beginning of an intense sound because of the considerable reflex delay. In contrast, protection by the muscular action is conceivable during the continuation of the sound, which might well be perceived as of lower

intensity than it would be otherwise, for example, during a transient exposure to the same intensity.

Let us finally note, anecdotally, a fact that may or may not apply to the human situation: In bats, the middle ear muscles contract immediately *before* they emit their orientation cry, and this makes the ear 10 to 20 dB less sensitive to their own sound output.

6 BONE CONDUCTION

Conduction of sound via the bones of the skull plays practically no auditory role in normal conditions of listening to airborne vibrations: the energy carried by that path to the cochlea is 30 to 60 dB less than that from the incident airborne sound. It is almost solely in the reception of one's own voice that bone conduction seems likely to be involved. In fact, one's own recorded voice initially sounds strange to one's ears; in particular, the low frequencies seem to have become relatively attenuated, since they had been well carried to the cochlea by bone conduction.

In contrast, the auditory role of bone conduction is of considerable interest in the clinic. It has therefore been the object of serious study, which we now summarize.

If a vibrating tuning fork is applied to the skull (at no matter what place), a certain amount of sound energy will reach the cochlea. Experiment has demonstrated that at a constant vibration amplitude, there is a certain frequency range (about 0.6 to 1.0 kHz depending on species) within which the general efficiency of stimulation passes through a maximum; this maximum is determined in humans by psychophysics and in animals by measuring the amplitude of the cochlear microphonic. The vibratory energy is transmitted through the bony walls of the skull at speeds that vary according to the place of application and also, it must be said, between particular researchers' reports (range 200 to 2000 m/s). In any case, this energy reaches the two ears with a time disparity that is less than the minimum delay that can be temporally resolved by the dichotic sound-localization system. In this situation, therefore, the subject is unable to localize the source and generally perceives the sound to be in the center of the head.

The ways in which the sound vibration is transmitted to the perilymph and to the receptors have been considered. For some time, two processes have been suggested (if only very much in outline): (1) a *compression* hypothesis, the vibration being transmitted by a direct compression/decompression of the cochlea, and (2) an *inertial* hypothesis, the vibration being transmitted via the middle ear ossicular chain, whose separate bones have unequal mechanical inertia.

Some modern work suggests that in fact the two mechanisms, one by the bony route and cochlear compression, the other by the so-called osteo tympanic route with its inertial mechanism, provide complementary transmission paths which seem to involve all three anatomical divisions of the ear—inner, middle, and external.

The *inner ear* can directly receive signals by the effect of fluid compression/decompression, this essentially for two reasons: First, the oval window has a smaller compliance than the round, so the latter will be deformed more easily than the stapes/oval window system. Second, the two cochlear chambers do not have the same volume, since the scala vestibuli is connected to the labyrinthine cavities. The net effect of fluid displacement would be a deformation of the cochlear canal.

There is a problem concerning direct excitation of the cochlea by the bony route. By what mechanism does the excitation, presumably acting at some point on the cochlea, finally end by setting up an apparently normal activity in the cochlear canal (even when the excitation does not begin, as normally, at the oval window)? This conversion to a normal excitation can be understood if we propose (and here we become involved with the physiology of the cochlea itself) that the different parts of its receptor surfaces are, by their own local properties (compliance, pass-band filtering), able to retain their capacity to respond preferentially to particular frequency ranges.

The *middle ear* plays a part also, and von Békésy thought up a cunning, if complex, experiment to study its role in humans: Mask one ear, in this case by white noise, making it nonfunctional (this is done because, as we have seen, bone-conducted sound reaches both ears); stimulate the other ear simultaneously by airborne and bone-conducted sound; then for the unmasked ear, attempt to annul the stimulation from the two signals (airborne and bony) by suitably adjusting the phase and amplitude of the bone-conducted sound with respect to the airborne sound. Such a cancellation is shown to be possible; therefore, it is clear that the two signals, airborne and by bone conduction, must eventually share a final common route, the middle ear. In animal work, a whole series of manipulations (e.g., changing the point of application of the cranial vibration, overloading the tympanum) have also convinced a variety of researchers (cf. Tonndorf 1976) finally to attribute a part of bone conduction to the mechanical inertia of the middle ear, tympanum, and ossicular chain.

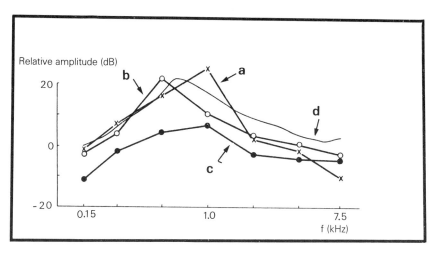

Figure 2.26
Bone conduction. Total bone conduction (d) and the components that are determined by the outer ear (a), middle ear (b), and inner ear (c) in the cat between 0.15 and 7.5 kHz. (From Tonndorf 1976)

[This point certainly remains controversial in humans, since clinicians have for long considered that loss of the middle ear does not affect hearing by bone conduction. The data from animal work manifestly disagree with this view.]

The *outer ear* also seems to play its part. A well-known observation holds that when a subject hears a sound by bone conduction, wherever the tuning fork has been applied, the source is localized "in the middle of the head" but, in contrast, if one external auditory meatus is (mechanically) occluded, the source is localized to the side of the occluded ear canal. A variety of explanations have been offered for this phenomenon, which is only observed below about 1 kHz. A recent suggestion (see Tonndorf 1976) involves the efficiency of the transmission of sound in the outer ear. When bone conduction occurs, not only the bony but also the cartilaginous partitions (the ear canal being one) equally play their part in transmission toward the tympanum but essentially in the manner of a high-pass filter above 1 kHz. They absorb low-frequency energy. When the ear canal is occluded, the high-pass filter effect will be minimized on that side, and so the cochlea on the occluded side will benefit from an increase in low-frequency input; thus the apparent sound source is localized to that side.

In conclusion (figure 2.26), the overall transmission curve for bone conduction, which as a whole peaks between 0.5 and 1.0 kHz (in a variety of species), is normally the result of conduction involving all three parts of the ear: The outer ear intervenes essentially at the lowest frequencies; the middle ear is concerned with mid-frequencies (with the resonance peak in the ossicular chain around 0.6 kHz); and the inner ear's transmission contributes more to the higher frequencies. The direct compression/decompression excitation of the cochlea only occurs in this frequency range.

IIB Sound Reception and Transduction in the Cochlea

7 AUDITORY SIGNALS IN PRIMARY NEURONS

Logically, we would attack the problems of transduction proper and of coding of auditory information in nerve impulse outputs in that order, first considering the excitation of receptors by the sound input they receive and then studying the resultant structure of the afferent auditory signaling. In fact, the detailed study of cochlear structure and cochlear receptor mechanisms, which has blossomed in the last decade, benefitted greatly from what had been discovered earlier about the cochlea's coding of auditory information. It is also easier to begin with a study upstream from the receptors themselves and then consider the nature of the messages borne by the cochlear nerve impulses.

It is only relatively recently that techniques for studying the activity in isolated nerve fibers became sufficiently refined to be fully exploited in this respect (Kiang 1965; Kiang et al. 1965). Several technical difficulties had to be overcome that we will not enumerate here.

We should note right away (and this matter will be referred to again more than once) that essentially, and probably totally, these results are concerned with nerve impulse patterns that originate from the *inner* hair cells; recall that in fact 90 to 95% of the auditory nerve afferents arise from those cells (Spoendlin 1970) and that the spread of their output (number of receptors exciting each fiber) is considered to be strikingly small. As a first approximation, unitary recording from each single nerve fiber demonstrates rather faithfully the output from one IHC (or a very small number of IHC). These outputs are generated in type I fibers exclusively. As for type II afferents innervating the OHC, as pointed out above, their very thin axons and their limited numbers have as yet prevented any particular proven physiological characteristics to be fully experimentally established. Whatever these are will no doubt be discovered one day.

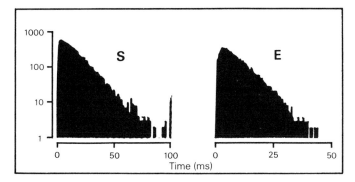

Figure 2.27
Interspike interval histogram for spontaneous activity (S) and for activity evoked by sound (E) in a cochlear nerve fiber. Sound signal is at the fiber's f_c, 7.84 kHz. Histograms for activity during 5 min (*left*) and 2 min (*right*). Notice the difference in scaling; 100 ms in S with bin intervals 500 μs, 50 ms in E with bin intervals 250 μs. (From Kiang 1965)

7.1 SPONTANEOUS ACTIVITY

In the absence of any sound input, most receptors generate spontaneous discharges in their afferents with very variable spontaneous discharge rates that depend on experimental conditions. In the anesthetized cat, for example, interspike interval histograms plotted for a whole series of fibers have always shown a skewed distribution of intervals with a large predominance of fibers with a low spontaneous discharge rate and with the mode of the spontaneous discharge rate being quite variable (between 5/s and more than 70/s) (figure 2.27). Liberman and Oliver (1984) have shown recently that according to their diameter—large, medium, or small (see chapter 1, 3.4) the type I axons in the cat show correspondingly different spontaneous discharge rates—high (>18/s), medium, or low (<0.5/s), respectively.

7.2 CODING OF FREQUENCY AND PHASE

One important characteristic of every fiber is the existence of its own *tuning curve*. If the *liminal* intensity for exciting a fiber is determined at each sound frequency, with this threshold response being defined as the smallest detectable change in its discharge rate, the resulting curve typically shows a minimal liminal intensity at a frequency variously referred to as optimal, preferred, or more often "characteristic" frequency (f_c), above and below which the excitation threshold is increased (figures 2.28, 2.29).

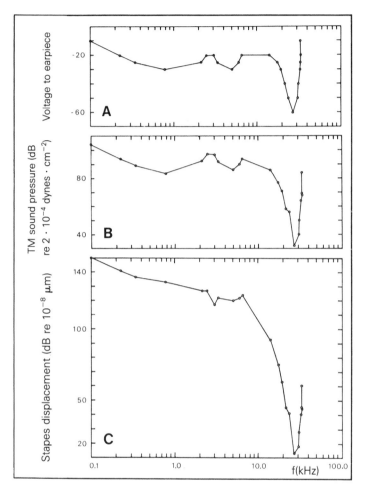

Figure 2.28
Tuning curves for a single auditory nerve fiber in the cat. Their shape depends on
the quantities chosen as the dependent variable (ordinate): A, Voltage applied to the
earpiece. B, Sound pressure at the tympanic membrane, in dB re $2 \cdot 10^{-4}$ dyne $\cdot$ cm^{-2}.
C, Peak displacement of stapes, in dB re 10^{-8} μm. (From Kiang 1965)

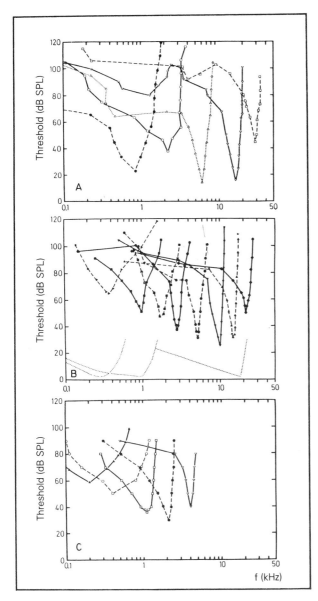

Figure 2.29
Frequency tuning curves for single cochlear nerve fibers of the cat (upper), guinea pig (middle), and *Saimiri* (lower). Below the curves for the guinea pig, in *B*, are the often generally accepted basilar membrane responses (dotted lines; arbitrary but analogous ordinate values). Note the difference between the band-pass characteristics of the fibers and of the basilar membrane. The basilar membrane mechanical selectivity shown by these curves requires modification in the light of later studies (see section 10 in this chapter). (From Evans 1982)

A proper understanding of these tuning curves calls for a certain number of comments. To define them we could, in principle, consider the pressure at the tympanum, specified in decibels with respect to the minimal audible sound pressure of 2.10^{-4} dynes $\cdot$ cm^{-2} (20 μN/m^2). In fact, some researchers have agreed that these curves are best obtained by also correcting for the transfer function across the middle ear between the tympanum and the stapes. Notably, Kiang (1965) did that, taking as the characteristic not the pressure at the tympanum but the peak to peak *displacement* of the stapes expressed as a relative value (in decibels) to the minimal effective value of this, estimated in the cat as 10^{-8} μm (decibels re 10^{-8} μm). We have seen above that the displacement of the stapes is not constant for a given tympanic pressure but varies with frequency (see figure 2.16). This correction is therefore clearly necessary. In fact, it may not even be sufficient in much of this work since (as we have already mentioned and will discuss in more detail later) the adequate stimulus at the oval window is the *pressure* exerted by the stapes, proportional to its velocity, therefore to the *first derivative* of its displacement.

These tuning curves are typically skewed: Threshold typically rises more rapidly with frequency above than below f_c. Usually the slopes of the rising thresholds are higher in those fibers with higher characteristic frequencies ($f_c > 2$ kHz), with the result that tuning is relatively sharper for such fibers than for those of lower f_c.

The skewed nature of these curves has a functional implication concerned with the fact that a fiber with a high characteristic frequency can also be excited by lower frequency sounds (or by the lower frequency components of a complex sound). The measured threshold for high f_c fibers at 1 kHz is a linearly increasing function of their f_c.

A variety of parameters have been used to specify the sharpness of tuning of these curves (and finally the bandwidth of the band-pass filters that, according to psychophysics, constitute the peripheral output (see chapter 1, 3.3). Physiologists have chosen to measure (1) the slopes in dB/octave for $f < f_c$ and $f > f_c$ or (2) a dimensionless ratio, called Q_{10dB}, defined as the ratio of f_c to the frequency band δf enclosed by the curve at an intensity 10 dB above the threshold for f_c, that is, as the inverse of the *relative* frequency spread: $Q_{10dB} = f_c / \delta f$. The higher the value of Q, the sharper the tuning curve and the more frequency selective the unit, therefore. As an illustration, we show in table 2.2 some values obtained from a variety of species. In

Table 2.2. Slopes in dB/octave and Q_{10dB} values for cochlear nerve fibers

Slope < f_c	Slope > f_c	Q_{10dB}	For fibers at
10–60	20–125	1–4	f_c < 2 kHz
90–180	200–600	3–15	$f_c \approx$ 8 kHz

general, selectivity so specified is better at higher frequencies (see also figure 2.30).

Other evaluations of selectivity are equally feasible. For example, we have above compared the *critical band* demonstrated by psychophysics with the *effective bandwidth* of the tuning curves. In this case, it is a question of comparing not a ratio but the frequency spread δf in hertz, usually chosen to be the frequency spread at 3 dB above the threshold at f_c. (This spread is about half the corresponding value for 10 dB.)

Apropos of such estimates from tuning curves, evaluations of Q_{10dB} have also been made on the vibration of the basilar membrane. These Q_{10dB} were found to have a flatter frequency variation, selectivity not varying very much with frequency. As we shall see in section 2.10.2 below, it is probable that this conclusion needs to be revised.

Other methods are currently employed to trace eighth nerve fiber tuning curves.

• Measuring, for a given sound intensity, the width of the frequency band that can generate a response in the fiber. These measurements are confirmatory in the sense that they show that the more intense the sound, the wider the frequency band δf over which the fiber responds.

• Determining for each frequency the intensity needed to generate a given selected reference response. These data form the basis of *isoresponse curves*. When it is a question of measuring from single isolated fibers, the criterion might be a certain discharge rate (or a certain increment above the spontaneous rate). This provides an *isodischarge* or, more commonly, *isorate* or *isofrequency* plot. If the response is analog (e.g., a graded receptor potential or a microphonic potential), not digital (e.g., nerve discharges), the plot is named *isoamplitude* (figure 2.31).

• Determining the magnitude of the response as a function of frequency, at a given sound intensity (Rose et al. 1971), yields an *isointensity* plot. If the phenomenon is graded, the isointensity curve can

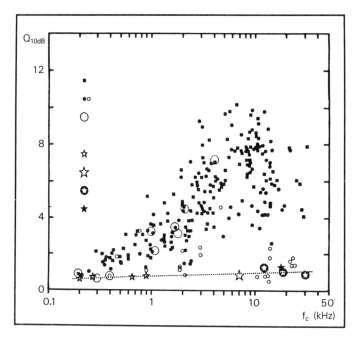

Figure 2.30
Q_{10dB} values for cochlear nerve fibers in cat, guinea pig, and *Saimiri*, as a function of the fiber's f_c. Symbols indicate nerve measurements: black squares, cat; small circles, guinea pig (filled, fibers in good condition: open, in poor condition). Large open circles, *Saimiri*. Star symbols show basilar membrane measurements by von Békésy in 1944 (see Békésy 1960) in guinea pig; by Rhode 1971, 1978 in *Saimiri*; by Wilson & Johnstone 1975 in guinea pig; by Johnstone et al. 1970 in guinea pig. (From Evans 1975)

be plotted by using the size of the response as the dependent variable (figure 2.32).

These various ways of specifying responses are not entirely equivalent and lead to different representations of the excitation of the fiber. Depending on the researcher and the research, one or another might be selected in describing the study of any of the diverse stages of the auditory system's operation.

[When establishing isointensity or isorate contours, it is equally necessary to make adequate correction to represent a constant stimulus over the whole frequency range by taking account of the tympanum/stapes transfer function.]

It is clear that, for a given fiber, the tuning of an isoresponse curve becomes sharper the more severe the response criterion selected, for

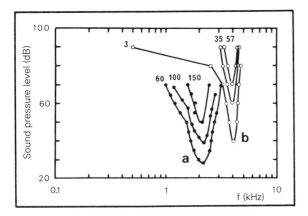

Figure 2.31
Isodischarge curves for two cochlear nerve fibers, (a) in cat and (b) in *Saimiri*. In each case the spontaneous discharge rate of the fiber was negligible. Mean frequency of discharge is indicated above each curve. (From Evans 1975)

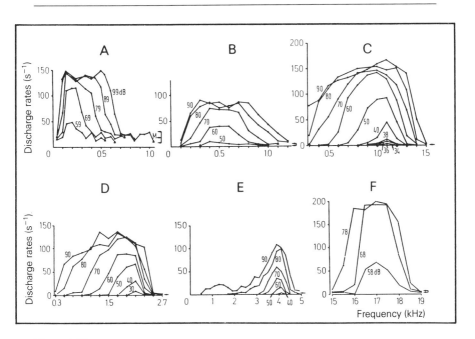

Figure 2.32
Isointensity curves. Curves of discharge rate of six cochlear nerve fibers in *Saimiri* as a function of sound frequency at fixed sound intensities indicated above each curve. (f_c values for each fiber are: *A*, 0.2 kHz; *B*, 0.4 kHz; *C*, 1.1 kHz; *D*, 2.1 kHz; *E*, 4.1 kHz; *F*, 17 kHz) (From Rose et al. 1971)

example, when the nerve discharge rate selected is high (see figure 2.31), whereas for isointensity curves only responses near liminal levels have a narrow tuning bandwidth limited to frequencies near f_c. As the test intensity criterion increases, the effective bandwidth increases, particularly toward the lower frequency side when f_c is high.

The minimal threshold intensity, which for each fiber exists at its characteristic frequency f_c, varies greatly from fiber to fiber. In fact, after carrying out a set of threshold determinations as rigorously as possible, coupled with an appropriate statistical backup and using an adequate number of fibers, it is seen that between 0.1 and 40 kHz the various thresholds arrange themselves along a curve which is essentially close to the behaviorally established audiogram for the species, though generally separated from it by + 10 dB (Evans 1982b). In other words, outputs from the receptor population behave like a homogeneous population, given a large enough sample. Whatever the frequency, 70% of the fibers have a threshold within 10 dB of the behavioral audiogram and 80% within 20 dB, although, in contrast, certain of them have a threshold that is as much as 70 dB above the corresponding behavioral threshold (Neff & Hind 1955; figure 2.33). Recent observations (Liberman & Oliver 1984), however, correct and complement these data: Type I fibers of large, medium, and small diameters, have low, medium, and high thresholds, respectively, and the small diameter fibers are found to have thresholds that are 90 dB higher than those of large diameter.

It is notable that unitary analyses of this sort yield curves that in general show *poorer* sensitivity than the global perceptual performance of the animal.

It cannot fail to be noted, finally, that this sensitivity curve is roughly parallel to the liminal sensitivity variation in the middle ear; this fact suggests that at least part of the cochlea's sensitivity variation with frequency has been governed by the frequency variation of middle ear's sensitivity (figure 2.30A).

Discharge rate coding can also be studied by measuring interspike intervals in the activity observed during the application of sound stimuli of given durations. The information might be displayed by two types of histograms, either in the frequency domain (interspike interval histograms, ISH) or in the temporal domain (peri- or poststimulus histograms, PSH, as the case may be). An ISH is plotted with the elementary intervals as abscissa and the number of events

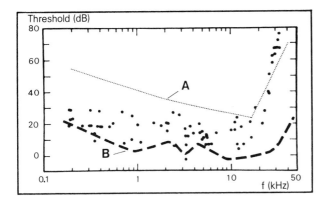

Figure 2.33
Comparison (in the cat) between behavioral thresholds (dashed curve B) and the thresholds of different cochlear nerve fibers. Each point represents the threshold of a single nerve fiber at its f_c. Behavioral values are due to Neff and Hind 1955. Curve A is the middle ear response, arbitrarily positioned in the ordinate, constructed from data like those of figure 2.21, of which it is the reciprocal; the threshold is judged to be proportionally lower the higher the measured stapes velocity at a constant sound pressure. (From Evans 1982b)

in each class of interval as ordinate; a PSH has time as the abscissa and, again, a measure of the density of activity as ordinate.

For units of high f_c, the ISH, plotted around f_c, is unremarkable; the general envelope of the histogram is rather like that of spontaneous activity, with the value of the statistical mode bearing little relationship to the period of the sound (see figure 2.24). Similarly the PSH, for its part, also reveals no particular periodicity.

In contrast, for units with $f_c < 5$ kHz we can see that over the whole frequency range in which the unit responds, there is a "frequency-locking" (Rose et al. 1971) or "phase-locking": The ISH shows, for each stimulating frequency, successive peaks that are spaced apart at practically the period of the incident sound—which effectively results in a display of many subharmonics (figure 2.34). There is one exception; the position of the first peak in the histogram can never be at less than a certain value (ca. 800 µs) that corresponds with the refractory period of the cochlear nerve fiber. Note that this frequency following effect does not occur only for units of low f_c but is also observed when fibers of high f_c are responding to low-frequency sound stimuli.

Finally, if we measure the discharge densities corresponding to

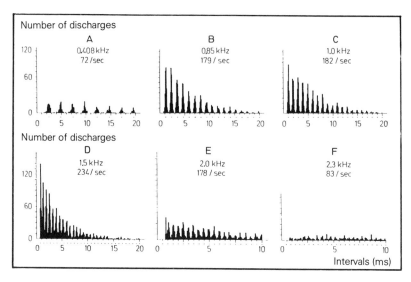

Figure 2.34
Interspike interval histograms (ISH) in *Saimiri* for responses in a single cochlear nerve fiber of low f_c (1.6 kHz) at different stimulus frequencies. Sound stimulus duration 1 s at intensity 80 dB. Each histogram (bin duration 100 μs) is from 10 successive stimulus applications. The dots below the abscissae mark whole multiples of the stimulating sound's period. The stimulus frequency and the mean rate of discharge are indicated above each histogram; note the difference in time base between E and F, and A to D. (From Rose et al. 1968).

each frequency at a given sound intensity, we obtain an isointensity profile that closely resembles the tuning curve for the unit.

Naturally, an observed frequency-locking leads to the expectation of a relationship between the discharge of impulses and the phase of the stimulus. At low frequencies (< 5 kHz), the frequency-locked discharge occurs preferentially at a precise part of the cycle. This is seen very well in peri-stimulus histograms (PSH) with the time abscissa confined to that of a complete sound cycle: The preferred region for the discharge depends on the particular fiber studied. As before, this phase-locking is not only seen for low f_c units but in high f_c units when they are stimulated at, and can respond to, low-frequency sounds (figure 2.35).

It has also been possible to demonstrate that the phase of the cycle preferred in the responses varies with f_c, at least for fibers with f_c < 8 kHz. For units with f_c > 8 kHz, the phase variation as a function of f_c no longer exists, which recalls a fact already recognized concerning

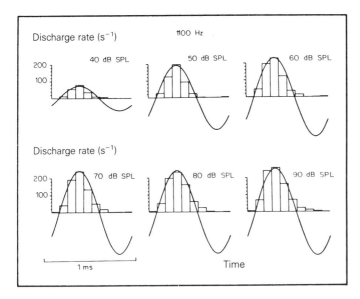

Figure 2.35
Response histograms for a fiber of low f_c (1.1 kHz) stimulated at f_c. Stimulus intensity is indicated above each histogram. The fiber responds for only half the stimulus cycle, with the discharge increasing and decreasing according to the 1.1-kHz waveform of stimulus intensity even when the magnitude of the peak discharge saturates above 70 dB. (From Rose et al. 1971)

cochlear mechanisms: When the cochlea is stimulated at low frequency but with high enough intensity, all the base of the cochlea, that is, the whole population of receptors with the highest f_c values, is set into activity synchronously.

The observations of phase-locking have an additional implication with respect to basic cochlear dynamics: They presumably indicate that excitation of the receptors is only effective when the pressure acting on the tympanum, and therefore on the oval window, is *in a certain direction* and that the inverse pressure is ineffective. We will return to this phenomenon below when discussing responses to a "click."

7.3 INTENSITY CODING

When the stimulus to a given unit is increased at a certain frequency (in particular at f_c), the discharge (measured as the total number of impulses or as the density of the discharge, depending on the experimental arrangements) is also increased and in most cases in a

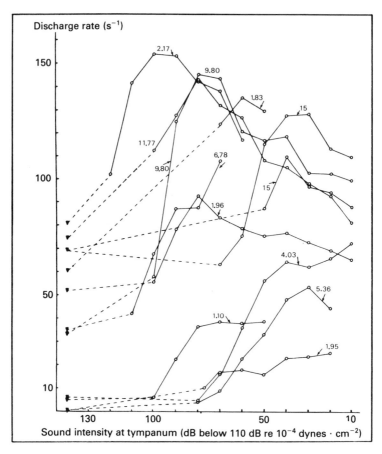

Figure 2.36
Relative discharge rates in cat cochlear nerve fibers as a function of sound stimulus intensity. Stimulation at the characteristic frequency of the fiber, indicated above each curve. The spontaneous discharge rate is indicated by the triangles to the left, each joined to the relevant curve by a dotted line. Notice that some of the discharge characteristics show a plateau and some a maximum. (From Kiang et al. 1965)

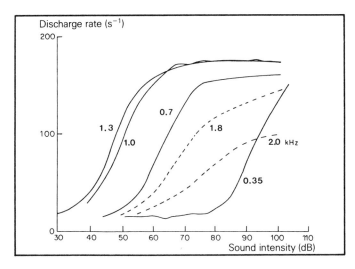

Figure 2.37
Intensity/discharge rate characteristics for an individual cochlear fiber for different stimulating frequencies (shown beside each curve). At f_c (1.3 kHz) the discharge rate passes from threshold to its maximal rate over a 30-dB increase in sound intensity. This dynamic range is greater for stimuli $> f_c$ (dashed curves). (From Sachs & Abbas 1974)

sigmoidal manner (Kiang et al. 1965; Sachs & Abbas 1974). In general it is found that the working range, between threshold and the final plateau (*dynamic range*), is somewhere between 20 and 50 dB (figure 2.36). [Notice that this dynamic range is much less than is observed in behavioral studies in animals or by psychophysics in humans.] In some rather rare cases the relationship between discharge and intensity passes to a maximum only to decrease again at higher intensities. Such "non-monotonic" functions are, however, rare in cochlear nerve fibers, although we shall see that they occur more frequently at more central stages. Notice also that the dynamic bandwidth of a given unit can be greater for a stimulating frequency greater than f_c (figure 2.37).

In contrast to the observation that the three classes of type I fibers have different thresholds according to their different diameters (see above), it seems that at f_c their dynamic bandwidths are all about the same. This observation might be important (see chapter 3, 10.3).

7.4 TIME COURSE OF NEURAL DISCHARGES

After presentation of a tone pip, most fibers respond with an initial high frequency transient in their discharge, followed by a plateau

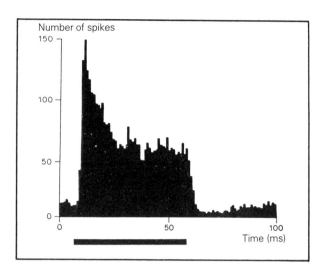

Figure 2.38
Response of a single cochlear fiber in the cat to a tone pip (indicated by the bar below). The figure shows a peristimulus histogram after summation of the discharges in the temporal domain during a large number of successive stimulating tone pips. Notice the large "on response" of the discharge at the beginning of the stimulus, followed by a decrease as the stimulus continues, followed by a temporary decrease in spontaneous rate ("off response") when the stimulus ceases. (From Kiang 1965)

lasting as long as the stimulus (figure 2.38). These units are therefore *phasic-tonic*. In rare cases the discharge is limited to the transient response only and the unit is therefore *phasic*. This relative simplicity contrasts with the complexity of response patterns that are observed in more central auditory relays, as we shall see.

Another situation, not yet considered here, is the result of stimulation with a *click*, a very brief stimulus (say 100 μs) with an extensive spectral spread of frequencies. Under these conditions a neuron of low f_c (<5 kHz) generates a repetitive response. Its PSH has many peaks, with intervals between them corresponding to $1/f_c$, and amplitudes that diminish progressively with time. In contrast, units of high f_c respond with a single discharge peak in their PSH (figure 2.39).

Given its brevity and precise timing, the click is very suitable for use in latency studies. Such measurements give latency values between 1 and 2.4 ms. For a given fiber, the latency is inversely related to its f_c (figure 2.40), and this presumably results from the transmission delay in excitation of the cochlear receptors between the base and apex of the cochlea. For units of basal origin, $f_c > 5$ kHz, this

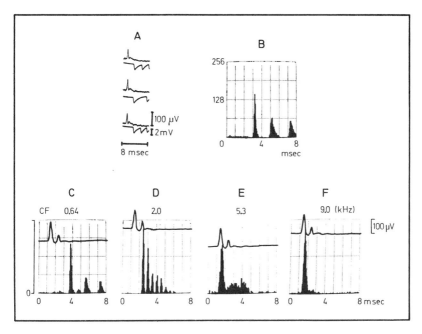

Figure 2.39
Response of a single cochlear nerve fiber to brief click stimuli. *A,* Oscilloscope traces for three successive clicks. In each case the upper trace shows the global evoked potential response to the click measured at the round window (as in figure 2.46) and the lower trace is the single unit fiber response (negative upward); note the repetitive nature of the responses. *B,* Poststimulus histogram (PSH) for the same fiber showing the resulting response characteristic, averaged over a long time, for 600 successive clicks. Fiber f_c, 0.54 kHz. *C* to *F,* Histograms of the temporal dispersion of the discharges of for four other fibers (f_c indicated above each PSH). Each of these shows above it an oscilloscope trace of the global evoked potential for the whole nerve measured at the round window. Ordinates: number of spikes (scales: C 258, D 128, E 64, F 128). All clicks had the same intensity and were presented at 10/s. Note the rhythmic discharge for fibers of low f_c (*B, C,* and *D*). (From Evans 1975 after Kiang 1965)

latency is like that of the N_1 component of the compound action potential of the eighth nerve (see section 8.4., below).

Using click stimuli also clearly shows the direction of basilar membrane movement that is effective for excitation. One can either use a *condensation click,* producing a positive pressure impulse at the tympanum or a *rarefaction click,* which applies a negative pressure impulse. Rarefaction clicks generate responses of *shorter latency* than condensation clicks, the peaks in the two PSH showing clear complementary patterns (figure 2.41). Thus the phase effective for excitation is a relative rarefaction, producing a pressure decrease at the oval win-

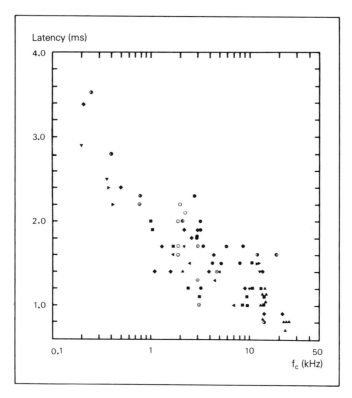

Figure 2.40
Click response latencies in single cochlear nerve fibers as a function of f_c in the cat
(filled symbols) and guinea pig (open symbols). For rarefaction clicks of 100 μs (cat)
and 50 μs (guinea pig) presented at 10/s at intensities 30 to 60 dB. (From Evans 1975)

dow and in the scala vestibuli and thus an *elevation of the basilar membrane toward scala vestibuli.*

8 BIOELECTRIC PHENOMENA IN THE COCHLEA

The analysis of the processes of transduction in the cochlea has
exploited a widespread range of techniques. It has been a matter
of using all possible means—not only bioelectrical but also
mechanical—to try to discover how the hair cells are excited by sound
waves. This preliminary discussion introduces the results of "global"
electrophysiological methods, that is, of those experiments that used
electrodes with rather large receptive ranges that could not therefore
selectively record from single units.

Having long since been applied to most compartments of the in-

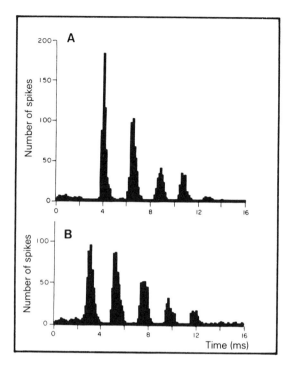

Figure 2.41
Poststimulus histograms for condensation (A) and rarefaction (B) clicks. Note the complementary positions of the maxima in the two discharge histograms. Fiber f_c, 0.54 kHz. (From Pickles 1982, adapted from Kiang et al. 1965)

ner ear, these methods have uncovered a variety of biological phenomena. The value and even the interest of these observations is somewhat mixed. Nevertheless, they pioneered, if only historically, the major future lines of attack needed to investigate cochlear mechanisms.

8.1 STEADY (DC) POTENTIALS

It is well known that there are steady and permanent potential differences between the various parts of the cochlea that are independent of any auditory stimulation (figure 2.42). First, the scala tympani is practically at the same potential as that of all nearby extracellular space and the body fluids in general. In contrast, the scala vestibuli is slightly positive (+ 2 to + 5 mv) with respect to the scala tympani. However, the most striking phenomenon is the existence of a considerable positive polarization (+ 80 to + 100 mv) of the scala media (the cochlear canal) with respect to the scala tympani.

Before trying to explain the origin of these potentials, it is worthwhile outlining briefly the origin and significance of the cochlear fluids (Sterkers et al. 1988).

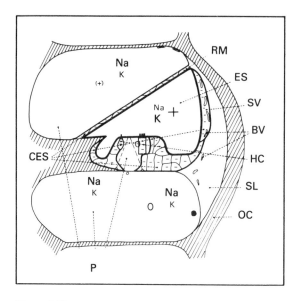

Figure 2.42
Distribution of the steady potentials in different parts of the cochlea. Scala tympani is taken as the reference zero. Scale vestibuli (SV) is slightly positive. There is a considerable positive potential in the endolymph space (ES) of the cochlear canal, scala media, with negativity in the intercellular space of the tunnel of Corti, which in this example was considered to be perilymph (but see text). The situation is more complicated in the stria vascularis. The intracellular potentials in the hair cells are considerably negative. P, perilymphatic space; OC, osseous cochlea; SL, spiral ligament; CES, cells of the endolymphatic space; HC, hair cells; BV, blood vessels; SV, stria vascularis; ES, endolymphatic space; RM, Reissner's membrane. (From Davis 1965)

Perilymph, which occupies the scala vestibuli and scala tympani spaces, is grossly an ultrafiltrate of plasma (K^+ 7 mM, Na^+ 140 mM, Cl^- 120 mM), although its composition is a little different and, in addition, the two perilymphs of the scala vestibuli and scala tympani are not absolutely identical (more potassium, glucose, amino acids, and protein in the scala vestibuli). What is more, the two perilymphatic fluids do not have the same source: Scala vestibuli plasma does originate in plasma (via an endothelial boundary), whereas scala tympani perilymph probably comes from cerebrospinal fluid (via a channel communicating with the fourth ventricle).

Endolymph has its source in the perilymph. It is known that Reissner's membrane is not totally impermeable but also that most exchanges at that boundary are chiefly in the direction scala vestibuli to scala media (Anniko & Wroblewski 1986). Yet analysis reveals a composition for endolymph (K^+ 150 mM, Na^+ 1 mM, Cl^- 130 mM) that is quite different from the perilymph. Also, the endolymphatic ionic composition in no way explains its positive polarization.

It is now established that the particular composition of endolymph is maintained by active processes, the site of which is in the *stria vascularis*. This tissue contains, particularly in its marginal cells, a very complex complement of enzymes (Na^+– K^+–ATPase; Ca^{2+}–ATPase; carbonic anhydrase; adenylcyclase). Note:

• Anoxia suppresses the positive polarization. It becomes negative (-30 to -40 mv) and persists at that value for several hours and then becomes related to passive exchange processes across the limiting membranes of the cochlear canal (Reissner's membrane, stria vascularis, etc.) whose ionic permeability is probably poor in normal conditions.
• After destruction of Reissner's membrane, endolymph and perilymph mix and only the stria vascularis itself demonstrates a positive polarity (Tasaki & Spiropoulos 1959).
• Stria vascularis is the site of intense ATPase activity. Ouabain, which is known to block enzyme systems, produces a decrease in the positive endolymphatic potential.
• Certain ototoxic drugs that act preferentially on the stria vascularis degrade the endolymphatic potential.
• The potential is not due to the organ of Corti itself; in fact, certain strains of mice (called "waltzing mice") congenitally lack an organ of Corti without thereby suffering a simultaneous lack of endocochlear potential.

In summary, it seems that the stria vascularis incorporates an electrogenic system (Na^+– K^+–ATPase) that is responsible for the steady polarization of the endolymph, and which reabsorbs sodium and secretes potassium against their concentration gradients.

von Békésy reported another steady potential of about -40 mv in the interior of the canal of Corti, but this potential has since been denied and explained as a potential resulting from cellular damage. *Cortilymph* is nowadays considered to be identical to perilymph, and the canal of Corti to be therefore part of the perilymphatic space.

8.2 COCHLEAR MICROPHONIC POTENTIALS

Wever and Bray (1930) were surprised to find that a metal electrode placed on the auditory nerve recorded a potential after amplification that faithfully reproduced the waveform of the sound stimulus. They thought they had recorded the integrated activity of the acoustic nerve but further study showed that this was wrong: The major signal that had been recorded was the result of an electrical activity that precedes the generation of nerve impulses in the transduction process. These potentials are the *cochlear microphonics* (CM).

The CM is most easily recorded by an *active electrode* near the round window with an *indifferent (reference) electrode* placed on nearby electrically quiet nonauditory tissue. It originates, as we shall see, in the massed activity of the receptor cells and is transmitted to the neighborhood of the recording electrode by the perilymph, which is a very good electrical conductor. Overall, the CM exactly follows the instantaneous amplitude of the stimulus and in that respect resembles the output of a microphone; it is practically without latency with respect to the stimulus, does not adapt or show any refractory period, and it is graded, not all-or-none as individual nerve impulses are.

One of its often quoted characteristics is the relationship between the stimulus intensity and the amplitude of CM (in millivolts). This *input/output* relation is a linear one between the log of the CM amplitude and stimulus intensity in decibels, this being obeyed up to about 80 to 90 dB. Saturation sets in above that intensity level, with in some instances a certain diminution following the maximal plateau value. But even at this level of saturation, the CM shows very little distortion (figure 2.43).

The cochlear microphonic is to some extent sensitive to anoxia. When an animal dies, the CM magnitude diminishes but does not disappear immediately. This has suggested the existence of two contributions to CM, one potential being *first order* (CM1) and requiring a normoxic environment, the other being *second order* (CM2), which can still be recorded for several hours after death.

ORIGIN AND SIGNIFICANCE OF THE COCHLEAR MICROPHONIC

This question, once CM had been discovered, was the inspiration of many and varied experiments and hypotheses. It is now known that the CM is generated by the hair cells. Recorded as above, it results from global activity of large amplitude that can be recorded at the base of the cochlea with ease. In those conditions the activity displayed can offer no spatial specificity, since it is a summation of the activity that has been elicited at a variety of places along the cochlea.

It is, however, possible to attain a *focal* or *differential* recording by

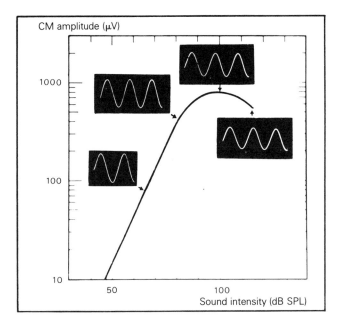

Figure 2.43
Input/ouput characteristic of the cochlear microphonic. CM recorded in the first turn of the guinea pig cochlea for a 7 kHz tone. Note the lack of distortion even at the maximal output. (From Davis 1960)

arranging two electrodes, one in the scala vestibuli and the other opposite to it in the scala tympani, placed symmetrically with respect to the organ of Corti. We shall see later that the cells in the organ of Corti constitute a transversally arranged dipole of activity that generates the CM; the arrangement just described preferentially records the contributions to CM from nearby dipoles rather than those that are generated more remotely. A step-by-step exploration of the activity at different levels of the cochlea is thus possible and shows that high-frequency sound gives the largest responses at the cochlear base and low frequencies at the apex (with, however, some movement of this latter response toward the base as sound intensity increases. This effect has not yet been fully explained).

Among the more significant observations on the origin of the CM are those (Dallos et al. 1972; figure 2.44) exploiting the remarkable properties of kanamycin, an ototoxic aminoglycoside antibiotic that destroys, almost exclusively, the OHC while sparing 90% of the IHC (Hawkins 1976). Having effected such a selective lesion of the OHC

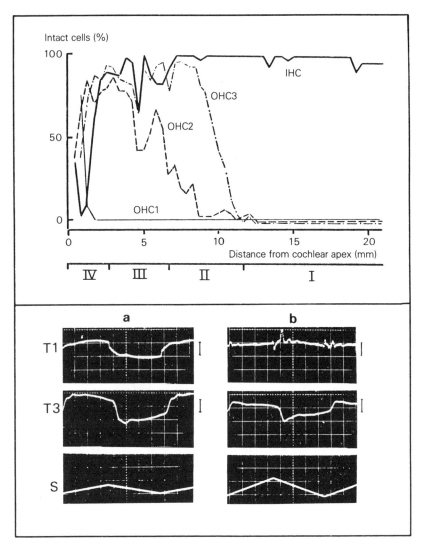

Figure 2.44
Effects of kanamycin on the cochlea. *Above,* Percentages of intact cells (ordinate) after kanamycin injection (guinea pig): IHC, in the single row of inner hair cells; OHC1, OHC2, OHC3, in the three rows of outer hair cells. The extent of each of the four turns of the cochlear spiral is marked I, II, III, IV. Neurophysiological measurements (see text) were made at the level of the first and third turns. *Below,* Cochlear microphonic potentials recorded (*a*) in a normal animal, (*b*) in a kanamycin-treated animal in T1, the first turn, and T3, the third turn, in response to the stimulus (S) showing stapes displacement (peak to peak amplitude 0.3 μm, frequency 73 Hz). (From Dallos et al. 1972)

of the first turn of the guinea pig cochlea, it was shown that the amplitude of CM was reduced to 10% of the normal, while continuing to obey the law of increase in CM with increasing sound intensity as in the normal case. It is occasionally suggested from these results that the whole CM is generated by OHC. In fact, this is almost certainly not strictly true, since 10% of CM can be accounted for by contributions from the IHC.

The exact nature of CM has been debated and still is in some respects. It had been suggested that a passive effect could account for it (e.g., piezoelectric effects in the cochlea) but also that it was chiefly explicable by ionic fluxes in membranes. Microelectrode investigations have localized its major source at the surface of the hair cell receptors, near the reticular lamina. This was achieved by mapping CM and finding the zone where its polarity reverses (always a good indicator of an electrical source, AC or DC). The results also lead to the conclusion that at least the first-order CM (observable in the living animal) is linked to the existence of a local dipole-like electrical generator at the hair cell surface. To anticipate a later discussion, it had for some time been postulated (Davis 1965) that the origin of CM might be connected with an ohmic resistance variation in the hair cells, or in the reticular lamina, synchronous with the stimulus. Given the existence of a considerable DC potential difference between the endolymph and the cytoplasm of the receptors (80 mv + 60 mv = 140 mv), it is in fact conceivable that this resistance change could generate a current that followed the stimulus, the magnitude of which would be compatible with the size of CM and also with its phase reversal between the scala vestibuli and scala tympani.

A whole series of recent studies on the cellular origins of CM have notably advanced our understanding of how the microphonic is generated. These will be discussed in section 9.2, below.

8.3 SUMMATING POTENTIALS

Apart from recording the CM, it is equally possible to detect at the oval window or from the cochlear canal a DC potential variation that lasts throughout the duration of a sound stimulus. In general, the change is such that the scala media becomes negative with respect to the scala tympani, but in many circumstances, such as during anoxia or for weak stimuli or during an artificially increased pressure in scala tympani, the change is the opposite (i.e., a positive potential variation; figure 2.45).

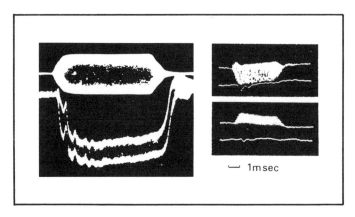

Figure 2.45
Cochlear microphonics and summation potentials. *Left,* A montage showing, in the upper trace, a cochlear microphonic recorded at the round window in the guinea pig and, in the lower traces, summating potentials (SP) at the beginning of which (to the left) can also be seen traces of the nerve action potential. *Right,* Upper traces: cochlear microphonic, including SP (seen as the steady mean level of the signal). Lower traces: nerve action potentials for (above) normal cochlea with SP negative; (below) after increasing the scala tympani pressure by serum injection, SP becomes positive. (From Davis 1960)

The origins and significance of this potential are still being discussed. One suggestion, following Davis' ideas about CM, is that consequent to a decreased resistance in the receptor layer, a DC current might be generated that creates a DC potential difference. According to that hypothesis, we would predict that the reticular lamina would be the site of an inversion in the sign of this summating potential (SP). In the structures immediately adjacent to the reticular lamina it is usually seen as a negative change in the scala vestibuli and the scala media and a positive one in the scala tympani. Recent intracellular investigations of the receptor cells, to which we will return (Russel & Sellick 1978, 1983), led to the suggestion that the summating potential is a nonlinear, rectifying attribute of the mechanisms that generate CM. But even that explanation of SP is probably too simplified. We have already mentioned that in some circumstances its sign in the scala media can become relatively more positive than in the scala tympani. In addition, two components have been discovered in SP (Honrubia & Ward 1969), one increasing with CM increase (and concordant with the rectifying nonlinearity suggested above) but with the other component progressively increasing with the duration of the sound stimulus. Such very slow components as the latter will probably be shown to be concerned with the progress of metabolic processes in the receptors themselves or perhaps even in other adjacent cells as well.

Honrubia and Ward also described the spatial distribution of SP along the cochlea, with its maximum at high frequencies being toward the base and at low frequencies toward the apex. A more detailed exploration (Dallos et al. 1972) combining spatial analysis with the use of an ototoxic drug selectively destroying the OHC showed that at a given place in the cochlea the scala media SP can be *positive* for *low* frequencies while being *negative* for *high* frequencies, in each case with reference to the scala tympani. This study also found that the use of kanamycin completely suppresses any positivity, the latter being therefore attributed to OHC, whereas the negative potential has part of its source in OHC and part in IHC.

8.4 ACTION POTENTIALS IN THE AUDITORY NERVE

The "global" compound action potential of the auditory nerve can also be recorded at the round window. This potential is the result of a summation of many individual impulses. It is particularly easily recorded by using a click stimulus which simultaneously excites a very large population of receptors. With that technique, the potential displays two or sometimes three successive negative excursions (figure 2.46), the latency of the N_1 peak being around 1 ms, N_2 and N_3 following N_1 1 ms and 2 ms later, respectively. The N_1 peak is due particularly to receptors in the basal turn of the cochlea.

When using stimuli of longer duration, such as tone pips, the compound action potential is absent except at the onset and termination of the stimulus; during most of the steady time course of the stimulus any response is less than the noise level. This could be due to a variety of reasons, one doubtless being the absence of synchronization of the activities of different individual nerve fibers during the continuing stimulus. [Recordings of action potentials such as these, whether following clicks or tone pips, need the simultaneous presence of CM, seen when recording from a single electrode, to be eliminated. This is best done by using a pair of focal electrodes, one being placed in the scala vestibuli, the other in the scala tympani, and the electrode pair employing a common, third, indifferent electrode as reference. In this way CM is cancelled (see figure 2.46) since it is recorded in antiphase between the two electrodes, whereas the com-

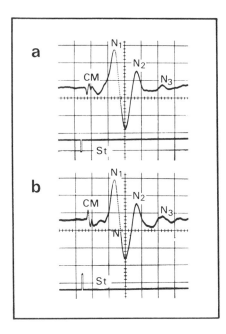

Figure 2.46
Cochlear nerve action potentials with their successive components N1, N2, N3, measured at the round window (cat). The major part of the cochlear microphonic has been cancelled by differential recording (except at the onset marked CM). The click stimuli (St) are recorded below each action potential (*a*) for a rarefaction and (*b*) for a condensation click. (Notice that while the click reverses the CM trace, the action potentials remain the same). (From Klinke 1972)

pound action potential is not eliminated. The two electrodes receive action potentials in phase since the spatial configuration of their source is not a suitably oriented dipole sited between the electrode pair. Being in phase they do not cancel.]

Such recordings, it must be admitted, hardly add much useful information on fundamental processes. However, in contrast to this, recording action potentials in the acoustic nerve and at more central levels of the auditory system can be invaluable during clinical investigations in humans.

9 COCHLEAR MECHANICS

We shall review here all the mechanisms by which an acoustic vibration reaching the oval window finally achieves excitation in the cochlear receptors themselves. These mechanisms are related to, among others, the elastic and hydrodynamic properties of the cochlea and particularly of the basilar membrane (BM).

9.1 BASIC FACTS AND HYPOTHESES

It has been generally agreed that each sound frequency affects a certain region of the cochlea between the apex and the base, at a place that depends on that frequency. Historically, two classes of hypothesis were proposed to explain this dependence between incident frequency and the part of the cochlea excited.

The earliest hypothesis for frequency selectivity seems to have been *resonance tuning*, for which von Helmholtz (1863) and later workers became enthusiastic. According to this theory, the basilar membrane comprises a series of resonant structures oriented transversely, each with its own resonant frequency and with high-frequency resonators being at the cochlear base, near the oval window, and the lowest frequencies near the apex, toward the helicotrema. The effect of a sound is to energize only the resonators that are tuned to frequencies corresponding with those that are present in the sound and, because of the regular sequential spatial sorting of resonant frequency, each separate place along the cochlea will respond best to a particular frequency. This theory relied heavily on *Ohm's acoustic law*, which originated in 1843 and stated that the ear is capable of resolving a complex tone into a Fourier harmonic series (see chapter 1, 1.1). It could also be regarded as an application of the *law of specific energies* (Müller 1838; see also Buser & Imbert 1982, Vol. II) which would predict that each tonal frequency ought to have, dedicated to its own detection, a limited number of fibers in the acoustic nerve.

Helmholtz' model very rapidly stirred up a whole series of theoretical difficulties, which we will only summarize. First, it is hard to imagine how a selective mechanical excitation of any one resonator could be attained by vibration of the stapes without a much larger stretch of the cochlea also being stimulated into oscillation. Second, to be highly frequency-selective a resonator also needs to be heavily damped; therefore on this theory a resonator would be slow to reach its maximal vibration amplitude and similarly would be equally slow to come to rest after the sound had ceased. In other words, hearing would be poor for sounds containing rapid changes in frequency and/or amplitude (e.g., speech and music). Third, the phase changes in such a resonator can only range between $-\pi/2$ and $+\pi/2$ at frequencies ranging from one side to the other of its resonant frequency. We shall see below that conditions are nothing like that since the phase shifts observed are much greater. Finally, there are other less direct arguments, for example, that Helmholtz' hypothesis cannot account for the auditory effects of certain sound summations, such as hearing the nonexistent so-called missing fundamental. We shall return to this discussion later.

THE TRAVELING-WAVE HYPOTHESIS

The other family of hypotheses suggests a quite different mechanism that is based on the existence of a propagating *traveling wave* that moves along the cochlea from base to apex. A very rough analogy might be that of a slack rope which, when one end of it is shaken, transmits a wave that travels along to the other end. The amplitude of this wave has to increase initially and then diminish in the course of its journey to the far end.

Such traveling-wave theories began with Hurst in 1894. They then found a sound experimental basis in von Békésy's work (from 1928 on) and were reinforced by many more recent experiments. Before discussing results we should understand the methods used.

von Békésy, who inaugurated this line of investigation, began by experimenting on models and then transferred his attention to freshly dead cadavers. An artificial stapes connected to an electromagnetic vibrator (hydrophone) was fixed to an artificial membrane that replaced the oval window (figure 2.47) and generated controlled hydrostatic pressure changes. Thanks to windows arranged in the cochlea and the use of stroboscopic illumination timed to the sound frequency, von Békésy was able to follow movements of different cochlear regions by exploiting water immersion microscopy aided by introducing local deposits of fine silver crystals on the structures concerned.

Unfortunately, he could only make tests at relatively low frequencies (up to 1.6 to 2.4 kHz) corresponding to apical regions of the cochlea. The limited resolving power of his apparatus did not allow him to study the much smaller, more basally situated vibrations that would be elicited at higher frequencies. However, various more modern methods do allow HF observations.

Interferometry is a classic technique for detecting small movements. In principle, it consists in combining waves emitted by two sources, one from a stationary reference and the other from the moving object whose displacement is to be measured. The apparatus can be designed to give an output essentially linearly related to the relative displacement of the two sources. Sensitivity of the method is vastly increased to being able to detect displacements as small as $3 \cdot 10^{-10}$ cm by using coherent (usually laser) light. Khanna et al. (1968), study-

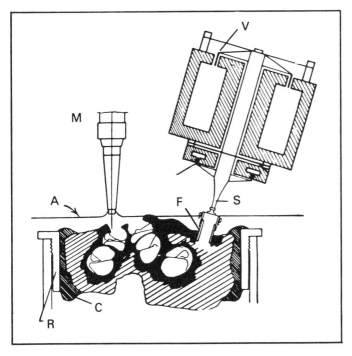

Figure 2.47
Classic arrangement used by von Békésy to examine cochlear vibrations. The temporal bone is dissected and cemented (C) to a rigid metal support (R). An opening is
made over the selected region of the cochlea and the movements (e.g., of the basilar
membrane) are observed microscopically (M) using a water-immersion objective since
the whole preparation is maintained in an aqueous medium (A). Oscillatory mechanical stimulation is attained with an electromagnetically controlled vibrator (V) moving
an artificial stapes (S), which in turn moves an artificial membrane sealed at (F) to
replace the oval window. All vibrations are observed in stroboscopic light. (From von
Békésy & Rosenblith 1951)

ing the cat, measured vibrations of order 10^{-5} cm by using as the
moving source a mica fragment weighing 1 μg sited on a surface and
acting as a mirror. Kohllöffel (1972), studying the guinea pig, used the
threshold of incoherence ("fuzziness") in interference ("speckled")
images formed by reflection of laser light from the basilar membrane
and was able to deduce both the amplitude and phase of movements.
Such measurements were an excellent complement to those of von
Békésy in studying the spatial propagation of the traveling wave.

    The *Mössbauer effect* was exploited by Johnstone and Boyle (1967)
and Rhode (1971) in which a radioactive source (stainless steel con-

taining ^{57}Co, decaying to ^{57}Fe plus a gamma ray) is placed in the cochlea at a given site, and a "daughter product" gamma ray absorber (^{57}Fe) is placed nearby in front of a gamma detector and counter. Absorption is tuned to the energy (and therefore the frequency) of the gamma emission, which is itself modulated by the velocity of movement of its source (by the Doppler effect). It is thus possible to measure the displacement velocity of the source (i.e., of the moving regions of the basilar membrane) absolutely and accurately.

A *capacitative probe* in which one electrode is placed immediately adjacent to the basilar membrane can also be used. The electrode–basilar membrane capacitance is deduced from impedance measurements at a given (radio-) frequency. The capacitance is a function of the distance between the basilar membrane and the electrode, from which the basilar membrane movement can be calculated (Wilson & Johnstone 1975).

Now let us summarize the theory of a traveling wave that propagates along the basilar membrane.

• Because of the incompressibility of the fluids of the inner ear, a pressure variation generated by the stapes brings with it a displacement of the endolymph with a compensatory displacement of the round window. These displacements cause a deformation of the cochlear partition in its basal region.

• This deformation then propagates as a transverse wave (perpendicular to the plane of BM) from the base toward the apex. The amplitude of this wave changes during its travel. It first increases progressively to attain a maximal value and is thereafter attenuated much more rapidly, to become very small or negligible at the apex (except at very low frequencies). The whole wave can be illustrated by a set of characteristic envelopes (figure 2.48).

• The speed of propagation decreases continually and uniformly as propagation proceeds from the cochlear base to its apex.

• Sounds of different frequencies produce traveling waves that reach their maxima at different places along the cochlea. Thus a disparity arises between the wave envelopes for different frequencies: For high frequencies the traveling-wave maximum is near the base, whereas for low frequencies the increase in amplitude is more gradual; the maximal displacement is reached closer and closer to the apex as the frequency decreases. In other words, the maximal vibration is local-

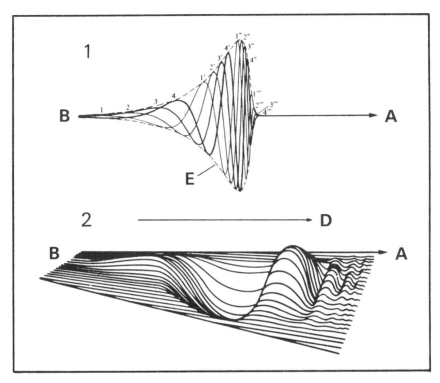

Figure 2.48
Displacement patterns of the basilar membrane traveling wave. In both diagrams the displacements have been magnified for the purposes of illustration; even at the threshold of pain, around 120 dB SPL, the vibration amplitude does not exceed 1% the breadth of the membrane. *1*, Two-dimensional representation of the positions of the traveling wave after successive intervals of 1/3 period (1, 2, 3, 4; 1', 2', 3', 4'; 1", 2", 3", 4"; etc.). *2*, Three-dimensional representation of the basilar membrane traveling wave at a given instant. Note: In each diagram the traveling wave propagates from the base B toward the apex A in the direction D. The displacement is maximal at a particular place on the membrane and thereafter diminishes steeply toward the apex. (From Tonndorf 1960)

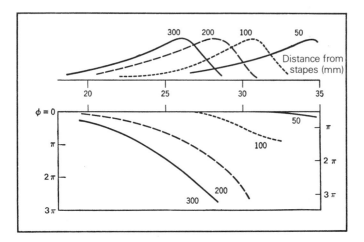

Figure 2.49
Relative amplitude and phase of vibration along the cochlea. Envelopes of the relative amplitudes of vibration (upper ordinate) and phase of vibration (ϕ) with respect to stapes velocity (lower ordinate) for places on the cochlea at different distances from the stapes and at different stimulating frequencies (marked above the corresponding curve). At 100 Hz, phase differences can exceed π and at 50 Hz practically all the membrane vibrates in phase. (From von Békésy & Rosenblith 1951)

ized to a particular place along the basilar membrane. This *spatial sorting* of maximal cochlear vibration (figure 2.49) is the fundamental process that eventually leads to pitch discrimination.

• Another, complementary way to represent the properties of the traveling wave is to measure the vibration *at a given point* along the cochlea as a function of frequency, for constant stimulus amplitude. Plotting these results at a given cochlear location yields an amplitude profile for the vibration as a function of frequency which shows a maximum response at a certain preferred or characteristic frequency, f_c. Different parts of the cochlea have different values of f_c (figure 2.50). [We have used the same symbol f_c for the preferred vibration frequency as for the characteristic frequency of the nerve fibers. This identity is not evident a priori. However, it becomes justified by recent data, which we shall describe below, showing how the basilar membrane acts like a band-pass filter, the selectivity of which becomes more like that of the afferent fibers, the greater the care that is taken experimentally to keep the functional state of the basilar membrane as untraumatized as possible.]

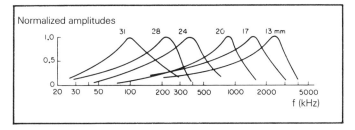

Figure 2.50
Frequency responses along the cochlear spiral. Responses as a function of frequency
at six places along the basilar membrane (distances from stapes between 31 and 13
mm indicated above the corresponding curve). Amplitude of the vibration measured
at each place at a variety of frequencies for constant stapes displacement. Amplitudes
normalized to unity value at the peak. (From von Békésy & Rosenblith 1951)

9.2 MORE DETAILED STUDIES AND RECENT DATA

When he analyzed the cochlea, von Békésy was scarcely able to explore beyond the apical region (i.e., not beyond the corresponding
low-frequency region), where he could generate vibrations sufficiently large to be seen. More modern techniques have allowed study
of the high-frequency vibrations of more basal regions and thus to
extend and, it must be said, generally corroborate von Békésy's early
measurements.

In addition, he saw the advantages of working on the fresh human
cadaver if one wished to make comparisons with the already well-
established data of human psychophysics. But the dangers are clear
that the "preparation," even if "very fresh," is not quite the same
as a living person. Some modern authors (e.g., Greenwood 1961;
Kohllöffel 1972; Rhode 1978) have not let pass an opportunity to
emphasize precisely these risks. Therefore much of the more recent
research has been carried out in living animals, notably the guinea
pig, less frequently the cat, and, most recently but not often, the
squirrel monkey (*Saimiri*); the differences between the results have
been attributed less to species differences than to disparate experimental conditions.

Many of these detailed investigations are still in progress and are
still likely to yield new approaches and to exploit technical innova-
tions. They have much increased our knowledge of cochlear mechanisms, whether concerning the mechanical properties of different
cochlear structures, or the relationships between stapes movements

and those of the basilar membrane or the laws of frequency sorting along the cochlear partition, or the speed of propagation of traveling waves, or the problems of the final transduction processes that these mechanical properties underpin.

MECHNICAL PROPERTIES OF DIFFERENT COCHLEAR COMPONENTS

Apart from studying the dynamics of the whole cochlea, there have also been investigations of the mechanical elasticity of different parts of the cochlear apparatus, chiefly of the basilar membrane which mainly governs propagation but also of the tectorial membrane and Reissner's membrane and of the cellular systems of the organ of Corti. [Studies of the mechanics of basilar membrane movement are probably vulnerable to revision as experimental techniques improve, particularly the detecting probes.] The following facts should be noted (von Békésy 1960; cf. Steele 1976):

• The basilar membrane is isotropic in its properties: Application of a punctate pressure deforms the membrane identically in all directions (except at the base).
• The basilar membrane is not normally under tension; a small cut made in it does not gape at the edges. The membrane behaves like a strip with a certain stiffness and not like an elastic membrane.
• The stiffness varies from base to apex, with a maximal stiffness (minimal compliance) at the base and a 100 times smaller stiffness (maximal compliance) at the apex. This difference in compliance is a factor that fundamentally controls propagation.
• The basilar membrane is so constructed that the direction of traveling-wave propagation is always from the point of minimal compliance toward a point of greater compliance, in other words from base toward the apex, *whatever the mechanism that has set the cochlea in motion*, whether via the stapes and oval window or via direct bone conduction (see above). It is in all cases the *compliance gradient* that determines the direction of propagation.
• Surprisingly, there does not seem to be any appreciable coupling between adjacent parts of the basilar membrane. Propagation does not depend on any such coupling. On the contrary, it is ensured by the cochlear fluids acting as an intermediary to transmit the pressure changes.
• However, the stiffness of the basilar membrane in a transverse direction does seem to be greater near the organ of Corti in the inner pars arcuata region than in the outer pars pectinata.

• These properties contrast with those of the other anatomical structures, Reissner's membrane, the tectorial membrane, the organ of Corti: Their elastic properties seem to remain constant throughout the length of the cochlea.

• Reissner's membrane is stiffer in the longitudinal than in the transverse direction.

INTRACOCHLEAR PRESSURES; FROM STAPES MOVEMENT TO BASILAR MEMBRANE MOVEMENT

Considering further the hypotheses for generation of the traveling wave, there is the problem of how a stapes movement is converted into a roughly perpendicular basilar membrane movement. Recently, some relevant experiments have measured the pressure differences between the scala vestibuli and the scala tympani using very sensitive detectors (Nedzelnitsky 1980). In these experiments the sound pressure at the tympanum is set to given levels.

At a *constant frequency*, a linear relationship is found between the sound intensity and the sound pressure in each scala. Moreover, there is a surprising lack of distortion in the fluid pressure variation relative to the incident sinusoidal sound wave. At a *fixed tympanic sound pressure*, the following effects are noticed when the frequency is changed:

• In the *scala vestibuli* the pressure increases rapidly, at 10 dB/octave, as frequency rises to 1 kHz and then decreases more slowly, at about 5 dB/octave, toward higher frequencies. The pressure wave phase change is initially $+90°$; this value then decreases progressively to $-225°$.

• In the *scala tympani*, the pressure scarcely changes, at least up to 0.5 kHz. At higher frequencies there is a slight increase. The phase angle is initially zero (in-phase), eventually reaching a $180°$ phase delay at 10 kHz. This almost absent pressure increase in the scala tympani might well be related to the large compliance of the round window, contrasting with the large impedance of the cochlea in the scala vestibuli.

These effects might play an essential role in cochlear dynamics, in that above 40 Hz all sound pressures at the tympanum will create *pressure differences* between the scala vestibuli and the scala tympani that are just the sort of transverse pressures needed to generate the special deformations of the basilar membrane along the length of the

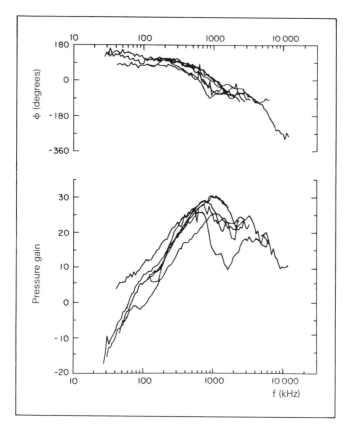

Figure 2.51
Pressure differences between scala vestibuli and scala tympani. A constant sound
pressure (P_T) is applied at the tympanum and the pressure difference between scala
vestibuli sound pressure (P_{SV}) and scala tympani sound pressure (P_{ST}) is measured as
a function of frequency. This differences represents the effective pressure difference
acting on the cochlear partition and the fraction ($P_{SV} - P_{ST}$)/P_T represents the pressure
gain of the system. The phase difference (ϕ) between the tympanic and cochlear pressures was also measured. (Modified from Nedzelnitsky 1980)

cochlea. These, described above, are the very basis of cochlear function (figure 2.51).

THE TRAVELING WAVE: AMPLITUDE AND PHASE

After von Békésy's work, theoreticians were confronted with the problem of understanding how the traveling wave, a set of transverse oscillations propagating longitudinally with a finite velocity along the length of a cochlear strip, might be generated by movements of the stapes. It is a matter not only of inventing equations to represent the phenomenon but at the same time to ensure the full involvement of two essential variables: $a(t)$, the amplitude of longitudinal vibration of stapes; and $b(t)$, the amplitude of transverse vibration of the basilar membrane. A whole variety of relationships might be devised in terms of the time variable t, or of the distance x of a point along the cochlear partition from base to apex, together with needing to represent how the traveling wave changes as a function of the frequency f of the vibratory stimulus and/or of its intensity. Thus, research has been specially aimed at determining:

• The value of b_m, the maximal vibration amplitude along the basilar membrane. This requires a plot of the envelope of the traveling wave all along the cochlear partition at a variety of different frequencies at a given time.
• The value of b_m at a given point on the basilar membrane, as a function of frequency.
• The phase Φ of the vibration with respect to the movement of the stapes as it varies with frequency; or alternatively, at a fixed frequency, how it changes with the position of the selected point along the basilar membrane. In all cases, these plots ought to be made while keeping the effective stimulus constant for all the frequencies investigated.

Mechanical Criteria for Setting the Basilar Membrane into Vibration
To analyze basilar membrane movements, it seems sensible to keep $a(t)$ constant throughout the frequency range; this is, in fact, how von Békésy's curves with normalized envelopes (see figures 2.49, 2.50) were obtained, namely, with a *constant displacement* of stapes. However, this method of stimulation is not appropriate, as we have already emphasized.

If we start from the premise that the adequate stimulus is a certain sound *pressure* at the oval window generated by the stapes, then we need to bear in mind that this pressure is proportional to the product of the *velocity* of the stapes [$d(a)/dt$] and the input impedance Z_c of the cochlea. Since the latter is practically constant throughout the length of the cochlea (see above), the problem is resolved by ensuring a *constant velocity* of stapes movement at all frequencies, while also taking into account the transfer function of the middle ear.

We have already seen above that if the sound pressure is maintained constant at the tympanum, the stapes *movement* is constant up to about 0.4 kHz but decreases at higher frequencies at a rate of 8 dB/octave. Thus to attain a constant stapes movement throughout the frequency range, the incident sound pressure should increase at 8 dB/octave beyond 0.4 kHz.

Finally, to attain a constant stapes *velocity* (the appropriate stimulus), the incident sound pressure at the tympanum should diminish by 6 dB/octave up to 0.4 kHz and then increase at 2 dB/octave above that frequency (Dallos et al. 1977; figure 2.52).

Correction of Experimental Curves
Agreeing that the amplitude of movement of the basilar membrane is not proportional to the displacement amplitude of the stapes but rather to its velocity, then when the amplitude of the stapes movement has been kept constant in an experiment, the displacement of the basilar membrane is expected to increase with frequency at 6 dB/octave, as would the stapes velocity itself in that circumstance. If, therefore, it is the aim to plot results for constant stapes velocity, it is necessary to introduce a correction factor decreasing the measured displacements at the rate of 6 dB/octave. In this way it is possible to recalculate traveling-wave envelopes of the displacement along the whole cochlear partition for the condition of constant stapes velocity.

Some curves thus corrected from those of von Békésy are shown in figure 2.53. Only the correction of 6 dB/octave at lower frequencies has been taken into account but, unfortunately, not the secondary correction of 2 dB/octave that rigorously ought to have been made at higher frequencies.

Movement of a Point on the Basilar Membrane as a Function of Frequency
In recent years, many researchers have remeasured the movements of the basilar membrane using a variety of sensitive detectors (9.1 above). Even after exploiting these elaborate techniques, the basilar membrane continued to be regarded for a considerable time as a series of low-pass filters, contrasting with the band-pass characteristics of the hair cells.

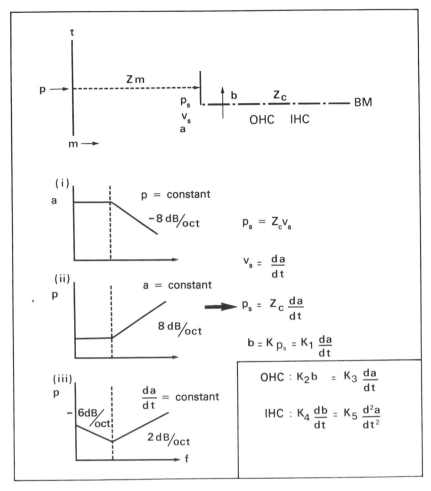

Figure 2.52
Schematic representation of modes of excitation for OHC and IHC. *Above*, *p*, sound pressure acting on the tympanum, t; *m*, resulting tympanum movement; p_s, v_s, a, respectively pressure, velocity and amplitude of movement of stapes and the oval window (ow) resulting from *p*; *b*, movement (transverse component) of the basilar membrane (BM); Z_m, Z_c, impedances of middle ear and cochlea. All functions *p*, *m*, *a*, p_s, v_s, *b* vary sinusoidally with time. *Below, left.* (i) Ordinate: characteristics of (*a*) when pressure (*p*) is maintained constant for all frequencies (abscissa). (ii) Pressures (*p*) that must be applied to the tympanum to attain a constant displacement (*a*) at all frequencies. (iii) Pressures (*p*) needed to attain a constant velocity of movement *da/dt* of the oval window. Formulae to the *right* and inset, *below right*: Specification of relationships between p_s, v_s, Z_c, *a*, introducing the fact that *b*, the transverse movement of BM, must finally be proportional to the velocity of stapes displacement *da/dt*. The adequate stimulus for OHC is the displacement *b* and for IHC is the velocity of displacement *db/dt*. (K, K_1, . . . , K_5 are arbitrary constants.)

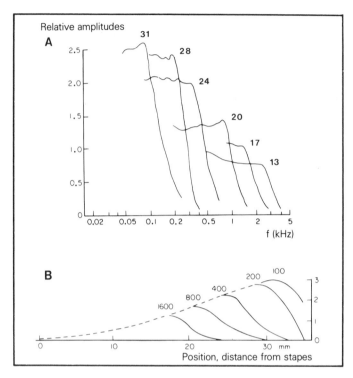

Figure 2.53
Displacement at various places along the basilar membrane for different stimulating frequencies, recalculated for a maximal stapes velocity that is constant with frequency. *A,* Relative amplitudes of movement at different places along the basilar membrane (marked above each curve) as a function of frequency. *B,* Relative amplitudes of movement at different frequencies (marked above each curve) as a function of position on the basilar membrane (abscissa). In *A* and *B,* position along the basilar membrane is specified as distance in millimeters from the stapes. (From Eldredge 1974)

Nevertheless, this view was revised after researchers gradually came to realize that the basilar membrane is an extremely fragile structure and that when more care is taken to avoid deterioration in its properties, then its measured characteristics approach more closely those of a band-pass system. They then show a peaked response (a sign of nonlinearity) and closely resemble the curves of transduction in the hair cells (Khanna & Leonard 1982; Johnstone et al. 1986; figure 2.54).

These results effectively demolished the prevailing version of the so-called second-filter theory, which was born from the discrepancies between the mechanical and nerve impulse tuning curves. It postu-

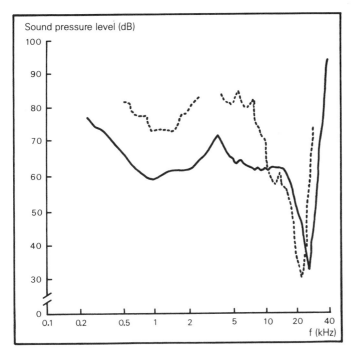

Figure 2.54
Mechanical and neuronal tuning curves. Solid curve, sound pressure level at the typanum needed to produce a basilar membrane (BM) vibration amplitude of 3.10^{-8} cm; dotted curve, neuronal tuning curve based on the isorate contour of 10 spikes/s above the spontaneous rate. The two curves have very similar characteristics near the peak (20 kHz). The major contrast is in the difference between the peak and plateau pressures for each curve, i.e., between 20 kHz and 1 kHz, being 44 dB for the neuronal tuning curve and 30 dB for the BM tuning curve. (From Khanna & Leonard 1982)

lated the need for an extra tuning arrangement between the basilar membrane and the transduction process that is sensitive to anoxia and to metabolic inhibitors.

(We shall return below to discussing a particular peculiarity in these mechanical curves and its significance. This is the existence of a second maximum at a frequency above f_c.)

Movement of a Point on the Basilar Membrane as a Function of Stimulus Intensity
Whether they used capacitative probes like Wilson and Johnstone's or the Mössbauer effect as did Rhode, most researchers agreed in reporting excellent linearity in the relationship between incident sound intensity and the vibration amplitude of the basilar membrane

at a given place, for a given frequency, up to high intensities around 120 dB (figure 2.55). This having been said, it must be added that when the behavior of the basilar membrane is examined in greater detail in the immediate vicinity of f_c, a certain nonlinearity is seen at intensities around 70 to 90 dB, where there is a reduction in the peak sensitivity (such as Rhode observed in *Saimiri*). Wilson and Johnstone also noted an inflection in some of their curves of amplitude vs. intensity (figure 2.55); this is also a sign of nonlinearity. We shall return to this aspect of cochlear dynamics briefly, below.

Phase Differences Between the Vibrations of the Stapes and the Basilar Membrane

First with the stroboscopic method and later with more refined techniques it has been possible to specify the phase changes seen along the cochlear partition between the local vibration and that of the stapes, at a variety of frequencies. Let us initially examine von Békésy's classic data as a preparation for discussing later modifications.

From the vicinity of the round window onward, the phase of basilar membrane movement is in advance of that of stapes by $\pi/2$ and therefore is in phase with stapes velocity and with the sound pressure (as would be expected from the above discussion). It is for this reason that we have added the right-hand ordinate scale to figure 2.49 showing phase angles with an initial phase difference of $\pi/2$, exactly representing the velocity of stapes.

Relative to a constant amplitude of vibration of stapes, the phase change *at a given point on the cochlea* varies apparently smoothly as a function of frequency between 0 and 3π.

Between base and apex, the phase shift along the cochlear partition increases more rapidly the higher the sound frequency, but it scarcely changes at all along the partition for the very low frequency of 50 Hz.

Considering instead the behavior at *points of maximal amplitude* of basilar membrane vibration at various frequencies, it is notable that near these maxima the phase shift with reference to the movement of stapes ranges between π and 3π (with a value that is generally near 2π). These results were not all obtained in von Békésy's earliest work. Indeed recent studies by Johnstone et al. (1970) and Rhode (1971, 1978), using the Mössbauer technique, have remeasured the phase of basilar membrane movements relative to the ossicular chain at places in the basal turn of the cochlea with $f_c \geq 6$ kHz. Beginning at low frequencies, the phase difference is $+ \pi/2$, as described above;

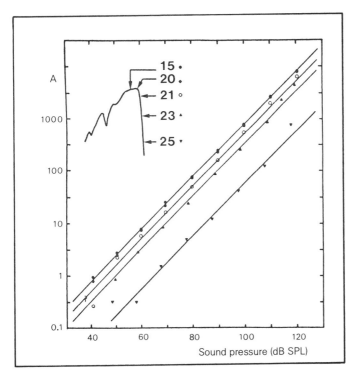

Figure 2.55
Relationship between amplitude of basilar membrane (BM) movement and sound pressure level. Mean square amplitude of BM movement (A) versus sound pressure for different frequencies above that for maximal BM displacement (inset, indicated beside a curve of BM amplitude as a function of frequency). Note the remarkably linear relationship except for a few points for 23 and 25 kHz at intensities > 110 dB. (From Wilson & Johnstone 1975)

thereafter the phase shift decreases, initially at about -3 rad/kHz then more rapidly, eventually at -10 rad/kHz, resulting in a total phase change as large as -7π to -9π, these values being much greater than any reported by von Békésy.

Some Absolute Values
We might at this stage wonder what are the absolute magnitudes of basilar membrane movements. A difficulty is that their determination is limited by the sensitivity of the available techniques. von Békésy, exploiting the optical observation of movements of deposited silver crystals and later using a more sensitive capacitative probe, had difficulty in measuring at any sound pressures less than $3 \cdot 10^3$ dynes ·

cm^{-2}, a value well above the normal physiological range. Extrapolating as he did from $3 \cdot 10^3$ to $2 \cdot 10^{-4}$ dynes $\cdot cm^{-2}$, that is, to the hearing threshold for 1 kHz, the extremely minute liminal displacement of $2 \cdot 10^{-4}$ nm! is suggested. The resolution of other methods, such as the Mössbauer technique, capacitative probes, and interferometry, is considerably better, while nevertheless remaining limited (e.g., for the Mössbauer methods the smallest radioactive crystal used in 1977 was $50 \times 40 \times 5$ μm). However, the necessary extrapolations become very much less hazardous than von Békésy's: They lead to a threshold magnitude of ≈ 0.1 nm at 20 kHz for the guinea pig (Sellick et al. 1982); for *Saimiri*, from measurements made at 70 dB and 7 kHz at the point of maximal displacement, a value 1.0 to 1.5 nm is suggested (Johnstone et al. 1970).

Movements of the tympanum have been estimated as 0.01 nm at threshold, 0.1 nm at 30 dB and 300 nm at 100 dB. Thus the vibration amplitude at the place of maximal basilar membrane displacement is about 30 dB more than at the handle of malleus.

Even if these values are eventually found to need revision they nevertheless illustrate what tiny movements are effective and therefore the extreme sensitivity of cochlear mechanisms. These movement amplitudes might be compared with the diameter of the hydrogen atom, which is on the order of 0.1 nm (10^{-8} cm) and with the 300-nm diameter of one of the hair cell cilia, 10^5 times larger than a threshold displacement.

Modeling the Cochlea
Models of the basilar membrane can be a useful aid to understanding the mechanics of cochlear mechanisms. Examining first the elements of basilar membrane movements, we recognize that at the oval window itself the displacements are longitudinal (i.e., tangential to the membrane). Thereafter they rapidly acquire a component normal to the membrane (transverse, therefore). This second component is related to pressure differences between the two scalae and initially suffers a phase shift of $\pi/2$ with respect to the stapes displacement and consequently is in phase with the *velocity* of the stapes vibration. The result is that, in theory, each point of the basilar membrane traces out an elliptical movement. The tangential component decreases monotonically between the base and the apex, whereas the normal component slowly increases along the cochlea to a point of maximal displacement and then decreases rapidly as the amplitude

of the envelope of the traveling wave diminishes toward the cochlear apex.

A variety of possible models have been considered for describing the basilar membrane's *transverse* vibratory properties.

• First, a simple model based on its static mechanical properties, considering them to be uniform across the whole breadth of the membrane.

• Alternatively, a system with two modes of vibration, one appropriate to the mid, more rigid, regions near the arches of Corti, the other relating to the lateral zone, the *pars pectinata.*

• Finally, a system with three modes taking note, in addition to the other two factors, of torsions in the bony support.

The second model on its own can encompass the description of a large part of the properties of the basilar membrane, provided, of course, that apart from the transverse variations other properties are included—such as the monotonic variation of compliance along the (31-cm) length of the membrane, being minimal at the base, where the breadth is 0.08 mm, and maximal at the apex, breadth 0.5 mm—and that due note is taken of the observed longitudinal frequency sorting, phase shifts, and propagation times.

The cochlea has long been considered to be well represented by a series of mechanical low-pass filters, the bandwidth of which decreases from the apex to the base. In fact, as we have noted above, more recent data suggests that this traditional concept of low-pass filtering will no doubt need a complete revision.

A NOMOGRAM FOR FREQUENCY DISTRIBUTIONS

By lumping together the data of von Békésy and the more modern information on more basal regions of the cochlea together with data from the electrophysiological analysis of cochlear outputs, it is possible to trace a function, f versus $\Phi(l)$, where f is frequency and l is the distance along the basilar membrane of the point of maximal vibration amplitude corresponding to that frequency. Many authors have published such curves (Von Békésy 1960; Kohllöffel 1971, 1972; Wilson & Johnstone 1975; Dallos et al. 1974, the latter using cochlear microphonics and Greenwood 1961 also). In all cases a roughly linear relationship has been reported between log f and the linear distance along the cochlea l of the point of maximal vibration (figure 2.56). According to Greenwood, some curvature can be observed in the cat near the apex (at low frequencies, therefore).

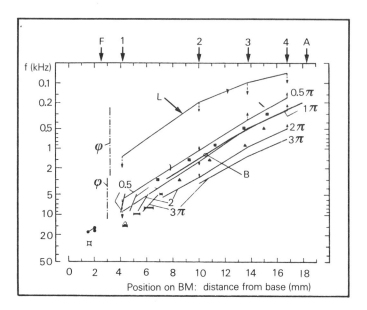

Figure 2.56
Nomogram for distribution of best frequency along the basilar membrane. The different curves show the results from different experimental methods. B, curve for von
Békésy's stroboscopic technique of 1944, plotting the places of maximal amplitude
as a function of frequency. Other curves were plotted according to differential CM
measurements at different places with respect to an electrode situated (at F) 3.2 mm
from the oval window. The location of these measurements is indicated by arrows at
(1) 4.1 mm, (2) 10.0 mm, (3) 13.7 mm, and (4) 16.8 mm along BM. Phase shifts of 0
(curve L) and of 0.5, 5, 1, 2, and 3π, which are indicated beside their appropriate
curves, are from Lissajou's figures measured by Tasaki et al. 1952 (the upper line Φ
marks the phase reference position). Phase shifts for 0.5, 1, 2, and 3π are also respectively marked beween 5 and 8 kHz. These come from stroboscopic laser illumination
techniques, the phase shifts being relative to a point at 3 mm along the cochlea (lower
phase reference line Φ). Squares, relationship between frequency/membrane position
from location of maximum of CM in scala media for 60 dB SPL (Honrubia & Ward
1968); triangles, same, but based on the negative summation potential in scala media
(Honrubia & Ward 1969); open circles, places of maximal CM amplitude at 13 to 14
kHz determined by CM (Kohllöffel 1971); rectangles, places of maximal response determined by laser interferometry (Kohllöffel 1972); curved box, optimal frequency shown
in a living animal by interferometry at 1.4 to 1.8 mm (Kohllöffel 1972); solid circles,
points of optimal frequency shown by Mössbauer technqiue (Johnstone et al. 1970).
(From Eldridge 1974)

The slope of the linear relation between log f and l has an obvious functional significance. It expresses the ratio between a relative frequency change $\delta f/f$ and the change δl in position of the maximal vibration. Its reciprocal represents a *mechanical resolving power* MRP $= \delta l \times f/\delta f$; the larger MRP is, the larger is the increase in cochlear distance δl corresponding to a given relative frequency change $\delta f/f$, and thus the better is the spatial frequency resolving power of the cochlea. In the case of the guinea pig, its magnitude is around 2.5 mm/octave. von Békésy, but surprisingly few more recent authors, calculated this MRP for a number of species showing:

• It does not change with frequency in the linear range of the function but it can at the extreme limits.
• In humans, unlike in other species studied, the MRP seems to be greater in the frequency band 1 to 3 kHz (which contains important components of the human voice).
• There are considerable phylogenetic variations, MRP being poor in the rat and mouse but high in the elephant, for example.

Lesions made in animal preparations, or discovered and defined postmortem in humans, that are small enough to influence only a limited part of the cochlea have been inspected for correlations between them and their effect on learned tonal discriminations in the first case or in deteriorating tonal perceptions in the second, within a limited frequency band. The expectation was that a unitary anatomical scale of frequency would be found which would support or confirm parallel data from electrophysiology or from mechanical analysis. However, such attempts have been very disappointing, whatever the lesioning technique used in animals, whether surgical or pharmacological (ototoxins like kanamycin). At most, we can regard as significant the findings that the loss of 40% of the outer hair cells at 30 mm from the basal turn produces a maximal loss of 40 dB in the frequency band in question (around 50 Hz), whereas at 7 mm from the base (where high frequencies are best represented), a 25% loss of outer hair cells causes a 30 dB deterioration and a 50% destruction lowers sensitivity by 50 to 75 dB at 8 kHz.

A very careful study by Engström (1983) describes morphological changes in hair cells after exposure to high intensity wide band noise. He particularly emphasizes that:

• Visible lesions are only observed in the inner, not the outer, hair cells; these appear to remain intact.

• It appears that the lesions essentially concern the cilia of the inner hair cells, either breaking the hairs or imposing an abnormal inclination upon them.

• The lesions are the same if the sound is applied after previously destroying outer hair cells by ototoxic drugs.

• Various physiological indices, as diverse as brainstem evoked potentials, reflex contractions of the middle ear muscles (see section 5.6, above), and the threshold for behavioral responses, all correspond well with the histology of these sound-induced lesions.

COCHLEAR MICROPHONICS AND COCHLEAR MECHANICS

In contrast to the somewhat disappointing correlations discussed above, *focal* measurements of CM have resulted in interesting conclusions not only about their own origin but also concerning the details of basilar membrane movements.

As already mentioned above, Dallos et al. (1972) observed focal cochlear microphonics after a kanamycin treatment in guinea pig that effectively destroyed the outer hair cells in the basal regions of the cochlea. When under these conditions low frequency *triangular* oscillations are imposed on the stapes, then, in the zones where outer hair cells are still intact (third and fourth turns) the CM has a "square" (in fact, trapezoidal) waveform. Remembering that the basilar membrane movement is proportional to sound *pressure*, namely, to the *velocity* of stapes, the fact that the CM itself is seen to be proportional to the first differential of the imposed stapes movement strongly suggests that CM is proportional to basilar membrane *displacement*. In contrast, the CM measured where only the inner hair cells are intact seems to be proportional to the velocity of basilar membrane movement, that is, to the second differential of stapes movement (see figure 2.44).

Another correlative study (Dallos et al. 1974) measured the amplitude of CM as a function of frequency at constant tympanum sound pressure, at constant stapes displacement, or at constant stapes velocity, again confirming the effective stimulus.

At constant *sound pressure level* (SPL) at the tympanum (figure 2.57), the CM amplitude increases at 6 dB/octave up to 400 Hz and thereafter decreases at 20 to 40 dB/octave as frequency increases. At constant stapes *displacement*, the plot of experimental values is exactly like that for basilar membrane displacement as a function of frequency, that is, the curve first rises (at 6 dB/octave), then falls very rapidly above the characteristic frequency. Finally, at constant stapes *velocity*, the

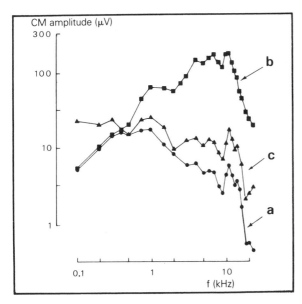

Figure 2.57
CM amplitudes in the first turn of the guinea pig cochlea as a function of frequency. Measured under three different conditions: (a) at a constant sound pressure of 50 dB SPL; (b) with sound pressures adjusted for a constant displacement of the stapes (10Å); (c) with sound pressures adjusted for a constant stapes velocity (25,000 Å/s). (From Dallos et al. 1974)

curve is flat right up to the cut-off frequency: This is what would be predicted from postulating that the effective stimulus is in fact the velocity of the ossicular system. (These data are correct for the guinea pig but have not necessarily been as clearly verified for other species, such as the chinchilla or the cat.)

Focal CM measurements can also confirm some features of the propagation of vibrations along the cochlea. The different behavior at different cochlear levels is clearly seen for a variety of stimuli at different frequencies and, for a given frequency, at different intensity levels. Thus figure 2.58 shows how wide frequency-band and low-pass filtered clicks, or low-frequency (500 Hz) and higher-frequency (4 kHz) tone pips differently affect the three turns of the guinea pig cochlea. These results agree with expectations from mechanical data and the theories of traveling-wave propagation (Eldredge 1974). The same agreement is seen in the data on spatial distribution of CM shown in figure 2.59, provided the stimuli are in the mid intensity

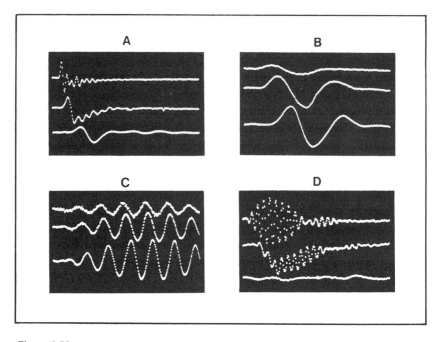

Figure 2.58
CM responses to different sound signals. CM responses measured in the first, second, and third turns of the guinea pig cochlea (upper, middle, and lower traces, respectively in each case) for four different sound signals. *A,* Wide-band click. *B,* Low-pass filtered click. *C,* Brief 500-Hz tone pip. *D,* 4 kHz tone pip. (From Eldredge (1974)

range ($<$ 70 dB). In contrast, at high intensities the peak CM amplitude is systematically displaced toward the stapes. This effect has only partly been explained (Honrubia & Ward 1968).

NONLINEARITY IN COCHLEAR MECHANISMS

In chapter 1, we introduced the study of perceived distortions of the incident sound that are possibly related to nonlinearities in the auditory system, this being particularly so for aural harmonics and combination tones. It is necessary to discover to what extent such effects are seen in the electrophysiological events accompanying cochlear excitation.

Cochlear Microphonics
Objective evidence for such distortions were soon found in CM investigations, whether global (via round window electrodes) or focal (using the more localized differential methods).

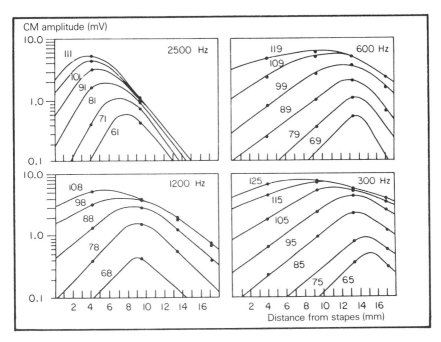

Figure 2.59
Spatial distribution of the cochlear microphonic. Based on measurements with four electrodes located at different distances from the stapes in the cochlear duct. Each figure is for one particular frequency (indicated) and at different intensities (dB SPL shown beside each curve). (From Honrubia & Ward 1968)

Subjective aural harmonics. Using a pure-tone stimulus, free of any objective harmonic, generates a CM that at feeble-to-moderate sound intensities is sinusoidal at the frequency of the incident sound. But at a given higher intensity, even before saturation is observable (already described and which is itself a sign of nonlinearity), a distortion arises resulting in the presence in the CM spectrum of harmonics 2, 3, . . . , the amplitudes of which increase as the incident sound intensity increases further (figure 2.60). Another important observation, which nevertheless is still the source of some controversy, is that the maximum amplitude of the second harmonic of f_c is localized at the same level of the cochlear spiral as its fundamental: It is therefore not the result of a propagating wave that has reached the appropriate place for $2f_c$ in the cochlea.

If, as in Dallos et al. 1974, the *saturation nonlinearity* at higher intensities is examined, it is notable that the amplitude vs. frequency

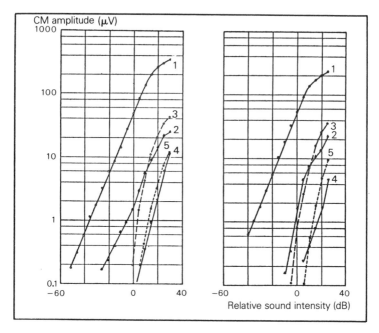

Figure 2.60
Subjective aural harmonics. *Left,* CM responses in the guinea pig for a 1-kHz pure tone. This generates a CM at the fundamental frequency but also harmonics of the order indicated beside each curve. Their amplitudes increase with incident sound intensity. *Right,* The same but with the sound stimulus replaced by mechanical vibration applied directly to the stapes. (From Wever & Lawrence 1954)

curves for CM (for constant stapes amplitude) measured in the basal turn of the cochlea are precise and well repeatable in fine detail, and for the most part they superimpose well, except for frequencies higher than f_c where differences appear that are a function of stimulus intensity (figure 2.61).

Combination tones. In these experiments, two stimuli with different frequencies are used, let us say 2.8 kHz and 1.0 kHz. The intensity of the 1-kHz sound is set at some fixed level, the intensity of the 2.8 kHz tone is progressively increased, and when this reaches a particular level an extra component arises in CM corresponding with the combination 2.8 − 1.0 = 1.8 kHz (figure 2.62). The increasing size of this component of CM (that corresponds to the *first order difference tone*) is parallel to the increasing CM generated by increasing the intensity of one of the primary tones alone. More complicated combi-

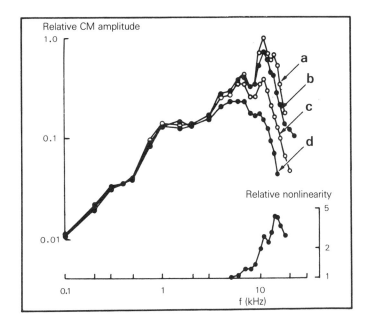

Figure 2.61
CM amplitude as a function of frequency. Recorded in the basal turn for different,
constant stapes amplitudes (in decibels relative to 1Å): (a) −10, (b) 10, (c) 20, (d) 30.
The lower curve is an estimate of the degree of nonlinearity, shown as the ratio
between the relative amplitudes for 1Å and 10Å. (From Dallos et al. 1974)

nation tones (whether difference tones or summation tones) are also
represented in CM (figure 2.63).

The cubic difference tone has been studied in particular detail with
results that, as we shall see, pose some problems. Dallos (1969),
studying the guinea pig and the chinchilla, applied two frequencies
f_1 and f_2 simultaneously as above and with $1 < f_2/f_1 < 2$. Recordings
from the first and third turns of the cochlea showed the existence in
CM of the difference tone $2f_1 - f_2$. But obvious problems arise from
distinct differences between these results and results from (1) psychophysics (see chapter 1, 5.2) and (2) analysis of the output of single
cochlear nerve fibers (see below). In fact, unlike these two latter
methods from perception and unitary neurophysiology, it was not
possible to cancel the CM difference tone by externally presenting an
extra tone of frequency $2f_1 - f_2$ that had an appropriately adjusted
intensity and phase. In addition, according to Dallos all the indications were that the cubic difference tone is a saturation phenomenon,

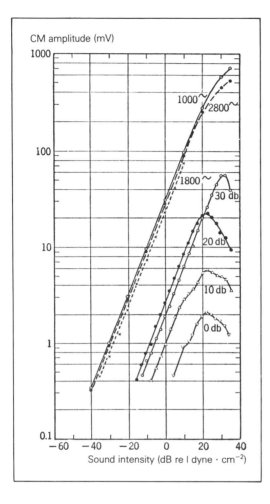

CM amplitude (mV)

Sound intensity (dB re I dyne · cm⁻²)

Figure 2.62
CM for a simultaneous two-tone stimulus. CM responses for the component corresponding to the difference frequency H–L, (1.8 kHz) for two simultaneous stimuli (H = 2.8 kHz, L = 1 kHz) applied monaurally to the same ear also for H and L applied singly in isolation, as a function of sound intensity. *Left*, Curves for the two primary stimuli and (dotted) for a tone at 1.8 kHz the first-order difference frequency. *Right*, Curves for CM responses at the difference tone frequency when the intensity of the 2.8-kHz tone is increased progressively, the 1-kHz tone being fixed at the different intensities indicated near each curve. (From Wever & Lawrence 1954)

like those predicted by Helmholtz' polynomials, rather than arising from essential nonlinearities as proposed by Goldstein. Moreover, using kanamycin lesions, Dallos asserted that to obtain a cubic difference component in CM, the *two separate regions* of the cochlea corresponding to f_1 and f_2 must *both* be intact (more exactly, their outer hair cells must be), whereas, in contrast, destruction of outer hair cells in the $2f_1 - f_2$ region does not affect the generation of the CM component. In other words, from these results the combination tone does not show its objective CM component in its own appropriate region of the cochlea.

Finally, CM measurements can also be related to another phenomenon due to interference between two tones (*two-tone suppression*).

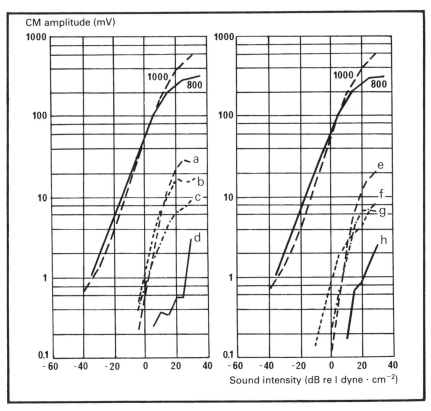

Figure 2.63
CM responses corresponding to difference tones (*left*) and summation tones (*right*) on stimulation by airborne sounds of 1 kHz and 2.8 kHz. Amplitude/intensity characteristics for the two primary tones ($L = 1$ kHz, $H = 2.8$ kHz) and for combination tones: (a) $2H - L$, (b) $H - 2L$, (c) $H - L$, (d) $2H - 2L$, (e) $2H + L$, (f) $H + L$, (g) $H + 2L$, (h) $2H + 2L$. (From Wever & Lawrence 1954)

When two sound stimuli f_1 and f_2 are close in frequency, with f_1/f_2 less than 1.5, the response to one sound, say f_1, can be diminished or even abolished when the stimuli are applied simultaneously. In the guinea pig, Legouix et al. (1973) have recorded differentially the CM for a given tone and observed how the response changes when a second tonal stimulus is applied simultaneously at other frequencies. With the test tone fixed near 8 kHz and intensity constant at 65 dB and the conditioning tone also set at constant intensity (70 dB) but at different frequencies between 5 and 12 kHz, they found regions, *on each side of the test frequency*, of near suppression or at least reduc-

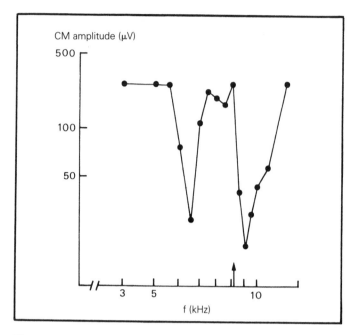

Figure 2.64
Two-tone inhibition shown in the CM. CM amplitude recorded in the basal turn of the guinea pig cochlea on application of two stimuli simultaneously. The frequency of the test tone is fixed near 8 kHz (arrow) and its intensity is 65 dB. The intensity of the interacting, suppressive tone is 65 dB; its frequency is indicated by the abscissa. (From Legouix et al. 1973)

tion of the CM compared with its response to the test frequency alone (figure 2.64). More recently, Dallos et al. (1974) also demonstrated inhibitory interference but did not find it in the frequency region above f_c.

Afferent Signals
Another way to investigate cochlear mechanisms is to record discharges in single isolated fibers of the cochlear nerve. A variety of researchers (e.g., Sachs & Kiang 1968; Goldstein & Kiang 1968; Arthur et al. 1971) using these techniques have been able to report objective evidence for interactions between sounds. Two examples are described below.

Two-tone suppression. A typical experiment consists in applying a test stimulus at the characteristic frequency f_c of a selected fiber (8.893 kHz in this case) so that the fiber responds with a continuous dis-

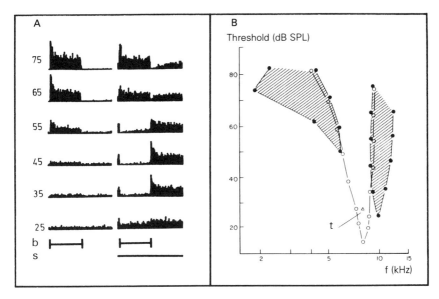

Figure 2.65
Two-tone suppression in a single cochlear nerve fiber. *A,* Poststimulus histogram for responses to a tone pip (8.080 kHz, duration 100 ms) applied alone (b, left hand column) and during a steady tone (s, right hand column) at the f_c of the fiber (8.893 kHz, 28 dB SPL). The intensity of the steady tone is kept fixed; the intensity of the tone pip is varied as shown (dB SPL values indicated in A) increasing from below to above. *B,* The curve marked by open circles delimits the fiber's excitatory response area for stimulation by a continuous tone; the hatched area shows the inhibitory flanking regions (in frequency and intensity) for effective two-tone suppression. "Effective" means diminishing the response to the test tone by 20% or more, as shown by the open triangle. (From Arthur et al. 1971)

charge. When a brief tone pip at a nearby frequency (8.080 kHz) is then also applied during the continuous sound, a suppression of the f_c response is observed throughout the application of the tone pip (figure 2.65).

Another method of observation is to apply the continuous f_c stimulus as just described, then to apply a sound of frequency f_v that *sweeps* across the whole audiofrequency range. When $f_v = f_c$, the two sounds reinforce and, provided the stimulus f_c is not already maximal, the response increases and a peak in the whole recording is clearly seen. In contrast, when f_v is either below or above f_c, there are regions where the response is relatively reduced, the suppression being greater when $f_v > f_c$ and not so great for $f_v < f_c$ (figure 2.66). Using an appropriate transformation of the data to plot an isodischarge

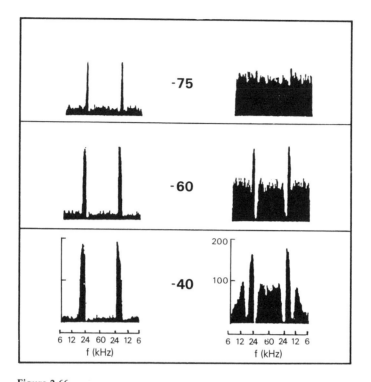

Figure 2.66
Two-tone suppression at f_c by a second sweep-frequency tone. Test tone at f_c and sweep tone have same amplitudes, as indicated. Recordings of single-fiber discharges were made in two stimulus conditions. *Left,* Variable frequency sweep tone (f_v) presented alone, frequency rising then frequency falling (between 6 and 60 kHz); a response is recorded in each passage of the frequency through the response area of the fiber around its best frequency (f_c = 22.2 kHz). *Right,* The same but in the presence of a continuous tone at f_c. In this case the continuous tone generates a discharge that is reinforced when the sweep tone passes through the fiber's response area but, in contrast, shows strong inhibitory interactions in flanking regions. (From Sachs & Kiang 1968)

response, this phenomenon of *lateral suppression* can be illustrated in the same way and as clearly as the data of figure 2.65 (see its legend, noting particularly that the criteria of suppression were based on a reduction of 20% in the discharge due to f_c being applied alone).

More recently, two-tone suppression has been demonstrated even in intracellularly recorded receptor potentials of IHC (Sellick & Russell 1979), thus firmly establishing their intracochlear origin.

Cubic difference tone. The same groups of researchers have investigated objective correlates of the cubic difference tone. A fiber is iso-

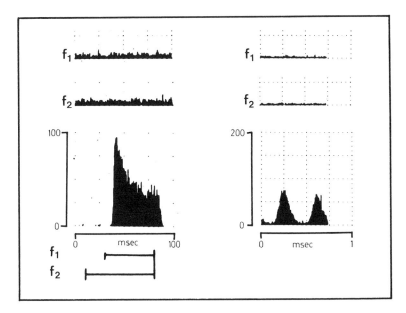

Figure 2.67
Excitation of cat cochlear nerve fibers by the combination tone $2f_1 - f_2$. In each case, impulse rate is registered as a function of time for (top) f_1 alone, (middle) f_2 alone, and (bottom) $f_1 + f_2$ combined. *Left column,* $f_1 = 10$ kHz (59 dB), $f_2 = 12.15$ kHz (69 dB); each sound in isolation has practically no effect, but when they are applied together (bottom trace, right portion) there is a very large response in a fiber with an f_c very near to $2f_1 - f_2$ (7.88 kHz). *Right column,* Similar experiment with $f_1 = 5.5$ kHz and $f_2 = 4.13$ kHz. In this case the simultaneous application of f_1 and f_2 leads to a *periodic* response in the fiber at its characteristic frequency f_c (2.76 kHz), which is also very near to the combination tone $2f_1 - f_2$. (From Goldstein & Kiang 1968)

lated such that its characteristic frequency f_c will roughly correspond with the cubic difference frequency $2f_1 - f_2$ generated when two stimuli at f_1 and f_2 are applied simultaneously. The result looked for is a clear-cut response to the cubic difference tone in its appropriate nerve fiber which also does not need the tones to be in a region of response saturation, this latter criterion being essential for establishing a proper link with psychophysical observations. In other words, the cubic difference response must not require exceptionally intense sounds, unlike the saturation mechanisms postulated by Helmholtz. They must be the result of an essential nonlinearity in the cochlear response. The differences in these nerve fiber data (figure 2.67) from the CM work are quite clear. This technique demonstrates that whereas the CM work could not show a cubic difference tone response at sites remote from either f_1 or f_2, there is nevertheless a cochlear nerve response in the fiber appropriate to $2f_1 - f_2$. What is more, unlike the data of Dallos et al. (1974) on CM, the single-fiber results of Goldstein and Kiang (1968) show that it is possible to suppress the cubic difference response in the fiber by a simultaneous external application of a third tone at the cubic difference frequency (suitably adjusted in phase and intensity). This illustrates a contradiction between the two methods and thus a problem to be resolved, as we have already suggested.

Presumptive Origins of the Distortions: The Basilar Membrane
It is now necessary to find where and how the sound distortions just discussed arise in the auditory apparatus. The distortions must arise in the inner ear, since middle ear transmission is so faithful even for relatively intense sounds.

When a frequency analysis is carried out on (1) the acoustic stimulus applied to the ear (supposed to be a pure sinusoid), (2) the stimulus as recorded in the interior of the meatus, (3) the round window vibrations, and (4) the cochlear microphonic potentials, it is quite clear that the size of harmonics other than the fundamental is always the largest in CM.

Naturally, the next assessment needed is to what extent the mechanical properties of the basilar membrane itself can account for the distortions. In this respect, successful research has been and is very dependent on the development of appropriately sensitive techniques for analyzing the very feeble movements involved. Using the Mössbauer technique which can measure the velocity of the displacement of basilar membrane (but only in a working range of not more than 30 dB) or alternatively using small capacitative probes, Rhode (1971) and Wilson and Johnstone (1975), following Johnstone et al. (1967, 1970), have provided a certain number of interesting conclusions.

In the basal turn of the guinea pig cochlea, the relationship between the movement of the stapes and the corresponding movement of basilar membrane is linear, according to Wilson and Johnstone, for sound intensities between 65 dB and as much as 115 dB. In contrast, recall that Rhode (1978) working near the second turn in *Saimiri*, discovered a large range of nonlinearity even at relatively lower intensities (70 dB). This *high sound pressure nonlinearity* is shown up by the gradient between the intensity in decibels and the log of the movement becoming less than unity at high intensities (figure 2.68). As a matter of interest, such a nonlinearity allows the cochlea to have an

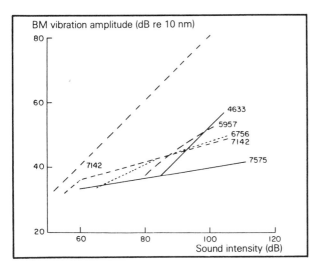

Figure 2.68
Basilar membrane (BM) movements in *Saimiri*. BM mechanical response determined
by Mössbauer technique at different stimulus frequencies (indicated) as a function of
stimulus intensity. The curve with a slope of unity represents the ideal linear situation.
The real curves have a lower slope showing that the BM movements are not increasing
in proportion to the stimuli (saturation nonlinearity). (From Rhode 1978).

extended dynamic operating range, of more than 120 dB. (Note that
this nonlinearity disappears as the condition of the preparation
deteriorates.)

When the Mössbauer technique is used (as by Rhode 1978) to measure the vibration at a point on the basilar membrane stimulated at
its appropriate characteristic frequency $f_1 = f_c$ and at a given fixed
intensity (e.g., 90 dB), it is observed that the simultaneous application
of a tone of frequency f_2 (such that f_1/f_2 is between 1.04 and 1.4)
reduces the amplitude of vibration due to f_1. The reduction depends
on the intensity of f_2: For $f_2 = f_1 = 90$ dB, it attains 8 to 10 dB. In this
respect then, two-tone suppression has a direct correspondence in
the functioning of the basilar membrane.

Using the same technique, results from research on the cubic difference tone are much less clear-cut. The problem here is to demonstrate
that when the preparation is presented with two tones at f_1 and f_2,
the audible combination tone $2f_1 - f_2$ finds its counterpart or not at
the cochlear place with that characteristic frequency or, if you like,
to demonstrate whether a traveling wave appropriate to the compo-

nent $2f_1 - f_2$ exists. The results of such tests (by Dallos and Rhode) have so far been negative. Some behavioral experiments (Dallos 1977) illustrate the difficulties well: Having made a very large kanamycin outer hair cell lesion in the chinchilla cochlea such that the animal ceased to respond over a wide frequency range, it was found that if two sounds f_1 and f_2 were presented simultaneously that were themselves within the zone of the animal's deafness but for which, in contrast, the cubic difference tone, $2f_1 - f_2$ lay *outside* the zone of deafness, then the latter was not in fact heard (which it should have been had its mechanical counterpart existed as a traveling wave). In other words, the behavioral experiment in no way suggested that the cochlear region corresponding with $2f_1 - f_2$ has any part to play in perception of the cubic difference tone.

It seems evident that some nonlinearities are generated beyond the level of cochlear mechanics. But this problem is by no means clearly resolved. Discussion continues concerning both the precise location and the precise mechanisms concerned in these distortions (e.g., rigidity of structures, mechanical coupling of stereocilia). Such arguments seem to us to be premature at present, particularly when taking into account the rapid progress that continues to be made in studying cochlear mechanisms (see below). Progress like this, as we have often emphasized already, strongly depends on developing new probes and methods of detection.

10 COCHLEAR TRANSDUCTION

We now need to consider the ways in which an acoustic stimulus is finally transformed into an excitation of afferent nerve terminals. Certain stages in the mechanisms of this transduction are known; others still need to be fully identified.

10.1 MEMBRANE PROCESSES THAT ACCOMPANY HAIR CELL EXCITATION

The biophysical properties of the cochlear and vestibular hair cells only began to be understood a few years ago. Nor were the mammalian hair cells successfully explored first but rather the saccular cells of batrachian amphibians (Hudspeth & Corey 1977), the turtle cochlea (Crawford & Fettiplace 1979), and only then the hair cells of the guinea pig (Russell & Sellick 1978; Tanaka et al. 1980; Dallos et al. 1982). It is certainly true that the cells studied are far from identical, but their phylogenetic lineage and structural similarities allow certain interesting predictions, conclusions, and contradictions to be emphasized.

Extracellular recording had already shown that saccular cells are polarized in the sense that deflection of the stereocilia in one direction (toward the kinocilium) produces an excitation and in the other direction an inhibition as evidenced by, respectively, an acceleration and a reduction in the receptor's spontaneous discharge rate (see also Buser & Imbert 1982). And it is in this relatively simple preparation that perhaps the most complete up to date information is available concerning the membrane processes that can accompany the excitation of hair cells (figure 2.69; Hudspeth & Corey 1977).

The intracellular potential varies as might be expected, with a depolarization (toward a more positive value) when the stereocilia are deflected toward the kinocilium and a hyperpolarization (to a more negative value) accompanying a deflection in the opposite direction.

The relationship between deflection of the hairs and intracellular potential is not linear but sigmoidal, showing a saturating maximal change (in each direction). It is also asymmetrical, depolarization exceeding hyperpolarization by about four times for equal and opposite hair displacements with respect to the vertical position. Consequently, a sinusoidal displacement about that equilibrium position evokes an asymmetrical response and therefore also introduces a DC component due to the resulting rectifying action.

Deflection of the hairs also generates a change in the transmembrane electrical resistance. This is demonstrated by applying small electrical test impulses at various phases of the oscillatory polarization and depolarization: Transmembrane resistance is decreased during polarization and increased during hyperpolarization.

Using an in vitro preparation of the saccular cells, it has been possible to measure the transmembrane current directly (most recently by whole-cell patch clamping) in the cells under voltage clamp and to follow its temporal changes during controlled manipulation of the cilia. Among the most important results are the following:

• Deflection of the cilia toward the kinocilium reduces the transmembrane resistance and generates an inward flow of cations, suggesting the opening of transduction channels.
• Superimposed on this global current flow there exist random current fluctuations that are interpreted as arising from opening and closing of individual ion channels. This electrical "noise" is estimated by the authors to arise from an effective number of individual active channels of about 200 per hair cell, or about 6 per cilium.

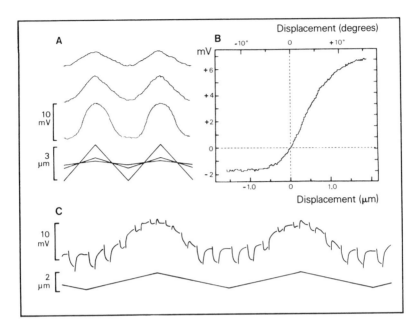

Figure 2.69
Receptor potentials recorded in saccular hair cells of the bullfrog. *A,* The mechanical
stimulating probe deflects the hairs to three different peak amplitudes with a triangular
time course (bottom trace) and the receptor potentials are recorded by an intracellular
microelectrode (upper three traces, each the mean of 32 responses, corresponding in
turn to the three levels of stimulation, weak, medium, and strong, all being subliminal
for nerve output. *B,* Response (in mV) versus cilia displacement (in μm and degrees)
from the rest position. Note asymmetry of response; greater amplitude for positive
deflections, toward the kinocilium, than negative, from displacements in the opposite
direction. *C,* Upper trace shows modification of transmembrane resistance of the cell
during two successive flexion/extension cycles (lower trace) at 1 Hz. Constant current
hyperpolarizing current pulses (70 pA, 45 ms) are injected at regular intervals and the
voltage changes induced are a measure of the transmembrane resistance. This becomes
smaller during depolarizations (upper parts of mV trace) than for hyperpolarizations
(lower parts of mV trace). (From Hudspeth & Corey 1977)

A systematic survey of various levels of the cell has demonstrated
that the electrical changes are greatest in the immediate neighborhood of the upper parts of the cilia, suggesting that the transduction
channels are situated in the tips of the hairs.

When the cell is depolarized by a stepwise current change, an
intrinsic phenomenon is revealed by the depolarization approaching
its final steady value in an oscillatory manner. This time course suggests that (even in the absence of cilia) the membrane of this type of
cell has certain self-contained oscillatory properties.

What ionic species take part in these phenomena? Natural stimulation, by deflection of the cilia, generates an initial entry of cations, presumably of K^+ since they are in high concentration in the endolymph. Remember the particular ionic environment of the hair cells; the hairs themselves are bathed in endolymphatic space (high concentration of K^+) and the rest of the receptor cell is surrounded by extracellular perilymphatic fluid (low K^+ concentration). The reticular lamina constitutes an impermeable barrier to ion flow.

In contrast, during artificial stimulation by applying a stepwise current to depolarize the cell to -40 mv transmembrane potential under voltage clamp, the current flow is *diphasic* with an initial entry of cations followed by a second phase showing an efflux of cations. By a variety of ionic substitutions and by the use of tetraethylammonium (TEA; see below) Hudspeth and Corey (1977) have identified the initial inward flux as being due to Ca^{2+}, the succeeding outflow being attributable to K^+ flux through potassium channels that are not very voltage dependent but are strongly Ca^{2+} dependent. Recently, Holton and Hudspeth (1986), also using whole-cell patch clamping and analyzing the noise due to the random opening and closing of transduction channels, confirm that the number of these channels per cell is 280 at the most and that the conductance of each channel is the order of 12 pS. The biochemical characterization of the channel structure has yet to be done.

It is now possible to envisage an at least provisional description of the ionic mechanisms likely to be concerned in the excitation of these hair cells: An initial, depolarizing entry of K^+ at the tips of the cilia following mechanical deformation activates the voltage-sensitive Ca^{2+} channels, which allows an entry of Ca^{2+} ions; these two influxes together generate the final depolarization. Then the resulting increase in $[Ca^{2+}]$ concentration provokes a secondary activation of other Ca^{2+}-dependent potassium channels that are sited in the basolateral parts of the cell, with the result that K^+ flows outward at this region of the cell, generating a repolarization. In addition, the increase in calcium ion concentration could be responsible for the eventual release of transmitter to act on the afferent nerve terminals. Recalling that the work of Hudspeth and his group also showed that the saccular cell membrane can develop an intrinsic rhythmicity via its membrane properties, it seems possible that this could arise from an alternating activation of the calcium and potassium channels (Lewis & Hudspeth 1983; Hudspeth 1985, 1986; figure 2.70).

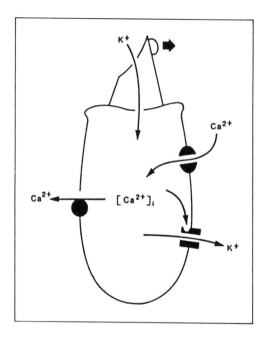

Figure 2.70
Schematic diagram of the proposed mechanism for resonant
tuning in the bullfrog's hair
cell. Depolarization of the cell
by a stimulus opens voltage-
sensitive Ca^{2+} channels. The
influx of Ca^{2+} regeneratively
depolarizes the cell: $[Ca^{2+}]_i$
then rises, activating Ca^{2+}-
sensitive K^+ channels. The resultant efflux of K^+ repolarizes
the cell to and beyond the
steady state potential. Ca^{2+}
within the cytoplasm is buf-
fered and rapidly extruded.
(From Hudspeth 1986)

A notable achievement in this area is the hypothesis proposed for
this causal chain of events by Corey and Hudspeth (1983). The experimental results are not compatible with two other models that had
earlier been proposed for other receptors because the transduction
latency can fall below values (<40 μs) that are too small for an *enzy-
matic mechanism* to be concerned, whether in a phosphorylating or
methylation reaction (protein-kinase or methyltransferase), a type of
reaction that had been proposed for some mechanoreceptors.

Similarly, the same argument justifies the rejection of hypotheses
in which a *second messenger* intervenes between the mechanical deformation and the conductance change, such as had been proposed for
photoreceptors (involving Ca^{2+} and/or cGMP; see Buser and Imbert
1987, 1992). In contrast, the authors suggest a *direct link* between the
mechanical deformation and the channel opening. Displacement has
its effect via the mechanical energy difference between the two possible states of the channel, open and closed (just as electrical potential
variation acts on voltage dependent channels). In the absence of mechanical stimulation, there exists (as we have seen) a "noise" due
to openings and closings that have occurred randomly. A positive
mechanical stimulus allows the channels *statistically* to spend more
time open than closed, resulting in a net continuous depolarization
in spite of the continuing random alternations between the open and

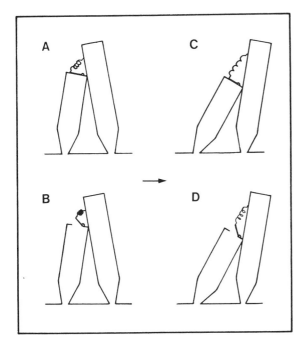

Figure 2.71
Pictorial representation of the mechanism proposed by Hudspeth to underly
mechano-electric transduction in hair cells. At any instant the transduction channel
at the tip of a sterocilium might be closed (*A*) or open (*B*) by thermal Brownian motion
in the nearby extracellular fluid (schematized by a spring expanded and contracted).
Constants are specified for the fractional open and closed durations, respectively k_{12}
and k_{21}, in the resting state. These openings and closings of the individual channels
are responsible for the "noise" in the system. When the hairs are subjected to a positive
force, i.e., excitatory and toward the kinocilium (see text) the fractional opening and
closing times are modified, k_{12} being increased and k_{21} being reduced. There results an
effective increase of inward current causing a relative depolarization of the cell, the
opposite deflection producing a relative hyperpolarization. (From Hudspeth 1985)

closed positions. Hudspeth (1985) pictures the mechanism as shown
in figure 2.71 (please read its legend), supported in addition by recent
data on mechanical linkages between adjacent cilia (see section 3.3,
above). When one cilium is deflected, its mechanical linkage to the
adjacent smaller one tends to modify the relative opening and closing
times of the transduction channels.

COCHLEAR HAIR CELLS IN THE TURTLE

Another interesting set of observations is concerned with the intracellular investigation of cochlear hair cells in the turtle (Crawford &
Fettiplace 1979, 1980, 1981, 1985). The turtle cochlea contains a set of

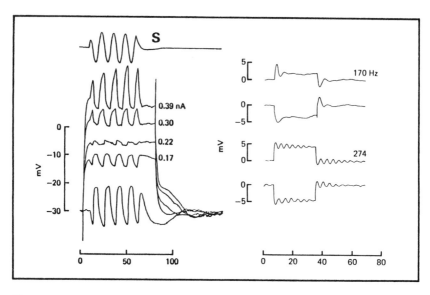

Figure 2.72
Hair cells in the turtle. *Left,* Effect of intracellular current injection (shown in nA) on the response of a cell to a tone pip S at the resulting (different) membrane potentials with respect to scala tympani (shown in mV). Note the value of the reversal potential, near zero (-3.5 ± 2.5 mV). *Right,* Examples of damped oscillations in membrane potential (mV) after injection of a stepwise current in two cells with characteristic frequencies, 170 Hz and 274 Hz, respectively. For the upper cell, resting membrane potential = -51 mV, current step = 0.08 nA; for the lower cell, -54 mV, 0.024 nA. Each trace is the mean of a few successive responses. (From Crawford & Fettiplace 1979)

hair cells along the basilar papilla (see section 3.3, earlier), each of which responds best to a particular audiofrequency and acts like a rather narrow band-pass filter, with a peak sensitivity at low audio-frequencies in the range between 50 Hz to 700 Hz.

Crawford and Fettiplace have investigated to what extent intrinsic properties of the membrane are responsible for this *frequency selectivity,* and one of the important criteria in deciding this is how the membrane behaves under the application of stepwise transmembrane currents (figure 2.72). Under these conditions, it is found, particularly near the lower end of the range of characteristic frequency, that the membrane potential exhibits a train of damped oscillations that are effectively near the frequency of the unit's best tuning, suggesting that the cell acts as a *resonant acoustic system,* which the authors model as an electric resonator containing elements of the type L (inductance), C (capacitance), and R (resistance).

Careful measurement of the phase of the cellular responses with respect to an acoustic stimulus shows that, near f_c, there is a phase shift of 180° with respect to the tympanum which shows, from what we know about the middle ear transfer function at that frequency, that the effective stimulus is a displacement of the basilar membrane toward the scala vestibuli (corresponding to a sound rarefaction).

Intracellular measurements during the presentation of a tone pip have also shown (figure 2.72):

• The existence of a response asymmetry, as in saccular cells, that signifies the presence of a rectification effect.

• A cancelling followed by a reversal of the responses under the influence of progressively increasing injected current. Cancelling occurs with a current injection of 0.3 nA. The reversal transmembrane potential is near 0 volts.

• The transmembrane resistance falls during the depolarization phase. This last change is not due to a nonlinearity in the current/voltage characteristic that exists in the absence of stimulation but rather suggests that during transduction the cell becomes depolarized by an increase in its transmembrane ionic conductance, with an equilibrium potential near zero.

Crawford and Fettiplace have also concerned themselves with the mechanisms of this conductance variation, exploiting tetraethylammonium (TEA), which blocks both calcium-dependent and voltage-dependent calcium channels. They claim that small doses abolish both the cellular tuning shown by stepwise current injection (see above) and the tuning revealed by acoustic stimuli. At high dosage the tonal tuning disappears, the cell becoming a low-pass system, and at the same time the oscillations following a current step are entirely abolished. In summary, here as in saccular cells, the cellular oscillatory responses involve increases in potassium conductances. There is still some doubt as to whether the variations in potassium conductance (gK) are voltage dependent or are calcium dependent as in the Lewis and Hudspeth (1983) observations on saccular cells.

MAMMALIAN COCHLEAR CELLS

Let us now examine the more important aspects of research into the cells of the mammalian cochlea, the guinea pig in particular (Russell & Sellick 1978; Tanaka et al. 1980; Dallos et al. 1982), noting that similar recent results have also been obtained from mouse cochlear cells in vitro (Russell et al. 1986).

Cochlear Microphonics, Summating Potentials, and Receptor Potentials
The model proposed by Davis some time ago might be summarized
essentially as follows: The acoustic stimulus evokes a change in the
transmembrane electrical resistance of the hair cells that cause the
entry of a depolarizing current. This picture remains generally true
today but it is very clear that recent work has added a great deal of
precision to it.

Intracellular measurements have been made in the basal regions of
the cochlea (first turn) the cells of which (IHC and OHC) are clearly
best stimulated by high-frequency sound but, if the stimulus is sufficiently intense, they respond to low frequencies also. It is interesting
to compare intracellular with extracellular measurement in their responses to low-frequency (300 Hz) and high-frequency (3 kHz) tone
pips.

In the *inner hair cells*, intracellular low-frequency responses are oscillatory at the stimulus frequency; in other words, have an *AC response* like the cochlear microphonic potentials. However, at high
frequencies the response is not at all oscillatory but comprises a continuous *positive* depolarizing *DC response*, which is somewhat like a
summating potential (SP), or at least like one of its components (see
below). Its amplitude is a function of the incident sound intensity.
The transition between the chiefly alternating and the solely steady
responses becomes obvious near 1 kHz. Nevertheless, a careful in-
spection of the 300-Hz response shows that even at this low frequency there is an asymmetry between the peak depolarizations
(positive) and the hyperpolarizations (negative) in the AC responses
(figure 2.73).

According to Russell and Sellick, the attenuation of the AC component (corresponding with CM) is related to the fall in the capacitative
component of transmembrane impedance as the frequency increases.
The ratio AC/DC (which might be compared with the ratio CM/SP)
is about 20% at 1 kHz and falls at higher frequencies by 6 to 9 dB/
octave, as it would in a passive resistance capacitance (RC) electrical
circuit (with a time constant of 0.50 ms). Figures 2.73 and 2.74 show
the rectifying effect and also the variation of the AC/DC ratio with
increasing frequency. Russell and Sellick are quite certain that the
depolarizing swings of the AC component and at higher frequencies
the DC depolarization are true receptor potentials for cells at the base
of the cochlea.

Measurements in the *outer hair cells*, still in the basal regions of the

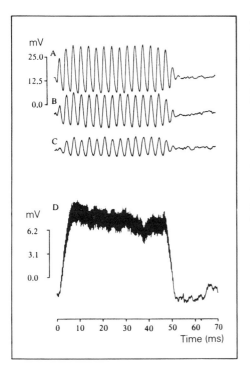

Figure 2.73
Examples of receptor potentials measured intracellularly in basal turn OHC of the guinea pig cochlea. *A* to *C*, Receptor potentials generated by 300-Hz tone pips at intensities (A) 90 dB, (B) 80 dB, (C) 70 dB. *D*, Responses to a 3-kHz tone pip. The rectification clearly observable in the AC responses, particularly *A*, is now seen as an effectively steady DC bias, free from AC oscillations. These have become short-circuited by the membrane capacitance (see text). (From Sellick 1979)

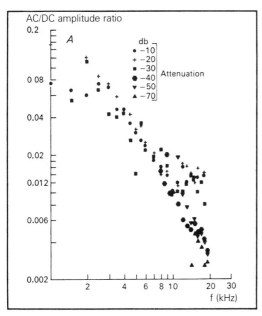

Figure 2.74
Ratio of the AC to DC components of the receptor potential of an IHC in the basal turn of the guinea pig cochlea. The AC component decreases considerably with respect to the DC with increasing frequency. (From Russell & Sellick 1978)

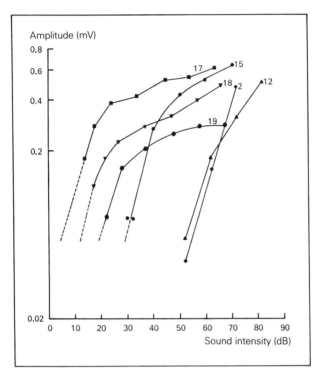

Figure 2.75
Amplitude of IHC receptor potential as a function of stimulus intensity. Frequency of each sound is marked near the appropriate curve, this cell being most sensitive at 17 kHz. The figure shows the AC component; the DC component has a similar general form (see text). (From Russell & Sellick 1978)

cochlea, by Tanaka et al. (1980), Cody and Russell (1985), and Russell et al. (1986) again yielded a whole series of depolarizing/hyperpolarizing AC responses to low-frequency sounds but this time without any sign of a rectifying effect. At high frequencies, no doubt because of this lack of rectifying effect, no DC component (summating potential) is seen in these cells. Its absence might also be due to the OHC transmembrane impedance being so much lower, from which arises not only the absence of rectification but also the more significant passive, electrotonic, spread of the cochlear microphonic type of response which is easily picked up by extracellular electrodes. It is known that OHC are the principal source of CM (see above).

This rectification difference between IHC and OHC has been partly challenged. Investigation of OHC in the third and fourth turns of the guinea pig cochlea (Dallos et al. 1982; Dallos 1986) detected an asymmetry which other experiments (Cody & Russell 1985; Russell et al. 1986) have only revealed in IHC. Future experiments will no doubt resolve this problem about the properties of OHC; they might depend on whether the cells are located basally or apically.

Russell and Sellick's intracellular measurements also gave data on the stimulus/response coupling of the receptor potential (amplitude in millivolts per stimulus intensity) for both the AC and DC components. The family of curves in figure 2.75 illustrates this function, which initially increases but eventually shows some saturation effect. The curves in figure 2.75 all relate to one cell and to the AC component; the parameter is frequency, which shows that the cell responds best at 17 kHz. Essentially the same form of response behavior is seen for the DC component.

These authors have also plotted tuning curves for individual IHC from both AC and DC receptor potential magnitudes. To make these directly comparable with prior and parallel studies on the discharge of appropriate afferent fibers, isoamplitude curves are plotted (stimulus intensity needed at each frequency to obtain a chosen level of response). These curves (figure 2.76) clearly show rather sharp tuning at low intensities, becoming more spread out at higher intensities. But the most important result is that at low intensities the Q_{10dB} for the intracellular potentials has essentially the same magnitude as for the nerve discharge tuning. Once again the tuning curves for AC and DC receptor potentials are alike.

What is seen if, in addition, the phase of stapes movements is compared with the basilar membrane vibration phase, with the phase of the time course of CM, and with the phase of receptor potentials? The observations of Dallos et al. (1972) cited above showed that the amplitude of the AC cochlear microphonic from the OHC is related to the amplitude of movement of the basilar membrane, whereas that from IHC is not only smaller but is related to the velocity of membrane movements. Intracellularly measured IHC potentials when compared with the local CM (essentially generated by OHC, as we have said) essentially confirm the above observations, in this case using a sound pressure wave that generates trapezoidal movements of the basilar membrane (Sellick & Russell 1980). In effect, the intracellular receptor potential corresponds to the first derivative of the

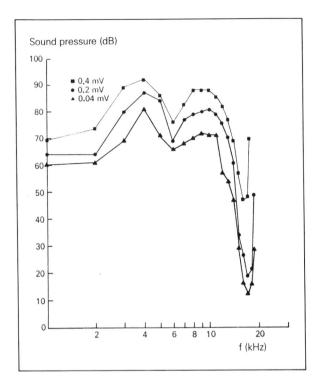

Figure 2.76
IHC tuning curves in guinea pig. Sound pressure generating a constant receptor potential amplitude (indicated for each curve) as a function of frequency. (From Russell & Sellick 1978)

global CM and thus to the second derivative of the sound pressure wave (figure 2.77).

The Cilia and the Receptor Potentials
We shall now describe the mechanisms by which acoustic stimuli are finally able to generate an excitation at the afferent nerve terminals. Unfortunately, although certain stages are known, there are others still to be worked out.

Analyzing membrane potential variations as a function of stereo-ciliar displacements toward and away from the basal corpuscle (the residue of a kinocilium) shows depolarization in the first direction and hyperpolarization in the second (Sellick 1979; Russell et al. 1986).

Symmetrical deflections of cilia to each side of their rest position generate larger depolarizations than the corresponding hyperpolar-

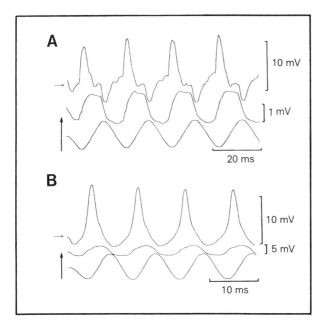

Figure 2.77
Intracellular receptor potential in IHC of the basal turn of the guinea pig cochlea in response to a triangular wave sound stimulus at (A) 52 Hz, 100 dB SPL and to a sinusoidal stimulus at (B) 102 Hz, 80 dB. For each recording: upper trace, receptor potential; middle trace, CM recorded extracellularly in immediate vicinity; lower trace, displacement of the tympanum. Horizontal arrows indicate the resting membrane potential (− 40 mV in A, − 30 mV in B). Vertical arrows show the direction for sound rarefaction. (From Sellick & Russell 1980)

izations (figure 2.78). This response asymmetry also introduces a DC depolarizing component that is superimposed on the AC output that mirrors the sound stimulus' waveform. In vitro studies of cochlear receptor cells have even established that the dynamic range of IHC is greater than in OHC: Saturation effects in IHC begin to be seen at 60 nm deflection of the extremity of a hair, whereas for OHC they are already present at 30 nm. In contrast, the sensitivities of IHC and OHC are apparently about the same, being around 0.4 mv/nm displacement of the tip of a hair. A similar sensitivity obtains in the turtle hair cells (see above) but, in contrast, saccular hair cell sensitivities are much poorer, 5 to 7 mv/μm (Hudspeth & Corey 1977). Finally, we must remember (see above) that in certain conditions the OHC can develop the same sort of asymmetry as seen in IHC but that this does not correspond with the results in vivo, where only

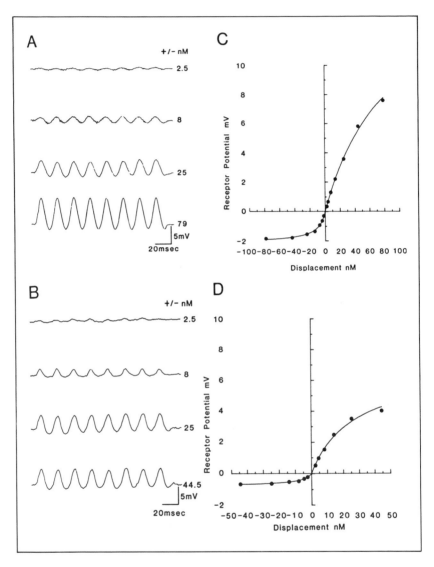

Figure 2.78
Responses to displacements of their stereocilia bundles for an IHC (*A*) and an OHC
(*B*) in a 4-day-old organ culture of the mouse organ of Corti. Displacement amplitudes
(nM) are shown against each trace. Displacement/receptor potential relationships are
shown (*C*) for IHC and (*D*) for OHC. The smooth curves through the points are for
paired rectangular hyperbolas, the constants for which were derived empirically.
(From Russell et al. 1986)

IHC (investigated solely in the basal turn, it is true) show the rectification phenomenon. As we have already noted, this constitutes a problem in making any final definitive conclusions about this functional aspect.

Hair displacement also generates a change in membrane conductance. However, when operating at high frequencies around 20 kHz, researchers have not been able to measure *instantaneous* resistance changes during the sinusoidal stimulus but rather have only been able to show that the *mean* resistance change is proportional to the intracellular depolarization (figure 2.79).

10.2 THE CILIA AND COCHLEAR MECHANICS

There remains another fundamental question, which is to decide how the cilia in the mammalian cochlea are set into motion by movements of the basilar membrane. If certain experimental results look promising, many details remain obscure nevertheless. Two aspects need to be considered; one is the coupling between the reticular lamina and the tectorial membrane, the other concerns the stiffness variations observable in OHC.

COUPLING BETWEEN THE RETICULAR LAMINA AND THE TECTORIAL MEMBRANE

Some argue, from mechanical and histological data, that the effect of a sound stimulus on the basilar membrane (and in particular on the recticular lamina) is to generate a rotational movement along an arc whose center of rotation is situated at the border of the bony spiral lamina. This movement can be dissected into a component normal to the basilar membrane and a tangential component. In addition, it is usually considered that basilar membrane displacements toward the scala vestibuli are responsible for excitation (which is certainly what results from comparing the effects of rarefaction clicks with compression clicks), but this point of view is still disputed.

The main present tendency is to regard the tangential component (parallel to the reticular lamina) to be the effective mechanical stimulus, since it produces a relative slippage between the tectorial membrane (TM) and the reticular lamina (RL). That hypothesis obviously raises the question of what are the links between the two strips (TM and RL) and, related to that, how are the hair cells anchored into RL.

The problem of the connections between the hair cells and TM has already been addressed above. The first early concept was that the cilia from all the receptor cells were firmly anchored into TM and the

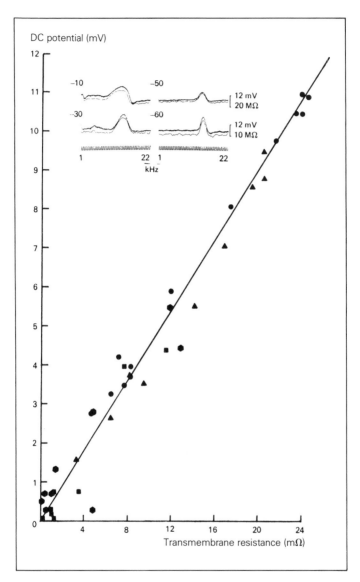

Figure 2.79
Linear relationship between DC receptor potential amplitude and variation of transmembrane resistance in IHC for increasing intensity of stimulation by pure tones.
The measurements were made at a variety of frequencies, each marked by a symbol.
Inset, Separate examples of the recordings made; in each case, the upper trace shows
the DC potential changes resulting from the resistance changes (trace immediately
below it) at four different intensities. These traces were obtained by sweeping across
the frequency range between 1 and 22 kHz. (From Russell & Sellick 1978)

resulting model was simple: Slippage between RL and TM generates shearing force that deflects *all* cilia and thus causes excitation at OHC and IHC afferent terminals.

The facts are now known to be quite otherwise (perhaps with the exception of certain IHC in the first turn), because only the hairs from OHC are firmly joined to TM (Lim 1986). The result is that the majority, IHC cilia, are only affected by fluid movements and resulting viscous forces. From this arises the hypothesis that is sometimes proposed suggesting that OHC hair displacement is proportional to basilar membrane displacement whereas IHC hair displacement is proportional to the velocity of basilar membrane displacement (Dallos et al. 1974).

Another important discovery is the essential role played by OHC in determining the tuning curves of IHC. Considering the distribution of axons between OHC (95%) and IHC (5%), there is not much chance that the latter contribute very much directly to the afferent output to higher centers, even if they actually possess an ascending axon to the central nervous system, which is still in doubt. All things considered, it is very surprising that kanamycin destruction of OHC, as we have seen, abolishes practically all of CM and distinctly modifies the tuning curves of IHC: The peak in the tuning around the IHC characteristic frequency is diminished and the fiber's relative response at frequencies $<f_c$ is improved (Evans & Harrison 1975; Liberman 1976; figure 2.80).

A minute analysis of the mechanical resonance curves led Zwislocki (1986) to suggest that the greater or lesser excitation of IHC, consequent upon a given slippage between TM and RL, depends on the greater or lesser rigidity of the OHC and the mechanical coupling between TM and RL. This is schematized in figure 2.81. When the OHC are very rigid (high stiffness), TM will be moved farther and its movement will deflect the OHC hairs in the excitatory direction; but when the OHC cilia are more flexible, TM will move much less above IHC, and the latter will be scarcely affected by the movement (or might even be affected in the opposite, inhibitory, direction).

Zwislocki (1984) also explains the puzzling effect of kanamycin destruction of OHC on the tuning of IHC by suggesting that the absence of OHC greatly reduces the radial movement of TM compared with that of RL and this, surprisingly, leads to a more effective shearing movement except in the region of tuning frequency, where the mass of TM plays the greater role.

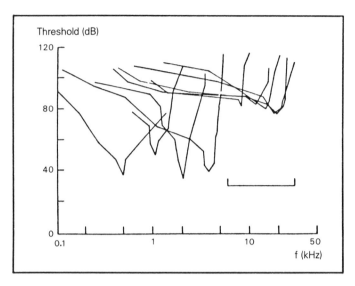

Figure 2.80
Tuning curves of cochlear nerve fibers after OHC lesions (guinea pig). The horizontal
bar indicates the region in which the peak of the tuning curve has been eliminated by
the action of an ototoxic drug. In this zone, corresponding to frequencies between 4
and 50 kHz, histology showed an essential destruction of OHC over their three rows
in the first 5 mm of the cochlea beyond the oval window. (From Evans & Harrison
1975)

THE CONTRACTILE ELEMENTS IN OUTER HAIR CELLS

Turning now to consider some more recent discoveries in cochlear
physiology concerning the contractile properties found in OHC, the
following are among the important new data.

Physiological investigations of single isolated hair cells made per-
meable by treatment with detergent and kept in an appropriate tissue
culture medium have demonstrated that they contract under the influence of a variety of manipulations: intracellular electrical stimulation; action of a medium rich in Ca^{2+} and ATP; presence of K^+ in
endolymphatic concentration (Flock & Cheung 1977; Flock & Strelioff
1984; Zenner 1980, 1986). This contraction involves the cell but not
the stereocilia themselves. It is suppressed by calmodulin inhibitors;
equally, in the absence of Ca^{2+} (by adding EDTA) ATP is no longer
able to release a motor response. These facts suggest the existence of
mechanisms in OHC that are not unlike those more familiar mechanisms involved in muscular contraction. Similarly, histochemically
finding a complex network of actin filaments, together with a certain

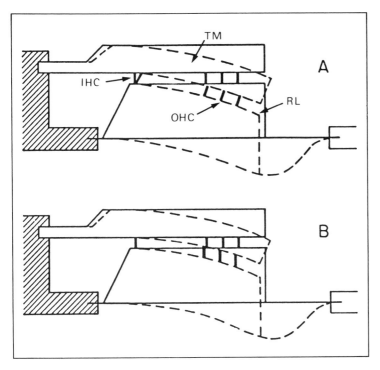

Figure 2.81
Schematic drawings of two fundamentally different modes of shear motion between the tectorial membrane (TM) and the recticular lamina (RL). *A*, It is assumed that the outer hair cell (OHC) stereocilia are very stiff and cannot easily be deflected. As a result, there is no shear motion at the OHC but a substantial shear motion at the inner hair cells (IHC). Their stereocilia are deflected away from the modiolus when the basilar membrane is displaced toward scala tympani. *B*, It is assumed that the tectorial membrane can slide freely over the recticular lamina at the OHC. Under this condition, there is little shear motion at IHC, the stereocilia of which are deflected toward the modiolus when the basilar membrane is displaced toward the scala tympani. In fact, an intermediate mode of motion should be expected. (From Zwislocki 1986)

amount of myosin and tropomyosin, in OHC (see 3.3, earlier) makes this possibility even more plausible.

A more detailed examination of the hair cell mechanics has led to distinguishing two types of movement (Kim 1986; figure 2.82). The movements that we have just described are slow (seconds or minutes), involve the cell body itself and structures throughout its length between the cuticular plate and the vicinity of the cell nucleus where subsynaptic cisternae are found. The movement is controlled by efferent fibers from the olivocochlear bundle. These fibers can themselves be excited by afferent signals from the cochlea (some of them proba-

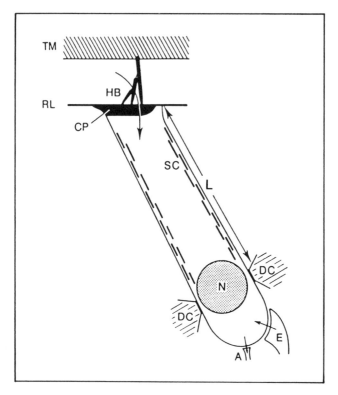

Figure 2.82
Schematic drawing of a mammalian outer hair cell (OHC). Two different types of
motile mechanisms are postulated in OHC: (i) a fast motile mechanism located in the
hair bundle (HB) and cuticular plate (CP) region, which produces an active force
operating laterally on the hair bundle; (ii) a slow motile mechanism localized in the
specialized elongated cylindrical portion of OHC. This changes the length, tension,
and stiffness in the longitudinal axis (L) of OHC. The OHC length and tension are
postulated to be under efferent control. TM, tectorial membrane; RL, recticular lamina;
SC, subsurface cisternae; N, nucleus; DC, Deiter's cell; A, afferent ending; E, efferent
ending. (Modified from Kim 1986)

bly carried in type II fibers from outer hair cells) and may therefore form a negative feedback system passing via the olivary complex and by this means control the structural stiffness of the OHC.

There is also a fast-acting system. An effectively instantaneous (microsecond) contraction of the cell can be generated by direct electrical stimulation which will follow even high-frequency stimulation (Brownell et al. 1985). This might well constitute a rapid-feedback mechanism in which distorting the cilia of OHC provoking a depolarization can also generate a *reciprocal transduction*, that is, a movement of cellular elements (particularly in the apical region near the cilia) caused by the depolarization that the cilia themselves have initiated. This sort of rapid feedback (based also on the nonmammalian work of Crawford & Fettiplace 1985, 1986) has been interpreted (Kachar et al. 1986) as a purely local electrokinetic effect tied to fluid displacements generated by the electric field, quite independent of energetic reactions and free from remote control. The existence of such a system modifies our conception of any resonance mechanisms; they are no longer to be regarded as simply due to alternately bringing into play different ionic mechanisms as imagined by Hudspeth (1985, 1986), but also involve active contractile processes.

An important phenomenon related to these movements of the cilia concerns an effect known for more than a decade but which has recently taken on a much greater significance. This manifests itself as *otoacoustic emissions* (OAE), first described by Kemp (1978) and later confirmed in various species (Wilson 1980; Zurek 1981; Horner et al. 1985; Kemp 1986). Sounds are emitted and can be detected by suitably sensitive microphones placed in the auditory meatus.

There are two sorts of emission, spontaneous and stimulated. Stimulated OAE are evoked by impulsive sounds (clicks or tone pips) after a latency of around 7 ms. They last between a few milliseconds and a fraction of a second; their amplitude at first increases linearly with stimulus amplitude but then saturates. In humans the threshold for evoking the effect can be lower than the perceptual threshold for detecting it, suggesting that the OAE is generated locally. Its sound spectrum embraces a large bandwidth, between 750 Hz and 2 kHz within which some narrow band peaks can be interposed (figure 2.83). Other evoked OAE can be recorded during the application of a continuous tone and in that case the stimulus frequency is also the dominant frequency component in the OAE.

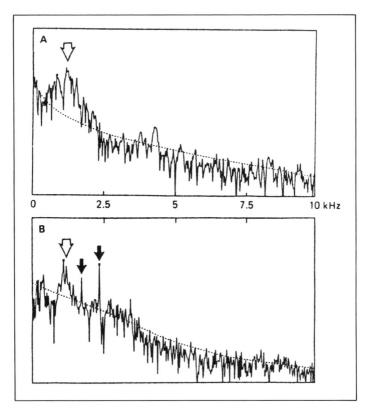

Figure 2.83
Two typical examples of evoked auditory emission (EAE) power spectra. *A*, An EAE
power spectrum that embraces a wide frequency band between 0.6 and 2.1 kHz (bandwidth 1.5 kHz) with a maximum near 1.45 kHz. This type of spectrum is present in
all EAE (white arrow). *B*, An EAE spectrum that contains a wide continuous frequency
band (white arrow) and some narrow band frequency peaks at higher frequencies
(black arrows). The dotted line represents the noise floor. Vertical logarithmic scale
(arbitrary units). (From Bonfils et al. 1988)

It appears evident that OAEs must originate in the cochlea. In
animal preparations they are affected by anoxia, by exposure to prolonged sounds, or after treatment with ototoxic drugs (Wilson 1984).
In humans they are absent in people suffering only a moderate hearing loss (Kemp 1978; Probst et al. 1987; Bonfils et al. 1988). This is
unlike spontaneous OAE, which are, in contrast, linked with significant cochlear lesions.

Apart from the diagnostic interest in measuring OAE, for which
we have no space to spread our discussion, these emissions are being
recognized as pointers to essential functional cochlear mechanisms.

They are also evidence for the existence of an *active contractile process* in the cochlear OHC.

Apart from this, there is a new and attractive suggestion that the contractions in OHC that generate OAE also have the effect of reinforcing the mechanical (tuning) selectivity of the basilar membrane according to the need, pointed out by Davis (1983), for a *cochlear amplifier*. The basilar membrane must thus be regarded as something more than the passive low-pass filter of von Békésy or the band-pass filter of more recent authors.

It is tempting, following the above analysis, to list the following set of stages to characterize the stimulation of the basilar membrane by an incident sound.

• The basilar membrane is brought into play with a zone of maximal displacement that is closer to the base of the cochlea the higher the sound frequency, resulting in the well-known tonotopic arrangement, but with a not very sharp tuning selectivity.

• Where it is displaced, the basilar membrane is thereby subjected to a rotary movement, which brings with it a tangential slippage between the TM and the RL.

• This movement of TM is responsible for deflecting the hairs of OHC, thus generating a depolarization that in its turn brings about a contraction in OHC.

• The effect of this contraction is to modify the coupling between TM and RL in such a way as to amplify the displacement of the basilar membrane locally in this restricted zone, thereby increase the selectivity of the mechanical filtering, and thus refine the tonotopic tuning.

• The hairs of IHC are in their turn mechanically distorted by the movement of TM, either directly or more likely by movements of the fluid immediately below TM. The final outcome is the generation of afferent nerve signals via the causal chain of hair deflection to depolarization in IHC, as discussed in detail above.

The Auditory Central Nervous System: Anatomy and Function

Some functional characteristics of the different levels of the auditory central nervous system (CNS) at which incoming signals are processed will be examined in this third chapter. This essentially physiological study will be preceded at each stage by a summary of the relevant structural features.

As a general introduction to the discussion, see figure 3.1, which is a very simplified sketch of the mammalian auditory pathways specifying the principal auditory structures that will be examined in turn: the cochlear nuclei (CN), the superior olivary complex (SOC), the nuclei of the lateral lemniscus (NLL), the inferior colliculus (IC), the medial geniculate body (MGB), and the auditory cortex (C).

From a neurophysiological point of view, it can be said immediately that each successive processing stage of the auditory pathways has undergone detailed single-unit investigations with the aim of specifying its individual processing characteristics in response to a variety of types of sound signals, whether classic ones such as tone pips and clicks or more complex ones such as frequency modulations or combinations of different sounds. The stimuli may be applied monaurally or, alternatively, binaurally when it is a question of studying aspects of the convergence and mutual interaction of the bilateral pathways.

It would be unnecessarily scrupulous to try to consider every aspect of the highly detailed measurements that have been made at each nucleus. We have thus limited the discussion to the essential operations at each main processing level.

Before beginning, two comments. The first remark, which applies equally well to all sensory systems, concerns the nature of the successive steps that occur during the elaboration of integrative processing. It is notable that as the subcortical integrative centers between the receptors and the cortex are traversed (1) the same stimulus can generate successively more elaborate and diverse responses and (2) more complex stimuli may eventually generate characteristic responses that

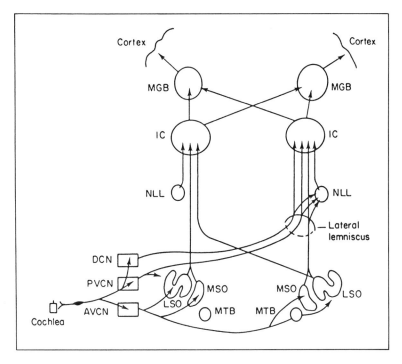

Figure 3.1
The central ascending afferent auditory pathways (schematic). AVCN, anteroventral
cochlear nucleus; PVCN, posteroventral cochlear nucleus; DCN, dorsal cochlear nucleus. Components of the superior olivary complex: MSO, medial nucleus; LSO, lateral
nucleus; MTB, medial nucleus of the trapezoid body; NLL, nuclei of the lateral lemniscus; IC, inferior colliculus; MGB, medial geniculate body. This sketch merely represents the general positioning of the nuclei; more details are available in later figures
(bulbar regions, figure 3.3; inferior colliculus, figure 3.15; medial geniculate body,
figure 3.24; cortex, figure 3.32 to 3.37. The arrows do not necessarily indicate direct
connections. (From Pickles 1982)

are specific for each individual stimulus. In all cases, the basic input
information is the cochlear output signal, which is then modified by
processing in the parallel pathways of the CNS. When recording from
a given unit in the CNS, the investigator must determine what part
of the response is effectively a simple relaying of an input that has
been modified during its ascent through the pathways and what part
has resulted from local processing in the nuclei of that central level
itself.

The second comment concerns the significance of the precise experimental method used. Until fairly recently, all investigations were

conducted using anesthesia, particularly barbiturates. However, it has become evident that these results can differ profoundly from the case of measurements made in the absence of narcosis in the awake unrestrained animal. What is more, some far from negligible advances have been made in this particular field of study, perhaps more so than in other sensory systems, by exploiting these new experimental arrangements.

1 THE COCHLEAR NUCLEI

1.1 STRUCTURE

The first synaptic connections are made in the complex of the *cochlear nucleus* (CN), which comprises three principal divisions: the *dorsal cochlear nucleus* (DCN), the *anteroventral cochlear nucleus* (AVCN), and the *posteroventral cochlear nucleus* (PVCN) (figure 3.2; see Osen 1969; Osen & Roth 1969).

Cytoarchitectonically the complex consists of a variety of cell types, whose distribution is shown in figure 3.2B: (a) large spherical cells, (b) small spherical cells, (c) "octopus cells" with long, straight dendrites, (d) giant cells, (e) globular cells, (f) multipolar cells, (g) granular cells, (h) pyramidal cells, and (i) dwarf cells. The disposition of these cells is not haphazard; as illustrated in figure 3.2, it is particularly clear that:

• In the *AVCN*, there is an anterior zone with large spherical cells, then small spherical cells are found more medially, while still more

Figure 3.2   ▶
Organization in the cochlear nucleus complex of the cat. *A*, Two parasagittal sections, one more lateral (*left*) the other more medial (*right*). Note the orientations: D ↔ V, dorsoventral; R ↔ C, rostrocaudal. AVCN, anteroventral cochlear nucleus; PVCN, posteroventral cochlear nucleus; DCN, dorsal cochlear nucleus which, because of its more medial position, is only seen in the right diagram. n. vest., vestibular nerve; n. coch., cochlear nerve; co.f., cochlear nerve fibers with the ascending branch (a.b.) and "descending" branch (d.b.). m.l., molecular layer in DCN; g.r.c.l., granular cell layer; h and l, high and low f_c cochlear nerve fibers; the dashed line on the left also shows the frequency gradient in AVCN. Horizontal hatching, central area of VCN; vertical hatching, central area of DCN. *B*, Section corresponding to A (*above, right*) showing the distribution of the principal cell types. (if), intrinsic fibers, between VCN and DCN. Cell types: (a) large spherical cells; (b) small spherical cells; (c) "octopus" cells; (d) giant cells; (e) globular cells; (f) multipolar cells; (g) granular cells; (h) pyramidal cells; (i) dwarf cells. cap, band of dwarf cells; o.c.b., olivocochlear bundle and (br.) its branches. (From Osen & Roth 1969; see also Osen 1969).

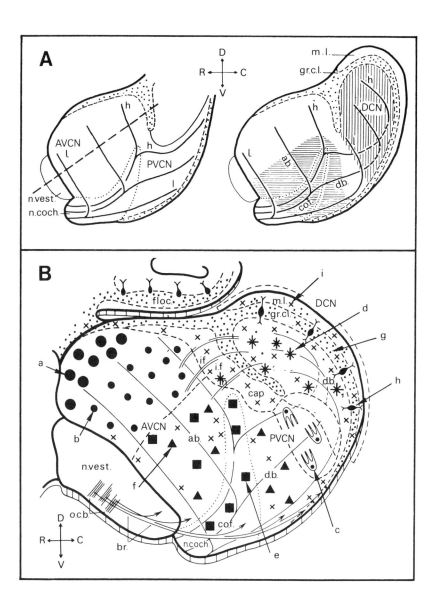

posterior regions show a mixture of globular, multipolar, and dwarf cells.

• In the *PVCN*, multipolar and dwarf cells are seen anteriorly with "octopus cells" posteriorly.

• In the *DCN*, there is a laminated arrangement (absent in the ventral CN) of three layers; one with giant, granular, and dwarf cells lies deep; the next more peripheral layer contains pyramidal (fusiform) cells, and finally there is a superficial "molecular" layer made up of the dendrites of the fusiform cells.

All afferent fibers from the auditory nerve terminate in the cochlear nucleus. At its entry into the (ventral) cochlear nucleus each fiber divides into an anterior (ascending) branch terminating in the AVCN, while its posterior (descending) branch innervates the PVCN, then turns dorsally to terminate in the DCN. The fibers terminate in an ordered way in each division of the nucleus, which suggests the possibility of a tonotopic arrangement. This has largely been confirmed by physiological experiments. This divergent pattern ends with a certain convergence, since each cell of the cochlear nucleus may be innervated by several auditory afferent fibers. Roughly speaking, for the entire cochlear nucleus there are three times as many cells as there are incoming auditory afferents.

The fiber terminations differ considerably in shape and size; in the VCN (from the ascending nerve branches) are found the wider terminals named *chalices* or *end-bulbs of Held* that innervate spherical cells. The other types of cells are innervated with the more commonly seen nerve terminations. Such "normal" terminals also innervate the spherical cells, though these might be the ends of descending fibers (see below). On the "octopus cells" there are seen two types of terminal boutons that differ in size.

In the DCN, auditory afferents terminate in the deeper layers and (at least according to certain experimenters) also in the most superficial layers.

The axons of the cells of the cochlear nucleus complex (i.e., second-order neurons in the auditory pathways) have three possible trajectories, all going contralateral, that is to say crossed: the *dorsal acoustic stria* (DAS), or stria of von Monakow; the *intermediate acoustic stria* (IAS), or stria of Held; and the *trapezoid body* (TB), a ventral tract (figure 3.3).

The distribution of the axons leaving the CN via these diverse tracts

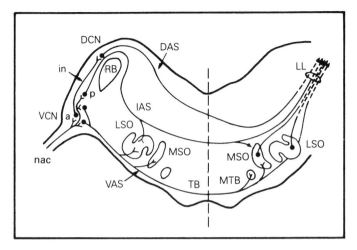

Figure 3.3
Trajectory of the pathways from the cochlear nuclei to the contralateral lateral lemniscus **(LL)**. nac, acoustic nerve sending fibers to the anteroventral (a) and posteroventral (p) divisions of AVCN and perhaps (not shown) to DCN; in, interneurons between VCN and DCN; RB, restiform body; DAS, dorsal acoustic stria; IAS, intermediary acoustic stria; TB, trapezoid body; MTB, medial nucleus of trapezoid body; MSO, LSO, medial and lateral nuclei of superior olive; VAS, ventral acoustic stria; refer to text. (Modified from Pickles 1982)

as well as their final destination are very complicated and not yet completely understood. Essentially, these axons might end in:

• The ipsilateral and contralateral *olivary complex* (the principal olivary nucleus, the accessory nucleus and the periolivary nuclei, see below).
• The *nuclei of the lateral lemniscus* (NLL), particularly the ventral division (VNLL).
• The *inferior colliculus* (IC); keep in mind that a fiber in this third tract might also send collaterals to either of the above.

A variety of studies (e.g., Warr 1982) suggest the following distribution: The axons of the DCN leaving in the dorsal acoustic stria do not go to either the ipsilateral or contralateral olivary complex but eventually reach the IC via the VNLL and collaterals. In contrast, axons in the intermediate stria, chiefly comprising outputs from the "octopus" cells of the PVCN, go to both ipsilateral and contralateral olives and to the NLL. Finally, the fibers of the TB containing output axons from VCN cells have different destinations depending on cell type: Globular and spherical cells essentially serve the ipsilateral and contralateral olives, whereas multipolar cells (although they do send collaterals to the olives) reach IC via the lateral lemniscus (LL).

In fact, not all the cells of the VCN (anterior or posterior) have long axons leaving the nucleus, but some act as *interneurons* serving the DCN and establish short direct connections between the two parts of the CN. Neurophysiological observations (below) confirm these connections.

1.2 FUNCTION

It is necessary to ascertain whether recordings made in the CN complex are truly postsynaptic and concerned with second-order neurons—and consequently give information on the nucleus' transfer functions—or whether they are not just a more remote record of cochlear coding from input afferents.

FREQUENCY CODING

In general, researchers are agreed that in the CN the neuronal tuning curves remain asymmetrical without any essential modification of what is observed in the auditory nerve. As in the nerve, the tuning curves seem to become increasingly sharper with higher f_c, that is, Q_{10dB} increases with increasing f_c (see Goldberg & Brownell 1973). Some researchers have nevertheless identified units in the CN, which they classify as type II, that have wide tuning curves and thus poor frequency selectivity (Rose et al. 1959).

An important discovery is the existence (figure 3.4) of a precise *tonotopic* arrangement of best frequencies in each of the three divisions of the CN; essentially, low frequencies are represented ventrally and anteriorly, high frequencies more dorsally and posteriorly. This tonotopic arrangement allows the definition of *isofrequency bands* that agree very well with the organization of fiber terminals and tracts from the auditory nerve into the various divisions of the CN (see above; Evans & Nelson 1973a,b). We might add that these results have been recently confirmed by histochemical techniques using 2-^{14}C-deoxyglucose, a tracer that indicates the local rate of cellular metabolism.

Phase locking of the neuronal discharge to the sound wave, seen in auditory nerve fibers for frequencies lower than 4 kHz, seems to be conserved after processing in the CN, particularly in the VCN, although such units are only rarely found in the DCN. Again, as in the auditory nerve, when locking to the tonal frequency is observed,

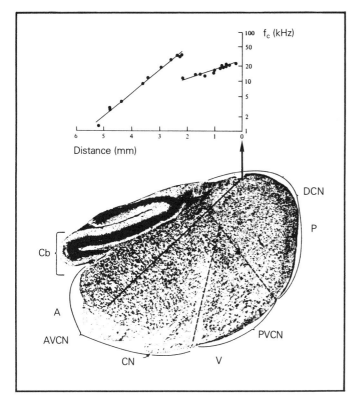

Figure 3.4
Tonotopic organization of the cochlear nucleus. *Below,* Parasagittal section (cell staining) of CN. A, anterior; P, posterior; V, ventral. As in figure 3.2, the cochlear nerve enters from an anterior direction (left) and ventrally. The dashed lines separate the principal divisions comprising VCN, subdivided into anteroventral (AVCN) and posteroventral (PVCN) nuclei, and DCN. *Above,* Curves showing characteristic frequencies of cells, f_c, encountered along a continuous anteroventral to posteroventral electrode penetration as a function of distance along track (mm) illustrating a strictly tonotopic organization. (From Evans 1975)

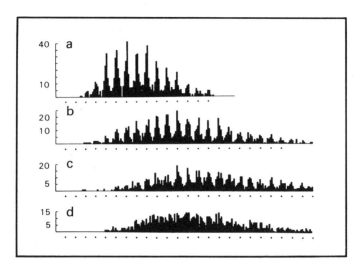

Figure 3.5
Interspike interval distribution for a DCN unit in the cat. Relative proportions of intervals in response to sounds of four different frequencies: *a*, 310; *b*, 610; *c*, 862; *d*, 1020 Hz. Intervals are normalized as multiples of the period (unity) for each frequency, the dots representing whole numbers. (From Lavine 1971)

the phase of the sound sinusoid at which a nerve discharge occurs is seen to change with frequency. A quantitative study of this case (Lavine 1971) suggests a linear relationship of the form $\Phi = af + b$ (figure 3.5).

Some different CN cell responses have been reported throughout the audiofrequency spectrum (Evans & Nelson 1973a,b). The cells show spontaneous activity, particularly in the absence of narcosis: Notably, cells with only a purely excitatory tuning curve response to a single tone (as in the classic tuning curves of the auditory nerve) become rather rare and, in contrast, most cells, particularly in the DCN, show flanking inhibitory effects for frequencies at either side of the excitatory zone. Others even show still more complicated responses with alternating multiple zones of excitation and inhibition (figure 3.6).

INTENSITY CODING

In general, the sound intensity/impulse rate relationship between stimulus and response is much more complex than in the auditory nerve (figure 3.7; Greenwood & Goldberg 1970). Evans and Nelson

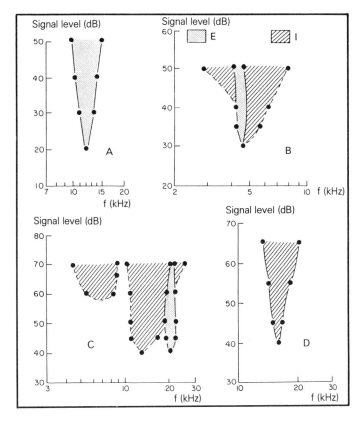

Figure 3.6
Examples of tuning curves encountered for DCN units in the cat. Purely excitatory
cells (*A*) are found in AVCN. Inhibitory flanking regions, more or less wide (*B*, *C*), or
even solely an inhibitory response (*D*) predominate in DCN. E, excitatory; I, inhibitory
zones. (From Pickles 1982; see also Evans & Nelson 1973a)

(1973) were able to distinguish three classes of cell responses in this
nucleus in the unanesthetized animal; type I corresponds to the classic sigmoid shape and has a purely excitatory response, and type V
has a purely inhibitory response, whereas cells of types II, III, and
IV, in contrast, show nonmonotonic responses with one excitatory
region but with more complicated inhibitory regions also. Consequently, the frequency tuning curves and the intensity relationships
are not independent. For the present, however, we need only inspect
the frequency response curves and their narrow intermingling zones
of excitation and inhibition (Young & Brownell 1976) to understand

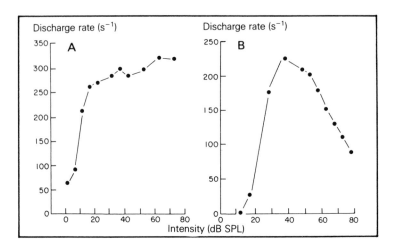

Figure 3.7
Discharge rate/stimulus intensity characteristics of two cells in CN. *A*, Monotonic
response; such cells show absent or feeble inhibitory flanks. *B*, Nonmonotonic response; such cells have very marked inhibitory flanks. (From Pickles 1982, after Greenwood & Goldberg 1970)

why such neuronal units have particularly rapidly changing relationships between the two parameters of frequency and intensity
(figure 3.8).

TEMPORAL CODING

It is in the temporal domain that we find the greatest variety of response characteristics in CN cells.

Responses to Tone Pips
It is generally agreed that there are four types of excitatory responses
to a tone pip in CN cells (figure 3.9; Pfeiffer 1966):

• Tonic excitatory responses, called *primary-like* because they are exactly like most responses in the auditory nerve.
• Purely phasic responses at the onset of a tone pip, this *on-response*
being followed by silence during the rest of the stimulus.
• *"Chopper"* responses with regularly spaced response peaks during
the stimulus, although these peaks do not correspond with the frequency of the stimulus except at very low f_c.
• Complex effects (*"pauser cells"*) with an *on-response* followed by a
pause and then a succeeding tonic response.

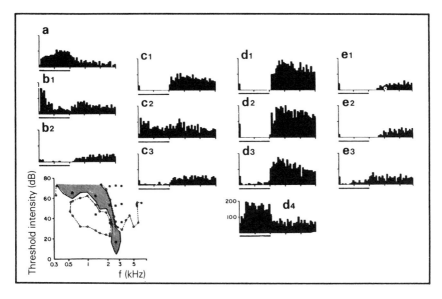

Figure 3.8
Responses of a type IV cell for different sound frequencies and intensity levels.
Above: a, 0.57 kHz 65.5 dB; b1, 1.30 kHz 62 dB; b2, 44 dB; c1, 2.16 kHz 71.5 dB; c2,
53.5 dB, c3, 35.5 dB; d1, 2.67 kHz 72.5 dB; d2, 52.5 dB; d3, 36.5 dB; d4, 16.5 dB; e1,
3.28 kHz 72 dB; e2, 54 dB; e3, 36 dB. *Below*: All the points corresponding to the above
values are shown in the graph. The shaded contour represents the excitatory zone and
the unshaded one the inhibitory zone. (From Young & Brownell 1976)

Note, however, that these response patterns can vary with the intensity of the stimulus in any one cell. Note also that although intracellular recording from cells of the cochlear nucleus has demonstrated
steady depolarizations during the discharge in cells showing tonic
responses (Romand 1978), there is no sign of a corresponding hyperpolarization in cells showing a pause (Romand 1978). The phasic cells
encountered at this first level of the central nervous system have a
special interest since they probably not only mediate the treatment
of messages related to sound transients but, equally importantly,
probably contribute to the eventual analysis of the amplitude and
frequency modulations that are basic components of most natural
complex sounds.

All response types are not necessarily present at any one location
in the nucleus. In particular, primary type cells are preferentially
present in the VCN and are at least to some extent associated with
spherical cells. On-responses are associated with "octopus cells,"

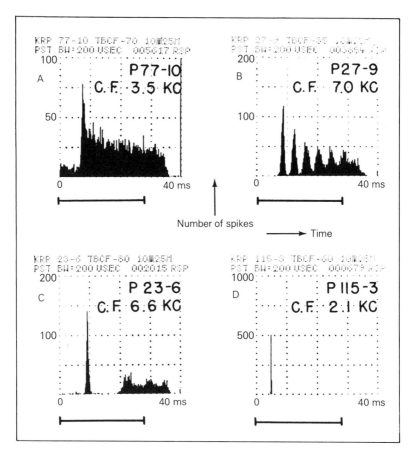

Figure 3.9
Types of response in cochlear units following a tone burst. Responses illustrated by poststimulus histograms: (a) primary response; (b) "chopper" response; (c) "pauser" response; (d) purely *on* response. Intensities about 20 dB. (Bar marks tone duration in each case). (From Pfeiffer 1966)

whereas "choppers" are chiefly found in posteroventral regions and in the DCN. Finally, "pausers" are predominant in the DCN and are the concern of the pyramidal and giant cells.

This list does not exhaust the range of response characteristics in CN. In fact, particularly in the awake animal, some cells (as we have seen above) generate an inhibition of their spontaneous activity during a tone pip, and this inhibition can itself be followed by an after-discharge, representing in some way an *off-effect*.

Responses to Clicks
Some studies on responses to click stimuli show that, unlike in the cochlear nerve afferents, the neural units of CN respond with only a single discharge peak even for low f_c.

Responses to Modulated Sounds
Many single units that respond in a special way to amplitude modulation in sounds have also been demonstrated in the CN. For most such cells (Møller 1974), their mean response rate when they are stimulated at their f_c varies with the intensity of the stimulus. But, more significantly, they are particularly sensitive to the instantaneous amplitudes of sounds with temporally varying amplitudes. Relatively small amplitude modulations generate much larger changes in discharge than the corresponding changes seen between different steady intensity levels.

Other CN cells show sensitivity to frequency modulation in sounds. For example, some interest has been shown in unit response patterns elicited by stimuli in which frequency varies about a certain central frequency (f_m), the frequency changes being ±1/8 octave and lasting for 200 to 1000 ms. The interest in such stimuli springs from their being more closely related than tone pips to sounds that are biologically behaviorally significant. This subject will be discussed in more detail in dealing with higher levels in the pathways.

Peristimulus histograms for CN cells have also been measured with the central frequency f_m being in each case fixed near f_c for the unit (Erulkar et al. 1968; Møller 1978). They show (figure 3.10):

• A symmetrical mirror-image response with respect to f_m which, given its bisymmetrical shape, implies that the unit responds equally well to a frequency variation below and above f_m, whatever the direction of the frequency change.
• Responses with a translation symmetry, the cell this time re-

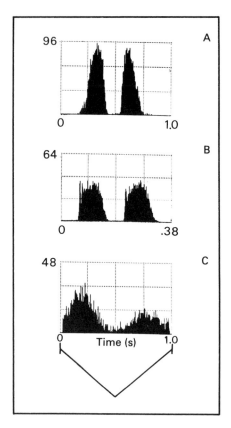

Figure 3.10
Responses of cochlear units to frequency-modulated stimuli. At zero time the sound frequency falls from f_m to $f_m - \delta f$ in 0.5 s then returns to the initial frequency in 0.5 s (diagram below). Stimulus histograms for each cell plotted for the total duration of each stimulus (i.e., 1 s). Three types of response are shown: (a) mirror symmetry; (b) same response for whatever direction of frequency change; (c) larger response for diminishing than for increasing frequency swings. (From Erulkar et al. 1968).

sponding differently to increasing and decreasing frequency whatever the position of f with respect to f_m.
• A bisymmetrical response, such that variation in one frequency region (e.g., $f > f_m$) generates a much larger response than in the other ($f < f_m$).

RESPONSE COMPLEXITY AND FUNCTIONAL DIVERSITY IN THE COCHLEAR NUCLEUS

Many researchers have emphasized the differences that can be demonstrated between VCN and DCN, particularly in the unanesthetized animal. In general, units in the DCN have more complex responses than in the ventral divisions of the nucleus, showing more clearly defined inhibitory fringes, tuning curves with multiple excitatory and inhibitory zones, and predominance of *on-cells* and *pausers,* that is, responses that are far different from the primary input. The idea arose that the VCN is a simple relay in the ascending pathways that preserves the information on time and phase provided by the cochlear output, whereas the DCN has more elaborate integrative capacity and recodes the incoming information for special purposes. It is also probable that the VCN exerts an inhibitory influence on the DCN via short-range interneurons (Evans & Nelson 1973b; Greenwood & Goldberg 1970).

Looking at responses from the point of view of how the three parameters of frequency, intensity, and duration might interact, it is fairly clear that these do not operate independently and that in detail the response patterns display a formidable complexity, particularly in the DCN. A given cell that responds, for example, by an excitation at threshold might develop an inhibition when acted on by a stimulus of the same frequency but higher intensity; another cell might have an on-response at threshold but become a phasic-tonic type at higher intensities. *It is impossible to deduce any generalized law of response after inspecting all such output variations.*

Some time ago, Katsuki et al. (1958) concluded from their experiments that tuning curves become systematically more sharply tuned in the successive subcortical neuronal processing areas (cochlear nuclei, inferior colliculus, medial geniculate) as the auditory pathways are ascended. Stated thus, the hypothesis is certainly excessively simplistic, as we shall see repeatedly below. There is a little more truth in it for the cells of CN that show inhibitory flanks: These have a higher Q_{10dB} than in the auditory nerve because the tuning curves have become steeper on the low-frequency side. But as we have even seen already, this is far from generally applicable.

2 THE SUPERIOR OLIVARY COMPLEX

2.1 STRUCTURE

Here we are concerned with a collection of nuclei (figure 3.11); the most prominent of them are specified below (see also Harrison & Howe 1974a,b).

• The two "authentic" olivary nuclei are the *principal, or lateral superior olive* (LSO), which in transverse section has an S shape, and the *medial accessory superior olive* (MSO).
• There is a cluster of nuclei known as the *nuclei of the trapezoid body* (TB) with a *medial nucleus* (MTB) and a *lateral nucleus* (LTB).
• Another cluster known as the *periolivary nuclei* has *dorsomedial* (DMPO), *dorsal* (DPO), *dorsolateral* (DLPO), and *ventromedial* (VMPO) regions.
• The *preolivary nucleus* is medial and ventral (MPO).

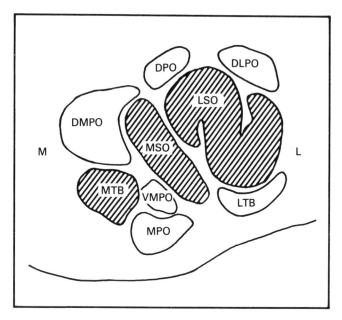

Figure 3.11
Topography of the superior olivary complex. The complex of nuclei is shown from a
frontal section in the cat with its medial boundary (M) to the left and its lateral one
(L) to the right. Nuclei receiving inputs from the cochlear nuclei are hatched. LSO,
MSO, the principal lateral and medial olivary nuclei; MTB, LTB, the medial and lateral
nuclei of the trapezoid body; DMPO, DPO, DLPO, VMPO, the dorsomedial, dorsal,
dorsolateral, and ventromedial periolivary nuclei; MPO, the medial preolivary nucleus.
(From Harrison & Howe 1974, after Morest 1968)

Certain of the olivary nuclei receive afferents from the cochlear
nuclei via the intermediate and ventral acoustic striae: these are the
nuclei LSO, MSO, and MTB. The MSO is innervated by both ipsilateral and contralateral fibers, whereas the LSO receives a direct input
only from ipsilateral afferents. The MTB, in contrast, only receives
inputs from the contralateral CN and relays them to the adjacent
LSO.

The preolivary and periolivary nuclei constitute the source of the
olivocochlear bundle, which we will return to below.

2.2 FUNCTION: TONOTOPICITY AND SOUND LOCALIZATION

As we saw in chapter 1, psychophysical observations suggest two
principal distinct mechanisms for localizing the direction of sound
sources: At low frequencies these operate on the basis of detecting

phase disparities between the sound waves that reach the two co-chleas, and at high frequencies they rely on interaural intensity dis-parities. These results require there to be neurons in the auditory pathways that receive binaural inputs and are sensitive to either phase or intensity differences and in this way provide a functional neuronal basis for dichotic sound localization.

The superior olivary complex (SOC) is evidently the first level where neurons exist that effectively receive signals from both co-chleas and can thus provide a coding of such binaural disparities.

Note first of all that in the cat the destruction of the trapezoid body, that is, an effective interruption of the interolivary commissure, significantly diminishes the animal's sound localizing capabilities. A typical neurophysiological experiment was that of Masterton and Dia-mond (1967), which consisted in training cats to distinguish between a sequence of click stimuli, one first to the left and then to the right (L-R) and alternatively the opposite sequence (R-L). The minimal in-terval disparity (δt) detectable by a normal animal is about 50 μs. After destruction of the trapezoid body, δt increases to 500 μs, a value far greater than any temporal disparities that normally can be shown to suffice for a good lateralization of a sound source. In con-trast, transection of the commissure between the inferior colliculi or of the corpus callosum that connects the cortical acoustic areas of each side brings with it no such gross deficit in this respect (Moore et al. 1974).

Single-unit researches have been made on a variety of species, dog (Goldberg & Brown 1968), cat (Watanabe et al. 1968; Guinan et al. 1972a,b), and kangaroo rat (Moushegian et al. 1975). The superior olive contains only about half the number of cells in the cochlear nucleus, which implies a certain convergence of the output signals from the CN.

Electrophysiological experimentation has clearly established the following:

• The existence of tonotopicity in both the principal and medial acces-sory olives and, apart from those, in the trapezoid body (figure 3.12).
• The presence of *binaural* cells, that is, those that respond to stimula-tion of both cochleas, of which certain cells are excited from both (*EE cells*) while others are excited by inputs to one ear and inhibited from the other (*EI cells*). Most often, but not invariably, it is the contralat-eral ear that is inhibitory.

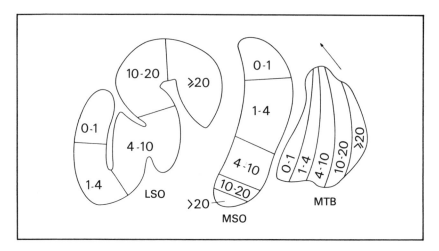

Figure 3.12
Tonotopic organization in the superior olivary complex. Boundaries of different frequency ranges (kHz) found in LSO, MSO and MTB: cf. figure 3.11. (From Guinan et al. 1972a)

• There is a complex arrangement of EE and EI cells, their respective proportions depending on what particular part of the olive they occupy (Goldberg & Brown 1968, 1969; Watanabe et al. 1968; Guinan et al. 1972a,b; Moushegian et al. 1975).
• The tuning curves of EE cells are similar for stimulation via either ear, including their flanking regions, like those seen in the CN.

Let us concentrate on binaural cells and their implications for sound localization (figure 3.13; Goldberg & Brown 1969). First consider the case of cells with high f_c (1.5 to 12 kHz). These neurons have different behavior depending on whether they are EE or EI. It is usual for EE units to respond to an increasing intensity by a sigmoidally increasing discharge rate. When stimulation is binaural, the resultant curve rises more rapidly than the curves for monaural stimulation, ipsilateral or contralateral.

To study the nature of the binaural interaction near f_c, we might, for example, fix the ipsilateral intensity (I_i) and study how the discharge rate changes while increasing the contralateral intensity (I_c). The result is a straight line, and different I_i values produce a family of straight lines that are almost parallel. From these curves we can easily predict either the change of discharge rate resulting from an increase in the intensity to both ears (common intensity) or the changes resulting from interaural differences in intensity (δI). We then observe that for EE neurons the curve for common intensity change has a steep gradient, whereas that for interaural intensity differences is practically horizontal; in other words, these EE neurons are very sensitive to differences in the common intensity but very insensitive to interaural intensity changes.

EI cells respond quite differently. The characteristic curves relating cell discharge to sound stimulus intensity are clearly different for inputs to the excitatory or to the inhibitory side; in this case the binaural curve lies between the two monaural curves, one of excitation, the other of inhibition. If we trace such curves, like those described in the last paragraph, for a given intensity of the excitatory input but now with a varying inhibitory intensity, we obtain a family of curves with a negative slope. If we then determine how the discharge varies for a common intensity change and for intensity disparities, the result is the opposite of that seen for EE cells: There is a very high sensitivity to changing interaural disparity and a feeble sensitivity to common intensity change. These EI neurons contribute to spatial localization of the stimulus that is based on intensity differences (figure 3.13).

Now consider the case of EE cells with low f_c. As in the cochlear nucleus, their monaural discharge rate increases with increasing intensity. In addition, the discharge rate varies with the phase of the incident sound wave, but in these cells the favored phase for an ipsilateral input does not necessarily coincide with that for a contralateral one. Such cells can therefore form a neural basis for localization by interaural (temporal) phase disparities.

Let us suppose that two stimuli are applied in such a way that for the cell being studied the successive peaks in response coincide. In this case, there will be a maximal discharge as a result of facilitatory interaction. However, it should be clear that simultaneity of responses does not necessarily imply simultaneity of the stimuli. To the contrary, in general there exists an optimal latency difference (specified by researchers as a *characteristic delay*) between the response of a cell to a stimulus applied to one or to the other cochlea. What is more, the characteristic delay also seems to vary little with the sound frequency; thus the cell cannot be said to be sensitive to *phase* but rather to a *time* disparity. Thus on displacing the two stimuli away from the characteristic delay, it is possible to find a disparity where the response, instead of being maximal, becomes relatively inhibited;

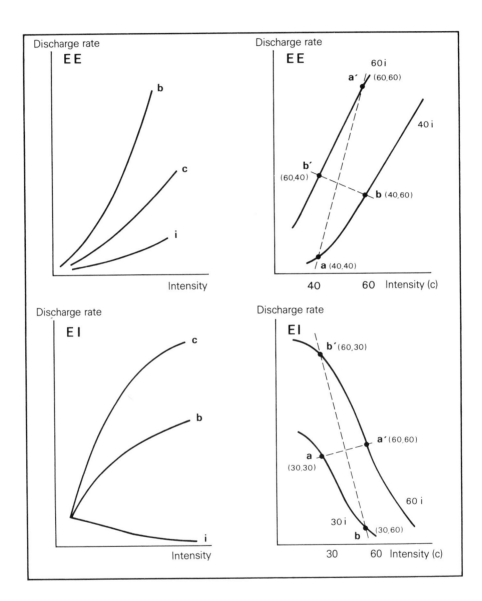

this applies for all delays between the characteristic delay peaks (figure 3.14). It is also notable that the position of the maxima and minima defined by these curves is rather insensitive to the intensity of the incident stimuli. Finally, it must be said that the participation of EI-type neurons in the perception of interaural phase differences has been disputed from the beginning, although it now appears to be accepted (even though only delays to one side might be effective). We do not want to dwell too much on this matter.

However attractive the hypothesis that such interactions constitute a neuronal basis for localization based on temporal disparities (for low-frequencies sources), one more difficulty is that the disparities for best excitation seen in these cells are often much greater than δt values created by real sources. There is a problem here in trying to relate the physiological data to psychophysical responses.

3 THE NUCLEI OF THE LATERAL LEMNISCUS

3.1 STRUCTURE

In the ascending tracts of the lateral lemniscus between the level of the pons and the inferior colliculus there are found clusters of nuclei referred to as the *nuclei of the lateral lemniscus* (NLL); three of these are distinguished as the *dorsal nucleus* (DNLL), the *intermediary nucleus* (INLL), and the *ventral nucleus* (VNLL). These nuclei receive inputs from auditory afferents but in a very complex way.

The *DNLL* receives fibers from the SOC and from the contralateral DNLL and also a few rare fibers from the CN. Therefore this structure is largely binaural, since the SOC itself, or a considerable proportion of it, receives afferents from each cochlea.

◀ Figure 3.13
Localization mechanisms based on interaural intensity differences. *Above*, EE type olivary neuron. Stimulus duration 100 ms at frequency f_c. *Left*, Discharge rate/intensity characteristics for contralateral (c), ipsilateral (i), bilateral (b) stimulation. *Right*, Parametric curves of discharge rate/intensity characteristics, for case of a fixed ipsilateral sound intensity (i) with the contralateral intensity (c) varying with abscissa value (dB). The two curves are for (i) = 60 dB and (i) = 40 dB. The straight line joining (a) to (a') corresponds with a *simultaneous* increase of the two intensities (i) and (c), i.e., passing from the condition 40 dB, 40 dB to the condition 60 dB, 60 dB. The straight line joining (b) and (b') corresponds to a reversal of the interaural intensity difference, i.e., passing from the condition 40 dB, 60 dB to the condition 60 dB, 40 dB. *Below*, EI olivary neuron. *Left*, Same stimulation conditions as above. *Right*, As above (but for (i) = 60 dB and (i) = 30 dB) and again with aa' representing simultaneously increasing (i) and (c), and bb' representing passage from one interaural difference to the opposite one. (After Goldberg & Brown 1969)

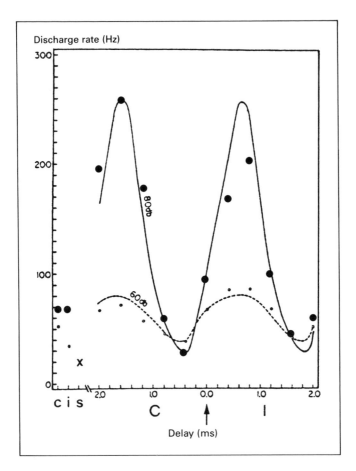

Figure 3.14
Mechanisms of localization based on interaural temporal disparities. Olivary cell, f_c = 444.5 Hz; stimulus duration 1 s; applied with different delays contralateral (c) and ipsilateral (i). The arrow marks zero delay; contralateral and ipsilateral delays to the left and right, respectively. The curves are for two stimuli at 80 dB (solid circles) and at 60 dB (open circles). The points to the left of the curves are for the corresponding *monaural* stimuli, and the cross shows the discharge rate for spontaneous activity (s). (From Goldberg & Brown 1969)

The *VNLL* is served by contralateral CN afferents, very few from SOC, and none from the contralateral NLL. This formation is thus largely monaural (contralateral).

The *INLL* receives principally from the medial nucleus of the trapezoid body (MCTB) and is equally essentially monaural and contralateral.

Lateral to the NLL nuclei is another region, the *sagulum,* which projects massively to the medial geniculate body.

3.2 FUNCTION

We will not linger very much over the response properties of the NLL; they are not very different from those seen at lower (SOC) and higher levels (IC). A few observations will suffice (see Aitkin et al. 1970; Moore et al. 1974; Glendenning et al. 1981):

• In monaural stimulation, low frequencies are represented more dorsally than high.

• Response patterns following excitatory stimuli are as variable as in the nearby centers, with both tonic and phasic characteristics existing.

• The frequency representation is also similar to that in nearby centers, with tuning curves more or less dissymmetrical with the low-frequency side less steep than the high.

• With binaural stimulation, cells mostly show EI responses. As in the SOC, there are cells sensitive to interaural intensity differences for cells of high f_c and to temporal disparities for cells of low f_c.

4 THE INFERIOR COLLICULUS

4.1 STRUCTURE

ARCHITECTONIC DIVISIONS

It has become the custom (Rockel & Jones 1973a,b), based on cytoarchitectonic studies exploiting Nissl staining or others using Golgi impregnation, to divide the inferior colliculus (IC) of the cat into a *central division* (ICC), a *pericentral division* (ICP) that brushes it dorsally and posteriorly, and an *external division* (ICX) that borders it laterally and anteriorly. The nucleus ICC is itself divided into a *dorsomedial division* (ICCDM) containing large cells and a *ventrolateral division* (ICCVL), where the cells are predominantly of moderate or small size (figure 3.15).

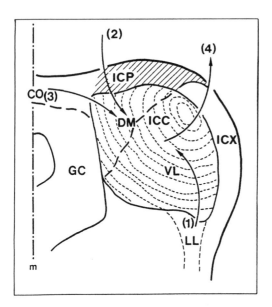

Figure 3.15
Organization of the inferior colliculus in frontal section. ICC, central nucleus with
its dorsomedial (DM) and ventrolateral (VL) subdivisions; ICP, pericentral nucleus;
ICX, external nucleus; LL, lateral lemniscus; GC, central grey; CO, intercollicular commissure. (1) Ascending projection through the lateral lemniscus; (2) descending fibers
from the cerebral cortex (corticocollicular); (3) fibers from the contralateral IC; (4) efferent projections from IC to the thalamus. Dashed lines show the concentric laminations
defined by the dendritic planes in ICC; m shows the midline. (From Rockel & Jones
1973a)

More recent work by Oliver and Morest (1984) confirms this organization while introducing an even larger number of subdivisions (figure 3.16). This more detailed segmentation rests on a reexamination
of dendritic organization and cellular structure. In a certain part of
the IC, disk-shaped cells predominate with their dendrites lying in a
plane. These cells are so situated that they constitute sheets of neurons (*fibrodendritic laminae*) along which are also found ranks of auditory afferent axonal terminals. Within a given subdivision of the IC
the fibrodendritic laminae are arranged parallel to one another.
    The ventrolateral part of the ICC (ICCVL) is subdivided into four
sections, medial (M), central (C), lateral (L), and ventral (V). In C and
M the fibrodendritic laminae are arranged parallel to one another
and inclined at about 50° to the horizontal plane. However, in L the
inclination of the laminae is at right angles to the others.

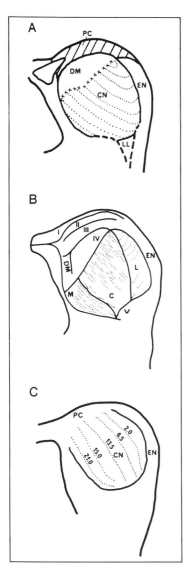

Figure 3.16
Comparison of structural models of IC (in frontal section). *A*, Rockel and Jones' model (figure 3.15) with the concentric lamination following the dendritic orientations. There is a different nomenclature in this diagram. Here PC represents ICP, CN represents ICCVL, EN represents ICX. *B*, Oliver and Morest's (1984) model showing the subdivisions of CN: L, lateral; C, central; M, medial; V, ventral. Note the differences in lamination of M and C compared with that of L. Note also that here the nucleus PC (ICP) shows lamination (layers I, II, III, IV). *C*, Recent data of Servière et al. (1984), showing isofrequency contours in ICC determined by 2-DG. (From Servière et al. 1984)

Above the ICC and lying dorsally and caudally there is a cortical zone (where four layers can also be distinguished but not necessarily with recognizably laminar dendritic arrangements) which in essence corresponds with the region usually referred to as the ICP.

ICC is surrounded by scattered *paracentral nuclei (ventral, lateral, rostral, and commissural)* without any typical lamination. Part of this constitutes the external nucleus ICX (or EN).

To summarize, these proposed new divisions do not fundamentally modify the older classification apart from one change that might be important: Rockel and Jones (1973a,b) had described in their study a rather different arrangement of laminated structures in the ICC, as being arranged concentrically and situated dorsoanterolaterally. We have just seen that the new study does not attribute a concentric arrangement to these laminae.

ORGANIZATION OF THE PATHWAYS

The connections in IC (ICC, ICP, ICX) are immensely complicated in detail. Three different categories of axons with different origins arrive there: (1) those that have passed along the ascending tracts in the lateral lemniscus, (2) others arising from the auditory cortex, and finally (3) those from the contralateral IC.

Afferent axons from the lemniscus are either second-order neurons from the CN or third-order neurons from the SOC or eventually from nuclei of the lateral lemniscus itself (VNLL or DNLL). These tracts, which serve effectively all three divisions of IC (central, pericentral, and external), can be either direct or crossed. Crossed inputs can involve either bulbar pathways (acoustic striae or trapezoid body) or, for some of the lemniscal fibers, arrival via the *commissure of Probst,* which cross-connects symmetrical groups of NLL nuclei. Finally, crossed connections can arrive from the opposite IC in the intercollicular commissure.

In the ICC, details of the very complex connections of the three principal characteristic types of lemniscal input have been examined above. These can come from (1) contralateral CN, (2) ipsilateral and contralateral LSO, (3) ipsilateral MSO, (4) ipsilateral DNLL, or (5) ipsilateral and contralateral VNLL.

This distribution poses a problem. Histological techniques (and equally, as we shall see, physiological recordings) suggest that these projections are arranged according to a *single* tonotopic scheme. Yet the sharing of these projections to the two divisions (ICCVL and

ICCDM) does not seem to be really identical: The lateral superior olive (LSO) projects to ICCVL, whereas the ipsilateral CN and the contralateral IC project preferentially to ICCDM (Brunso-Bechtold et al. 1981). Therefore, the whole status of the IC seems to have been arranged so that in spite of a single global tonotopicity there exists at the same time many *parallel paths* which have far from similar properties (in particular with respect to their laterality, as well as some being monaural and others binaural, and so on). In other words, in the IC a certain segregation of different auditory processing mechanisms is established in spite of a common global tonotopicity (Roth et al. 1978).

Apart from its projections to the medial geniculate body, the ICC sends fibers to the superior colliculus (SC), to the cerebellum, to pretectal regions, and to the mesencephalic reticular formation.

ICX connections are much more complicated. Effectively, these neurons receive, in addition to lemniscal inputs, a certain number of projections from the auditory cortex, others from the principal nuclei of ICC, and, above all, somesthetic afferents arising in the dorsal column nuclei. These in turn project to the medial geniculate body (but in rather limited numbers), to the superior colliculus, and finally to pontine nuclei for relay to the cerebellum and the mesencephalic reticular formation.

4.2 FUNCTION

We shall select from the multitude of IC functional studies only those results that describe phenomena other than a simple relaying of afferent information and that therefore demonstrate the particular functions of this nucleus.

The IC, as described above, is essentially arranged in three divisions, the central nucleus (ICC) with the pericentral and external areas ICP and ICX. The physiological data also essentially correspond with these three levels (Aitkin et al. 1975).

THE CENTRAL NUCLEUS

The central nucleus (ICC) is the principal processing station for outputs to the medial geniculate body. Its particular functional response properties are as follows:

The tuning curves of ICC cells tend to be sharper than at lower levels, even though their sharpening (attributed to lateral inhibition) is not as universal as earlier authors have suggested (figure 3.17).

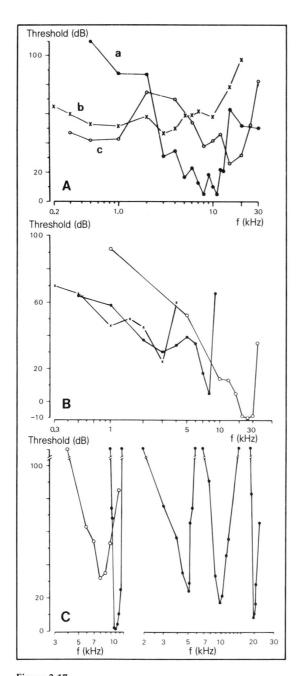

Figure 3.17
Tuning curves in different nuclei of inferior colliculus. *A*, From ICP (a) and ICX (b, c). *B*, wide and *C*, narrow ICC tuning curves. (From Aitkin et al. 1975)

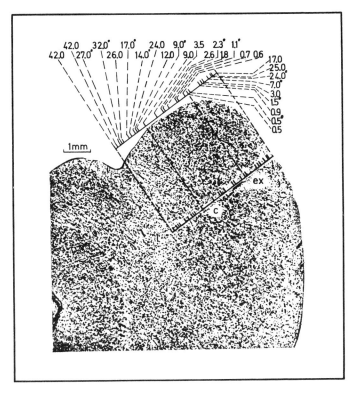

Figure 3.18
Tonotopic organization of IC in the cat (in frontal section). The continuous line shows electrode track. The f_c values marked with a dot are for single units, the others show the f_c of the maximal response measured in a simultaneously recorded *group* of neurons. Note the existence of a double tonotopicity, one corresponding with ICC (c), the other with ICX (ex). (From Rose et al. 1963)

The tonotopic organization, that is, the systematic mapping of preferred frequency of neural units, is relatively complicated. Generally, it might be described as globally in the dorsal-ventral direction with low frequencies more dorsal and high more ventral (figure 3.18; see also Rose et al. 1963).

However, the arrangements are more subtle in detail, since units of similar f_c are arranged along a horizontal plane from the medial side but this *isofrequency surface* curves ventrally and at the same time laterally and anteriorly. This arrangement is even more complex for units of low f_c (situated dorsally in the ICC) than for the high f_c surfaces (situated more ventrally) and is such that an electrode enter-

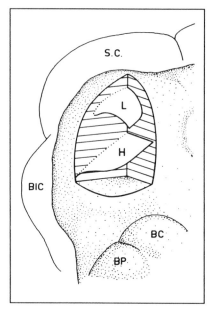

Figure 3.19
Isofrequency surfaces in IC of the cat. Diagrammatic representation of a low-frequency (L) and a high-frequency (H) isofrequency sheet viewed within the left IC from an anterolateral direction. BIC, brachium of the inferior colliculus; BP, pontine brachium; SC, superior colliculus. (From Semple & Aitkin 1979)

ing in a direction anterodorsal- to -posteroventral in a parasagittal plane will cross successive isofrequency layers (Semple & Aitkin 1979; Servière et al. 1984). These results are shown in figure 3.19.

Traditionally, the IC has been regarded as dedicated to sound localization. Much powerful and interesting experimentation has been carried out in this respect (figure 3.20; see also Rose et al. 1966; Semple & Aitkin 1979).

The well-used classification for SOC (into EE and EI cells) has accrued such complexity and diversity after more recent investigations into the binaural characteristics of cells at all levels (but in IC in particular) that it is not always easy to find one's bearings with respect to earlier descriptions. Some researchers have adopted the following classifications (note that all the special responses used to specify cell type come from observations taken at f_c).

• *EO cells* respond from one ear only. There is no influence during monaural or binaural stimulation from the other ear; most are excited by a contralateral stimulus.
• *Characteristic-delay cells* stimulated binaurally are influenced by interaural phase disparities; among these cells, some are excited by monaural stimulation from either ear and others only from one ear (ipsilateral for some, contralateral for others).

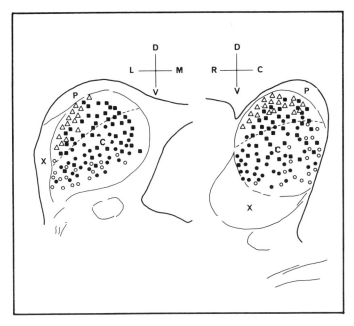

Figure 3.20
Binaural cells in the inferior colliculus. Relative proportions of different types of cells in the C, P, and X divisions of IC shown in frontal section (left): L, lateral; M, medial; D, dorsal; V, ventral; and in longitudinal section (right): R, rostral; C, caudal. The dashed line indicates the isofrequency contour for 3 kHz. Squares, EE cells; full circles, delay cells; open circles, EO cells. (From Semple & Aitkin 1979)

- *EI cells* are excited from one ear (generally the contralateral); stimulation of the other ear itself generates no response but profoundly inhibits the response from the opposite ear.
- *EE cells* are excited from either ear separately, and there is no essential change in the binaural response when either the interaural temporal or intensity disparity is changed.

This is the classification that will be used here. (Various groups of IC researchers have adopted different schemes, based on different criteria specifying the cells' monaural, binaural, summation, and inhibition characteristics, among others, in determining their different responses—see, e.g., Imig & Adrian 1977; Phillips & Irvine 1983—but it is not possible to consider all of these in detail now.)

In the examples already quoted with respect to superior olive cells, it was recognized that there are EE cells at high f_c that are sensitive to intensity changes that are *common* to both ears, whereas EI cells at high f_c are sensitive to *differences* in interaural intensity. These can therefore provide localization information at *high* frequencies. The characteristic-delay cells mentioned as a special class in IC equally demonstrate a mechanism for interaural δt discrimination at *low* frequencies. Figure 3.21 illustrates one case that concerns a cell of *low* f_c (which consequently has a discharge locked to the stimulus frequency) and is of the type EE. Even though it can respond at a variety of frequencies, it presents a maximal response at one particular interaural time disparity between the ipsilateral and contralateral stimuli (160 μs in this example).

Moving on to consider the distribution of different types of cell in the ICC (using the classification adopted above) we find a grouping of cells according to class: EO units responding only to contralateral stimulation are sited caudally, ventrally, and laterally; characteristic-delay cells are concentrated rostrally and dorsally; EE and EI cells have maximal concentrations at different but overlapping parts of ICC with the EI cells spreading more rostrally. These distributions are to some extent "logical"; for example, cells sensitive to delay δt are localized in low-frequency regions and those sensitive to intensity disparity (EI) in high-frequency regions. But for other groupings the logic is not so apparent. Figure 3.20 summarizes the data. Experimentally, it has been shown that the relative proportions of the different cells are EE 57%, EO 25%, and EI 18%.

This type of organization in the ICC, while being very interesting, poses some problems concerning the arrangement of the projections at this level. On the one hand, there is evidently a global absence of discontinuity from the point of view of tonotopicity but, on the other hand, the distinctly different binaural responses imply segregation of function inside the nucleus. Similarly, when anatomical data are considered, they show that many different and distinct regions direct their outputs to IC (see above) of which each enjoys its own tonotopic organization but which differ from one another in their degree of binaural connections. All this leads to a dilemma: In one sense it can be asserted that these different projections are organized in such a way that a global tonotopicity makes the IC look like a homogeneous continuum, whereas the different degrees of binaural involvement establish the existence of many different pathways in the IC, each no doubt attaining its own type of decoding of incoming auditory spatial information. This reinforces the hypothesis dominating this whole

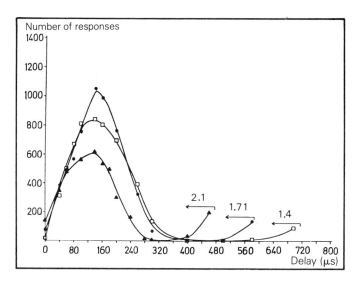

Figure 3.21
Response of a "critical delay cell" in IC of the cat. Binaural stimulation with right ear stimuli delayed with respect to left for three different frequencies (1.4 kHz 40 dB, 1.71 kHz 48 dB, 2.10 kHz 50 dB) duration of stimulation 10 s. Each point represents number of responses during the 10 s. The cell responds maximally for a critical delay of about 150 μs, whatever the frequency or intensity of the sound. In each case the periodicity of the response is equal to that of the stimulus. (From Rose et al. 1966)

discussion that there must be a multiplicity of auditory afferent pathways operating in parallel (Semple & Aitkin 1979).

One of the general problems posed by sound localization in external space is to know whether there is a representation of acoustic space in the IC. However, at present, there is no clear experimental proof of the existence of such an organization at this level, for example in the form of a topographic mapping of active collicular cells according to the location of the sound source. We shall see below that for the superior colliculus (a center considered heretofore as being chiefly visual), there is some evidence in that nucleus of a certain representation of auditory space.

In the absence of anesthesia, the ICC is found to be rich in tonic cells that discharge throughout an acoustic stimulus. But cells have also been recognized at this level that are responsive to AM or FM modulations of stimuli (Nelson et al. 1966 in the cat; Evans & Wilson 1973, Rees & Møller 1983 in the rat). The responses to modulated sounds are not always predictable from responses to pure tones.

Modulation characteristics significantly determine their response. Thus, for a given carrier frequency (say, f_c) a cell may respond very differently for different modulation rates, with a response that is optimal at some rate and is much reduced at others.

AREAS SURROUNDING THE ICC

The zones ICX and ICP, peripheral to the ICC, show response characteristics that are even more complicated (see figure 3.17).

The External Area (ICX)

Cells respond with tuning curves that are so broad that the specification of an f_c value becomes hardly possible. As in the DCN, responses with inhibitory areas are seen. In the absence of anesthesia, the variability and variety of response patterns increases yet more, to such an extent that it is scarcely possible to extract either the pattern, preferred modality, or any other simple parameter for classifying the cells into response type.

Any tonotopic arrangement there might be is practically nonexistent. Most cells have a phasic characteristic, that is, show only a transient response at the beginning of a prolonged stimulus. Most cells have a binaural input.

Some cells are influenced by somesthetic inputs, more precisely by tactile inputs (or by electric stimulation of the dorsal columns), mostly from those contralateral forelimb and hindlimb afferents that show large receptive fields (Aitkin et al. 1978; figure 3.22). Some cells are *bimodal*, responding equally to somesthetic and auditory inputs; others are *monomodal*, being either somesthetic or auditory. In bimodal cells the auditory responses are often excitatory and the somesthetic inhibitory.

The Pericentral Area (ICP)

The responses here are in some respects like those at the ICX in the sense that tuning curves are wide, the specificity to type of acoustic stimulus is poor, and the responses are essentially phasic.

Nevertheless, a certain tonotopic arrangement is distinguishable and, apart from that and unlike those of the ICX, these cells are monaural and lacking somesthetic inputs. Also in contrast to ICX, the cells of the ICP receive a host of centrifugal inputs from the auditory cortex. This is not the case in the ICX.

In our descriptions of tonotopic organizations, we have adopted the three traditional architectonic divisions ICC, ICP, and ICX, one

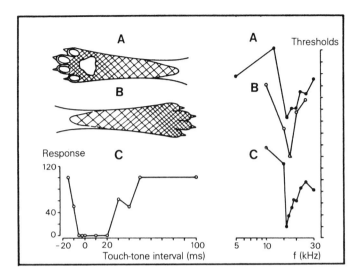

Figure 3.22
Somesthetic and auditory responses in ICX. Cells A & B: left, receptive field of their somesthetic responses; right, tuning curves of effective auditory stimuli. Cell C: left, inhibition of response to sound by previous tactile stimulation; right, auditory tuning curve. These cells were recorded respectively 2.00, 2.00, 2.05 mm below the surface. (From Aitkin et al. 1978)

reason being to allow a certain systematic approach and a synthetic view of the diverse functional properties of the auditory pathways. However (and we shall touch on this below in our discussion of tracer methods), it is probable that new physiological studies will be performed before long to discover more clearly the correspondence between neurophysiology and cytoarchitectonics, using sectioning and detailed histological fine-structure analysis by methods such as those recently proposed by Morest and Oliver (1984). The price paid for this effort might well be the need to modify many of our present views.

Finally, anatomical data show the presence of projections from the two nuclei ICP and ICX to the mesencephalic and bulbar reticular formation and from the ICX to the lower bulbar and spinal levels; people have tried to attribute functions to these pathways that are quite distinct from those of the principal auditory tracts. In particular, there are two possible ways in which they might be involved;

• The ICX, being an audio/somesthetic integrator, might contribute to a certain class of audiomotor reflexes.

• Similarly, the ICX and ICP, thanks to their connections with the reticular formation (that is, with an ascending activating pathway), might serve some of the areas that control diffuse alerting responses to auditory inputs.

CELL MARKING BY ¹⁴C-2-DEOXYGLUCOSE

We have already emphasized the importance of this autoradiographic method: 2-DG is absorbed by nerve cells—the more active they are the higher the absorption. 2-DG is then phosphorylated but not metabolized by isomerase (Buser & Imbert 1982). This cell marking therefore provides a real quantitative estimate of the amount of activity in a set of neurons under the influence of a given form of stimulation.

The method has been applied to a variety of cases in the auditory system. It is at the IC level and below that the most significant results exist for description; here and now is a good time to discuss them.

Cochlear Nucleus
Anesthetized cats exposed for a considerable time to monaural sound stimulation at 0.5, 4.0 and 15 kHz and tested by 2-DG marking have shown:

• For a given frequency, two zones of activation are 2-DG–marked, one in DCN the other in PVCN.
• At 15 kHz, these bands are most marked in the most dorsal division of each nucleus, the transverse orientation of each band corresponding with the corresponding distribution of incoming auditory fibers.
• At the lowest frequencies, the bands appear in more ventral positions (Webster et al. 1978).

IC of the Anesthetized Cat
In the anesthetized cat, 2-DG marking of the IC has been observed by Servière et al. (1984) using prolonged stimulation by pure tones. Their results show that:

• For a given frequency, a marked band of neurons is observed the orientation of which, in frontal section, is ventrolateral- to -dorsomedial.
• For a high-frequency stimulus (15 kHz), this band is relatively more medial and for low frequencies more lateral.
• These parallel isofrequency bands extend throughout the central nucleus (in its central, medial, and lateral regions) but equally overflow into the dorsal cortex (a part of the zone that we have designated above as ICP) and also into the dorsomedial nucleus.

• This arrangement does not agree with the scheme proposed for ICC in 1973 by Rockel and Jones (i.e., a concentric distribution of neuronal layers, considered to be isofrequency) but at least partially agrees—for the central and medial parts of ICC—with the more recent tracer work of Oliver and Morest (see above). They proposed a particular common orientation in fibrodendritic laminae for both the dendrites of IC cells and the terminals of the afferent axons that influence them.

• At high frequencies, 2-DG marking only occurs for contralateral stimulation (this corresponding with the dominance of EI cells at high f_c).

• At low frequencies, in contrast, marking occurs for binaural stimulation, corresponding with the EE cell type, which seems to be the most common in this frequency range (Webster et al. 1978).

• There is a problem posed by the fact that at high frequencies, depending on the organization of the EI cell, an ipsilateral stimulation is most often inhibitory; is it therefore possible to distinguish inhibition from excitation in 2-DG marking? Experiments using continuous monaural stimulation by white noise to the *contralateral* ear together with a simultaneous monaural *ipsilateral* pure tone stimulus at a given frequency have shown that when there is an ipsilateral inhibitory effect there is a corresponding zone of feeble marking that contrasts with the intense marking observed in the rest of IC at the same time (Webster et al. 1984a).

IC of the Unanesthetized Rabbit
Using an unanesthetized rabbit, it has been shown that a long-duration pure-tone stimulus has caused marking not of a single band but of many, these all being parallel to isofrequency lines predicted by the distribution of axons and by electrophysiological recording (Jones & Disterhof 1983). Clearly there are differences between the cell actions in the anesthetized and conscious animal; the differences could be due to anesthesia suppressing quite a series of projections that are presumably indirect (from the reticular formation, across the cortex, and so on).

IC of the Alert Monkey
Studies in awake monkeys by Webster et al. (1984b) should be mentioned. They show essentially the expected results with cell marking for low frequencies in dorsal regions and for high frequencies in ventral regions of IC, together with a dorsomedial- to -ventrolateral orientation of isofrequency bands at 20° to 30° to the horizontal.

Gerbil Auditory System
In this case, one cochlea was destroyed (Woolf et al. 1983). 2-DG treatment (and necessarily moanaural acoustic stimulation) showed that this ablation caused cell marking to be deficient in the ipsilateral divisions of the CN (AVCN and DCN) and also in the contralateral DNLL, VNLL, and IC. The olivary complex showed no significant metabolic difference between one side and the other.

These experiments were complemented by another series, not after cochlear ablation but after interruption of the *middle ear conduction system*. The results are somewhat surprising. Effectively, a relative *increase* of metabolism was seen in some neurons that were part of the pathway that had been deafened by conduction block. Metabolism, in fact, increased in the ipsilateral AVCN and DCN, in the SOC, and in the contralateral DNLL. This observation prompted a possible explanation from clinical experience where it is known that certain forms of conductive deafness (see appendix A) are accompanied by buzzing or humming sensations (tinnitus). A sustained neuronal hyperactivity provoked by conduction deficits could provide an explanation for this effect. However, the etiology of tinnitus is more complex (and not yet explained by 2-DG marking experiments); in particular, it is also present in sensorineural deafness (see appendix A).

Higher Levels of the Central Nervous System
It must not be forgotten that none of the above studies has demonstrated a significant 2-DG cell marking in higher levels of the auditory pathway, neither in the medial geniculate body nor in the auditory cortex. Probably the relative changes in metabolism and the present limited differential sensitivity of 2-DG cell marking are not sufficiently discriminating to be successfully exploited at these higher levels.

5 THE SUPERIOR COLLICULUS AND ACOUSTIC SPACE

We have just considered the incontrovertibly important functions of the IC in transferring acoustic signals to the medial geniculate body, in its being an integrative center and, in particular, its involvement in the localization of sound sources. There is, however, another midbrain structure that is now recognized as a site where a "topography of acoustic space" appears to be present, though this was not necessarily to be expected. This nucleus is the *superior colliculus* (SC), a center that participates in the integrative mechanisms of the visual system; we refer readers to the detailed discussion of this aspect in

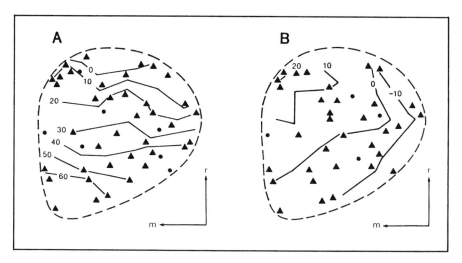

Figure 3.23
Surface maps of the right superior colliculus of response properties of cells of the intermediate gray layer following tonal stimulation from localized sources; free-field stimulation. *A*, For azimuth of the sound source, from zero to 60° contralateral. *B*, Source elevation: +, upwards; −, downwards. The lines show contours corresponding to the triangles that represent elevations for maximal response. The dots show sites differing by 10° to 20° from values predicted by the data for triangles. m, mediolateral; r, rostrocaudal directions. (From Middlebrooks & Knudsen 1984)

Buser and Imbert (1992). Apart from its very obvious visual projections, the SC also enjoys auditory (and somatic) inputs in its middle and deep layers. [In bats, who certainly benefit by being able to exploit a very special and complex system for avoiding obstacles by untrasonic echo sounding, the SC (and IC) show acoustic responses in cells of f_c between 30 and 80 kHz. It has, however, yet to be shown that the bat SC is particularly involved in the spatial skills achieved by its sonar.]

Middlebrooks and Knudsen (1984) recently studied the problem of space representation in the cat SC (figure 3.23). They found that cells responding to free-field sound stimuli are present in the mid and deep layers of the SC. These cells respond poorly to pure tones and when they do, it is with a 40-dB elevated threshold and a very wide tuning curve, no well-marked frequency selectivity.

The most effective adequate stimulus is a "noise burst" for which the threshold is only 10 dB above that determined in the same way for IC neurons.

In contrast to IC, each SC cell has a *spatial receptive field* that is, a range of spatial locations of a sound source within which it can be stimulated. Some fields are *frontal* (situated in front of the ears); others are *hemispheric*, extended over a whole auditory hemisphere, half in front of and half behind the vertical interaural plane; others are *omnidirectional*. However, each cell has an *optimal response* when the source occupies a *well-defined spatial position* not only *in azimuth* (angular distance from the sagittal plane, between 0° and 180° to left and right, with 90° representing the vertical plane passing through the ears) but also *in elevation* (positive or negative angular distance with respect to the horizontal interaural plane). This preferred direction is within a rather restricted area referred to as the *best area* for the cell. These spatial characteristics (receptive field and best area) do not depend on stimulus intensity.

Best areas are distributed in SC in such a way that azimuths 0° (straight ahead) and 80° (near the interaural axis) are respectively mapped toward the front (0°) and rear (80° contralateral) of the SC. Positive elevations (+ 20°) are found to be medial in the SC and negative elevations (− 10°) more lateral; the optimal representation is for cells responding best within about 35° around the horizontal plane.

Units quite often respond to both visual and auditory stimuli, and when they do the visual and acoustic receptive fields appear to coincide. SC thus contains an audiovisual representation of external space.

6 THE MEDIAL GENICULATE BODY

6.1 STRUCTURE

Most axons leaving the IC reach and terminate in the medial geniculate body (MGB) of the thalamus. This projection flows bilaterally to the two MGB, some pathways crossing via the intercollicular commissure, though the ipsilateral projection seems to be the more important one.

Traditionally (Morest 1964; Harrison & Howe 1974a,b), the MGB has been separated into three main divisions, the principal ventral region (MGBv), the principal dorsal region (MGBd), and a medial magnocellular region (MGBm). A number of subdivisions have also been agreed on, which we will discuss below. In addition, recent peroxidase retrograde tracer studies have clarified the precise interconnections from the IC into the three principal divisions of the MGB (figure 3.24; see also figure 3.25).

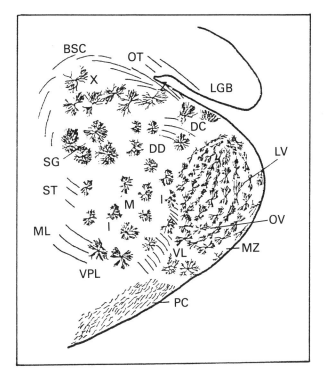

Figure 3.24
Frontal section of MGB complex in thalamus of the cat. Sketch of typical distribution
of major classes of cells in the principal divisions of the nucleus. Dendritic orientations
from Golgi-Cox method (cat 15 days old). The MGBV comprises a lateroventral zone
(LV), a more medial zone (OV), and below that the ventrolateral zone (VL) and the
marginal zone (MZ). The MGBD comprises the superficial or caudal dorsal nucleus
(DS) and the deep dorsal nucleus (DD). M, magnocellular medial nucleus MGBM; SG,
suprageniculate nucleus MGBsg; PC, cerebral peduncle; VPL, ventroposterolateral
thalamic nucleus; LGB, lateral geniculate body; OT, optic track; BSC, brachium of the
superior colliculus; ST, spinothalamic tract; ML, medial lemniscus; X, lateral posterior
nucleus. (After Morest 1964)

The *ventral division* (MGBv) has small cells (parvocellular division) within which two areas can be distinguished, one lateral (MGBvl) and one ventromedial, pars ovoidea (MGBvo). The central region of the inferior colliculus (ICC) projects massively to MGBv.

Lateral and ventral to MGBv, the *ventrolateral nucleus* (MGBvl), unlike MGBv, receives inputs from the peripheral inferior colliculus (ICP). At the lateral boundary of MGBvl it is also possible to identify a particular region, the *marginal zone* (mz).

The *medial (magnocellular) region* (MGBm) also receives projections from the IC, but some are from the ICC and others from the external nucleus (ICX). Apart from that, this region also receives inputs from the superior colliculus and the somesthetic system. The anatomical data suggests that this region may well have a multisensorial function.

The *dorsal division* (MGBd) consists essentially of two parts, the one deep (MGBdd), the other caudal or superficial (MGBdc or MGBds). Histological tracer methods suggest that the dorsal deep regions receive from ICC and the dorsal caudal from ICP.

Another division of MGBd, called the *suprageniculate nucleus* (MGBsg) receives from the superior colliculus, from the visual cortex, and from the somesthetic pathway, hence is clearly a multisensorial region.

To complete the picture concerning the thalamic projections of the IC we must mention that some fibers from the ICC project to a nucleus immediately adjacent to the MGB that belongs to the *posterior group* (PO) of the thalamus, in this case to its *lateral division* (POL).

Based on all this data, some researchers suggest that the system of projections IC → MGB comprises in fact many *parallel pathways* (Andersen et al. 1980a,b):

- ICC → MGBv (vl and vo) and ICC → MGBdd
- ICP → MGBdc and ICP → MGBvl
- ICC and ICX → MGBm
- A supernumerary pathway, not yet mentioned, leading from deep SC and the interstitial nucleus of the brachium of IC toward the suprageniculate region of MGB (MGBsg) (figure 3.25; see figure 3.26).

Horseradish peroxidase retrograde tracer studies of Calford and Aitkin (1983) have confirmed these paths but have also shown the situation to be even more complicated in detail.

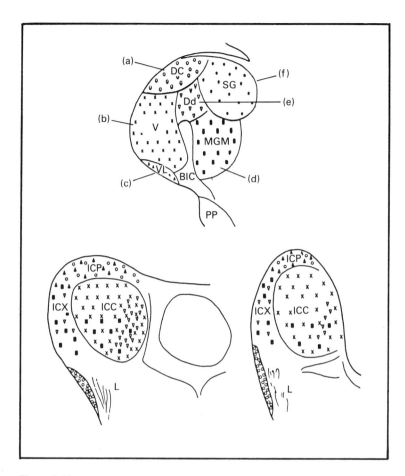

Figure 3.25
Summary of midbrain connections with the thalamus. *Above,* Frontal section across
MGB with its subdivisions: (a) DC, dorsocaudal; (b) V, ventral; (c) VL, ventrolateral;
(d) MGM, magnocellular; (e) Dd, deep dorsal; (f) SG, suprageniculate nucleus. *Below,*
Dorsal ipsilateral midbrain section, showing two frontal sections separated by 1.0 mm
together with the positions of ICC, ICP, ICX, and the nucleus of the lateral lemniscus
(L). Each MGB cell has its own class of symbol and the same symbol is used at the
midbrain level for cells marked by retrograde HRP transport after injections made in
the appropriate MGB site. (From Calford & Aitkin 1983)

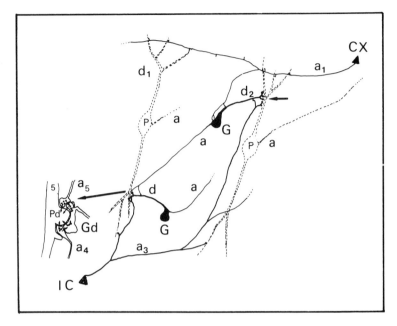

Figure 3.26
Some of the major synaptic connections in ventral MGB. Axon (a_1) descending from
an auditory cortical cell (CX) terminates on distal dendrites (d_1) of principal cells P and
on proximal dendrites (d_2) and the soma of type II Golgi cells G. Axons (a_3) from
inferior colliculus cells (IC) make contact with distal and intermediate dendrites of G
and P cells. In these arrangements can be distinguished particular zones called "axonal
nests" (or glomeruli) which in EM (left inset) correspond to "synaptic nests" (arrows).
In these structures a dendrite Gd of cell G connects dendrodendritically to a dendrite
Pd of a principal cell P. Some axons of collicular origin (a_4) and others of unknown
origin (a_5) connect with these two types of dendrites creating triads of the type $a \rightarrow$
Pd, $a \rightarrow$ Gd, Gd $\rightarrow$ Pd. (From Morest 1975). Refer also to figure 3.27.

It is in the MGBv that the fine structure of the thalamic auditory
relay has been best identified (Morest 1964, 1965, 1975). There we
see the *principal* thalamocortical *cells* (PC), which make up 50% or
more of this structure. They have bushy, widely branching dendrites
(PCd) and long axons (PCa) with very few collaterals. The PC dendrites are typically spatially oriented in a particular direction, in
marked contrast to the dendrites of cells in the dorsal and magnocellular divisions of MGB. *Type II Golgi cells* (GC), which make up 30%
to 40% of this structure, are interneurons with branching dendrites
(GCd) but with short axons (GCa) that remain internuclear.

Like the lateral geniculate body (LGB), MGBv contains systems of local, so-called *synaptic nests*, or *glomeruli*, comprising particularly dendrodendritic connections and that are often arranged as triads.

Optical and electron microscopy (figures 3.26 and 3.27) have each yielded precise data on the relationships between cell types and the two classes of inputs to MGB, that is, afferents from IC (ICa) and inputs efferent from the auditory cortex (CXa), these latter particularly being found in the glomerular nests:

• ICa afferents terminate both medial on the PCd dendrites and dorsal on the GCd cells.
• GCd cells make dendrodendritic contacts with PCd cells.
• Some GCa cells terminate on PCd cells, some on GCd cells.
• The axons of PC cells, in contrast, have no recurrent collaterals and make no synaptic contacts in the glomerular region.
• Corticofugal axons (CXa) send terminals to proximal dendrites and soma of GC, in contrast to ICa outputs, which contact GC distal parts and also the distal dendrites of PC cells.
• There are no terminals from PC on GC; neither are there axo-axonal connections between them.

6.2 FUNCTION

Response properties in cells of the thalamic auditory relay have been chiefly studied in the anesthetized animal but also in the freely moving, awake animal; the results from the latter experiments sometimes confirm and sometimes contradict those obtained under anesthesia.

We noted above that the MGB comprises several distinctive cell groupings of which the largest is MGBv and that each of several subgroups receives to some extent its own afferent input pathway from the IC. At present, functional investigations have concentrated more and more on understanding the significance of this multiplicity of different areas in the nucleus and have tried to establish an inventory of the particular functional responses of each "subnucleus" in terms of different stimulus parameters.

FREQUENCY SELECTIVITY AND TONOTOPIC DISTRIBUTIONS

We can conclude the following from the point of view of tonotopicity and frequency selectivity (Aitkin & Webster 1972; Webster & Aitkin 1975; Calford & Webster 1981):

A very good frequency selectivity is observed in MGBv (lv and ov), a moderate one in MGBdp, and a very poor one in the other divisions MGBdc, MGBsg, MGBm, and MGBvl. To summarize, in the whole

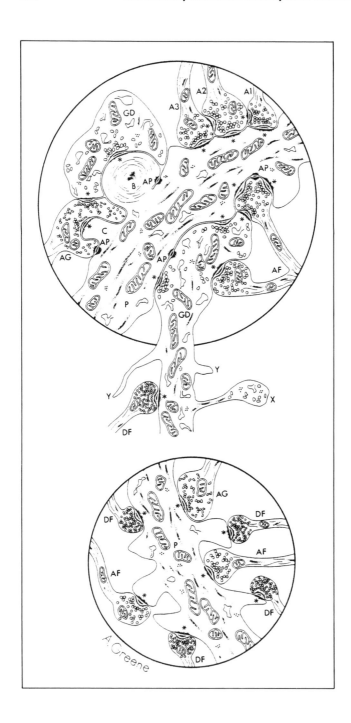

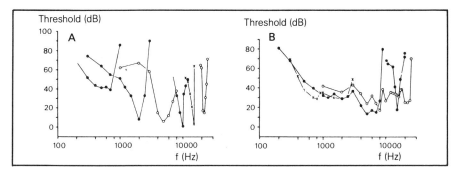

Figure 3.28
Tuning curves of MGB cells. *A*, Ventral division. *B*, Medial division. (From Webster & Aitkin 1975)

MGB there exist regions of very good frequency selectivity along with other regions that are very poorly tuned (particularly in the MGBm). It is suggested that cells that are auditory but poorly selective probably receive convergent inputs from many collicular cells, particularly from the ICP.

In the MGBv, the selective cells show, as elsewhere (see above), narrower tuning curves with better frequency selectivity corresponding to higher f_c. The increase of Q_{10dB} with increasing f_c shows no discontinuity, which suggests that MGBv is homogeneous from this point of view (figure 3.28).

The only subnucleus where tonotopicity is clearly seen is MGBlv, where each frequency has a two-dimensional representation as an isofrequency sheet. The different laminae corresponding to different frequencies are roughly parallel to the lateral surface of the MGB and arranged roughly concentrically from laterocaudoventral regions for

◀ **Figure 3.27**
Above, Organization of a synaptic nest. P, principal cell dendrite with "ball" and "claw" appendages, the former (B) containing whorls of neurofilaments and a central dense body, the latter (C) containing filamentous and finely granular material; GD, Golgi type II cell dendrite with pre- (X) and post- (Y) synaptic, filiform appendages just outside the nest. AF, acending axonal endings; AG, axon of Golgi type II cell or of an undefined extrinsic source; A1, A2, A3, sequential axo-axonic and axodendritic synapses involving small, large, and medium-sized afferent axons, respectively, and the principal cell dendrite. Asterisk, postsynaptic sites; AP, attachment plaques; DF, corticogeniculate axon. *Below*, Distal dendrite of principal cell with typical hatchet-shaped and dentate appendages. (From Morest 1975)

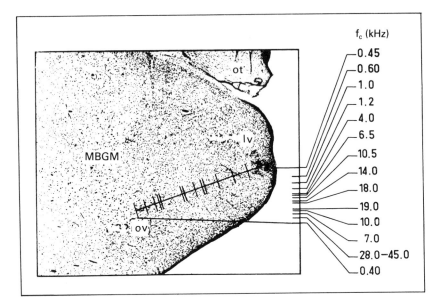

Figure 3.29
Frontal section of the anterior third of MGBM in the cat. Tonotopic distribution of f_c along a lateromedial electrode track: Note the regular progression of f_c values in the lv zone of MGBV, which becomes much more irregular in zone ov. (From Aitkin & Webster 1972)

low frequencies to mediorostrodorsal parts for high frequencies. Because of the not very simple arrangement of the isofrequency sheets, a large number of electrode tracks from various angles are necessary to establish what tonotopic arrangements there are in the nucleus (figure 3.29).

In nucleus "ov" the tonotopicity is in the opposite direction to that in "lv" and considerably more compact, though the selectivity of the cells remains good. In other nuclei it has not been possible to delineate such arrangements as these; in MGBdp scarcely any representation of other than high frequencies has been found.

Finally, in the absence of anesthesia, a state that is favorable to continuous spontaneous activity in neural units, it has been possible to identify inhibitory fringes in the tuning curves, as in other nuclei, but they are particularly common and well marked here.

RESPONSE PATTERNS

Probably this aspect of the MGB most clearly demonstrates its particular nature with respect to other levels.

Clicks or tone pips with steep onset profiles generate ON-responses that are well suited to measuring response latencies. These are quite small (7 ms minimum) in MGBv (lv or ov), a little longer in MGBdp, and very long (25 ms) and also very variable in all the zones of poor frequency selectivity (MGBdc, sg, m, and vl).

For long-lasting tone pips, most cells only respond to the stimulus onset. They behave as transient or phasic units. A rather small number are tonic, and there are relatively more of these in the magnocellular nucleus (MGBm).

Click stimuli generate particularly complex patterns (figure 3.30; Aitkin et al. 1966).

In the alert, unanesthetized animal, the number of tonic cells is considerably increased (68%) and, what is more, they show a notable diversity of response patterns (e.g., excitation, inhibition, OFF-effects, and rather complex combinations of these; see Aitkin 1975, 1976). In the absence of anesthesia, the intensity/discharge rate characteristics are generally not monotonic but show maxima.

Taking into account all these various factors, it is not difficult to predict that some response patterns will be particularly complicated, involving different combinations of excitation and inhibition all of which change as a function of frequency and intensity (figure 3.31; Webster & Aitkin 1975).

One of the questions posed by these responses particularly relates to the inhibitions seen in MGBm. Certainly some of these have their counterparts lower in the pathway and thus the nucleus could be acting more or less like a relay of afferent inputs. Nevertheless, certain data argue for local intrageniculate inhibitions: (1) In this nucleus there is a complex network of short range interneurons, as already described above, which might well be inhibitory. (2) Electrical stimulation of the pathway directly afferent on the MGB (providing simple input volleys without previous synaptic interactions) nevertheless generates not only excitatory responses in MGB but also inhibitory ones which are necessarily local in this case (Aitkin & Dunlop 1969). It is thus quite possible that many of the response patterns in the MGB are related to local inhibitory processes, and specifically this may explain why the majority of cells in the nucleus have a phasic response.

Finally, cells have been found in the MGB that respond to complex sound patterns (such as vocalization or other behaviorally significant sounds), whereas they do not respond to pure tones. Such cellular

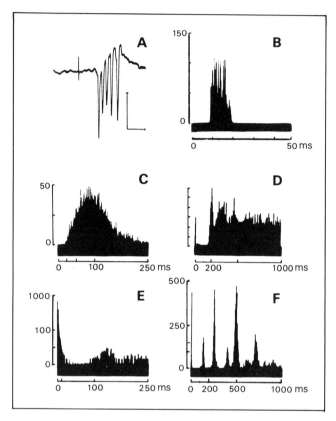

Figure 3.30
Complex responses to clicks of three MGB neurons in the cat. *A,* Unit response to a 1-ms click; note the repetitive response (time scale 10 ms). *B,* The corresponding poststimulus histogram for 662 responses of that sort (time in ms). *C,* Response of a different unit shown as spike interval histogram in the absence of stimulation (spontaneous activity). *D,* Effect of a 1-ms click. Note inhibition of the activity for about 200 ms. *E,* Spontaneous activity for a third unit; activity in bursts. *F,* Suppression of spontaneous activity by click followed by repetitive activity with peaks separated by about 200 ms. All stimuli monaural; ipsilateral in *A* and *B,* contralateral in *D* and *F.* (From Aitkin et al. 1966)

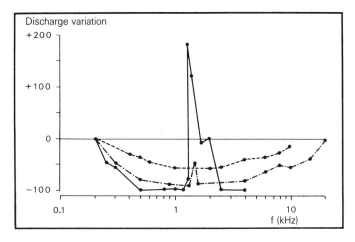

Figure 3.31
Discharge variation as a function of the frequency and intensity of a sound in MGB unit with a W-shaped response curve. Changes in total number of spikes following a tone burst of constant duration as a function of frequency for two different sound intensities; solid line, 75 dB; dots/dashes, 65 dB; dashes, 35 dB. (From Webster & Aitkin 1975)

"pattern detectors" as well as others that prefer novelty inputs (sounds that are unexpected or unknown to the animal) constitute evidence for some new integrative processing at this thalamic level in the auditory pathways.

After this brief analysis of MGB responses we can, like Calford and Aitkin (1983), devise a provisional scheme for summarizing the response properties of the principal divisions of MGB (see figures 3.24 to 3.26; table 3.1).

BINAURAL ARRANGEMENTS

Various studies have concentrated on binaural interactions in MGB cells. A large proportion of these were found to be sensitive to stimulation in either ear, some being of type EE and others of type EI, while there also exist some EO cells for which there is no influence of any sort from one ear. Globally, the relative proportions of these cell types are about the same as in ICC (EE 57%; EI 18%; EO 25%). Low-frequency EE cells are sensitive to interaural δt disparities; others of type EI are sensitive to δI differences for $f_c > 6$ khz.

Calford and Webster (1981), comparing binaural effects in MGBlv and MGBdc, showed that at low frequencies the two nuclei behave

Table 3.1. Properties of the principal divisions of MGB

MGBv (lv and ov)	Good frequency selectivity
	Short latency responses
	Good tonotopicity (certainly for lv)
MGBvl	Poor frequency selectivity
	Long latencies
MGBm	Poor frequency selectivity
	Variable latencies
	Presence of tonic responses
MGBdc	Poor frequency selectivity
	Long latencies
	Responses to novel stimuli
MGBdp	Moderate frequency selectivity
	Moderate latencies
	Predominance of high f_c
	Predominantly tonic responses
MGBsg	Bad frequency selectivity
	Long latencies
	Irregular responses

similarly with predominantly EE cells whereas, in contrast, at high frequencies "dc" contains only EE cells but "lv" includes in addition some EI and EO types.

Perhaps the most interesting of the MGB studies concerns the correlations between orderly topographic arrangements of different binaural responses found at the thalamus and at the auditory cortex at the level of AI. These experiments, based on electrophysiology with simultaneous careful histological control and mapping, are discussed in section 7 on the cortical auditory areas, immediately below.

7 THE AUDITORY AREAS OF THE CORTEX

7.1 FUNCTIONAL TOPOGRAPHIC ORGANIZATION

The final output from the auditory pathways is in the acoustic radiations from the thalamus to the auditory cortical areas. For all mammals the auditory cortex is in a subsylvian position. In the carnivores, it is largely spread over the convex surface of temporal regions; in primates, it is more or less buried in the sylvian fissure. Because of the coexisting direct and crossed connections in the auditory pathways, each cochlea is apparently universally represented bilaterally in the auditory cortex.

We shall examine below some of the functional properties of the auditory cortical areas, first from the point of view of topography and tonotopicity and then dealing with other functional factors, for a variety of species.

To repeat the principles already implicitly presented above, it is generally agreed that:

• Audiofrequencies are projected in a regular, serially ordered way to the auditory cortex.
• The cochlea also is rerepresented point by point in the auditory cortex.

These first two observations are clearly correlated but, strictly speaking, each does not necessarily imply the existence of the other.

• Many serial representations coexist within the auditory cortical areas, globally, at least in the species that have been most studied in this respect.

AUDITORY CORTICAL AREAS IN THE CAT

General Topography
Many auditory cortical areas have been recognized in the cat, each mutually interconnected with the MGB cluster of nuclei. Their responses as considered below are drawn from the cytoarchitectonic data of Rose (1949) and especially the electrophysiological work of Rose and Woolsey (1958). This is not the place to critically assess the fine detail in cytoarchitectonic data; such studies point out, in particular, the importance of cortical layers III, IV, and V. For those who are interested, more detail can be found in Winer (1984), among others.

Over time, the following areas have been mapped: area AI and area AII (both ectosylvian), an anterior and dorsal region called the suprasylvian fringe (SF), a posterior ectosylvian area (EP), and a variety of more ventral regions such as area AIII and the insular area (INS). Nowadays, different divisions and, above all, different nomenclatures have been proposed that we shall adopt here. This newer classification for the auditory areas is based on a whole series of new data, both physiological from electrical recording and histological, using cell marking techniques (figure 3.32; Reale & Imig 1980).

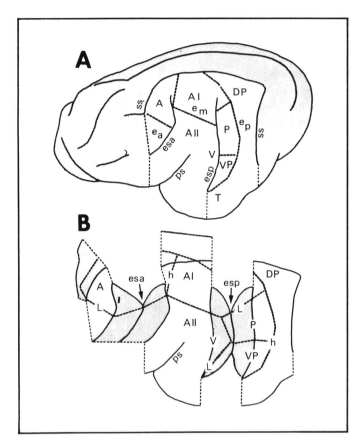

Figure 3.32
Cortical auditory areas in the cat. *A*, Positions of areas on left temporal cortex. A, AI, P, VP: anterior, primary, posterior, and ventral posterior areas. These four have a clear tonotopic organization. DP, T, V, AII: dorsal posterior, temporal, ventral, and secondary areas with broader less definite tonotopic arrangements. *B*, "Exploded" view with the posterior ectosylvian (esp), anterior ectosylvian (esa), fissure opened showing the extremities of the tonotopic arrangements for high frequencies (h) and low frequencies (l) in A, AI, P, and VP. ss suprasylvian fissure. ps, pseudosylvian fissure; EA, anterior, EM, medial, and EP, posterior ectosylvian gyrus. (From Reale and Imig 1980)

• Area *A* is the most anterior area and is situated on the anterior ectosylvian gyrus (EA).
• Area *AI* extends over the medial ectosylvian gyrus (EM) and a part of the border of the posterior ectosylvian fissure (efp).
• Areas *P* and *VP*, situated caudally and ventrocaudally, are situated essentially on the caudal bank of the efp with an extension to its rostral bank and to the posterior ectosylvian gyrus (EP). These areas occupy a part of area EP in the old conventional nomenclature. [Some authors use a more cumbersome terminology, AAF, PAF, and VPAF—AF signifying auditory field—instead of V, P, and VP].
• Area *AII* lies ventral to AI between the anterior (efa) and posterior (efp) ectosylvian fissures.
• Area *DP* is dorsal and posterior to AI.
• Area *V* is posterior to AII on the ventral border.
• Area *T* is still more posterior and ventral.

The areas DP and V correspond more or less with the areas AIII and INS in the earlier nomenclature. [Quite recently, Winer 1984 has reintroduced areas AIII and INS as entities while retaining the other newer divisions and their nomenclatures. A saga to be continued, we wonder . . .?]

Studies with histological markers (both anterograde and retrograde) have identified the ways in which ascending afferents from the various divisions of the MGB connect with these cortical areas (Imig & Morel 1984). The scheme is as follows:

• A and AI both receive afferents from various divisions of MGB (MGBlv and MGBov, the deep dorsal nucleus MGBdp, nucleus MGBm) and apart from MGB proper, from nucleus POL. The other areas P and VP have essentially the same sort of connectivities.
• In contrast, areas AII, DP, V, and T, which form (as we shall see) a sort of surrounding belt showing poor tonotopicity, are connected to the dorsocaudal nucleus MGBdc and to the medial magnocellular region MGBm.

We must conclude, therefore, that in some cases (A and AI particularly) many subnuclei of the MGB send axons to a given cortical site. This organization was recognized by Rose (Rose & Woolsey 1958) when he discovered that certain thalamic nuclei only show degeneration after ablating several cortical areas (evidence for what he called "multiple (*sustaining*) projections"), whereas other nuclei seemed to be strongly dependent on the integrity of a single site (*"essential projection"*). Not surprisingly, the elimination of all cortical areas known to receive auditory inputs (called at that time AI, AII, SF, EP, AIII, INS) brought with it a massive degeneration of almost the whole MGB.

More recently, Morel and Imig (1987) reexamined the thalamic projections to cortical areas with sharp tonotopic mapping, A, AI, P, and VP. They showed that each of these areas receives, at the same time, projections from thalamic nuclei showing sharp tonotopicity and from those with broad tonotopicity, the pattern of projections being characteristic for each site. This distribution, with convergences and divergences (which suggests the possibility of treatment of the information in parallel by several areas), does not seem to exist in the guinea pig (Redies et al. 1989). In the latter species, a point by point thalamocortical correspondence seems to be the rule. Probably there is an interesting story on phylogenetic evolution to be followed up here.

Present data obtained from cell marking have thus extended but also complicated the general notion of multiple dependence between the cortex and the thalamus. It is now seen to be present in the auditory connections.

To summarize, therefore: All the data on the auditory pathways' projections to IC, from IC to MGB, and finally from MGB to cortex, can be collated into a hypothesis, already mentioned above, suggesting that certainly in the cat the ascending auditory pathways constitute *at least two different afferent systems acting in parallel.* One is *cochleotopic,* with a good frequency resolution, and serves areas A, AI, P, and VP; the other is a *diffuse* system with poorer tonotopicity, ending especially in AII. We shall see how certain physiological data begin to confirm this synthetic view; yet in spite of its simplicity, there is not yet full agreement (Andersen et al. 1980a).

Tonotopic Arrangements
The clearest justification for distinguishing divisions between the different auditory areas in the cat arises from the existence in some of them of a particular tonotopic frequency distribution. To delineate the boundaries between these different areas needs the measurement, using tone pips, of an f_c and tuning curve for each neural unit encountered. In most cases, the animals are anesthetized, which as we shall see below seems to assume major importance (Merzenich et al. 1975, 1976) even for this sort of study.

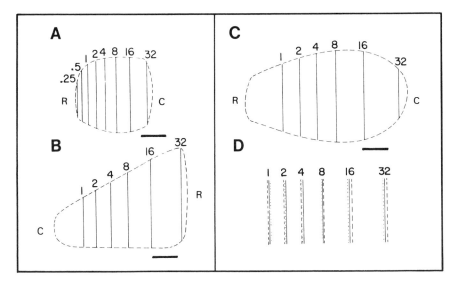

Figure 3.33
Tonotopic organizations in AI of squirrel (*A*), cat (*B*), and macaque (*C*). Gradation of frequency along the anterior-posterior axis; rostrocaudal from left to right for squirrel and monkey; caudorostral for cat. Horizontal bar under each example gives the 1-mm scale. (*D*), The tonotopic spacing of the octaves has been normalized so that the arrangements of the frequency contours can be compared directly. The relative abscissa scaling is ×2.1 for cat, ×1.2 for squirrel, ×1.0 for macaque. Note: The representations have the same proportions for each species. (From Merzenich et al. 1976)

Area AI. (See figure 3.33.) [The description "primary auditory cortex" sometimes adopted for AI should be forbidden, it seems to us. The importance of this observation will appear later.]

Exploration of AI reveals an extremely precise tonotopicity when the cells recorded from are in the mid layers (III and IV) of the cortex.

• The apex of the cortex (i.e., low frequencies) has a posterior representation (posterior ectosylvian fissure) and the base (high frequencies) is anterior (anterior ectosylvian fissure).
• Tuning curves are generally sharp, illustrating a good frequency selectivity for these units.
• Selectivity depends on f_c. It is relatively better the higher f_c (Q_{10dB} increasing, quite rapidly, as a function of f_c).
• When an electrode penetration is normal to the surface of the cortex, the tuning curves of the cells encountered have f_c values that are very close to one another. This suggests a columnar organization.

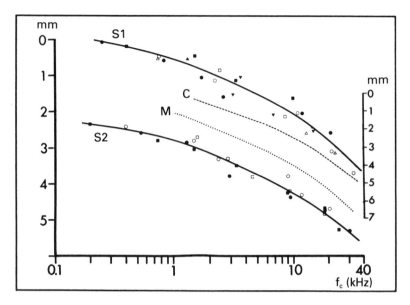

Figure 3.34
Frequency representation across AI, for squirrel (S1 and S2), cat (C), and macaque
(M). Distances are measured along rostrocaudal axis (left, squirrel; right, cat and macaque). The curves have been displaced vertically with respect to each other for ease
of reading. (From Merzenich et al. 1976)

• In contrast, the breadth of the tuning curves around f_c can vary
within a given "column"; see below.
• Each frequency is represented in an *isofrequency band*, the orientation of which is mediolateral and thus perpendicular to the direction
of the low frequency to high frequency progression.
• High frequencies are better represented in the cortex than low,
judged by the relative width of their isofrequency bands.
• Using the correlation between the frequency bandwidth δf for different f with corresponding distances along the cochlea (e.g., by
using Greenwood's formula) one can arrive at a ratio between millimeters along the cochlea from the apex and millimeters along its
corresponding cortical representation. The relationship is not strictly
one-to-one; widths of cortical bands representing equal widths of
cochlear bands are relatively more extensive for the basal projection
(i.e., for high frequencies) than for the apical projection, for low frequencies (figure 3.34; Phillips & Irvine 1981).

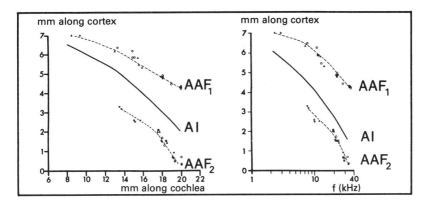

Figure 3.35
Tonotopic organization of anterior area A (here specified as AAF) studied in two animals (AAF₁ and AAF₂) and compared with area AI. *Right,* Lower curve obtained by mapping characteristic frequency at right angles to the AAF-AI border in a rostral direction. Upper curve, displaced upward by 4 mm to assist comparison with AI arrangement (middle curve), distances are now in the caudal direction from the AAF-AI border and again, for clarity, displaced by 2 mm. *Left,* Cochleotopic representation deduced from curves on the right. Abscissa, mm on cochlea obtained from nomogram like figure 2.56. (From Knight 1977)

We have already examined the essentials of the connectivity of the various divisions of the MGB to AI, in particular for the nuclei "lv" and "ov." By means of electrophysiological recording and cell marking, it has been possible to carry this much further and to specify the extremely complex relationships between a given isofrequency sheet in the MGB and the corresponding isofrequency strip in AI. From this we now know that a given "point" on the thalamic sheet is distributed to a number of points along a cortical isofrequency strip (a divergent organization) whereas, contrariwise, a restricted area of a cortical isofrequency strip benefits from several convergent projections from many points on the thalamic isofrequency sheet. We shall see below the importance invested in this organization in the arrangement of binaural characteristics of the cortical cells (Middlebrooks & Zook 1983).

Area A (or AAF).   In a general way this area, placed anterior to AI on the medial and anterior ectosylvian gyrus, has characteristics that are very like those of AI (figure 3.35; Knight 1977; Phillips & Irvine 1982).

• The tonotopic map is the mirror image of that in AI so that the high frequencies are dorsoventral, contiguous with the high-frequency

bands of AI, and the isofrequency bands start dorsoventrally and then proceed anteriorly, corresponding with lower and lower frequencies; they then curve inward to follow the curvature of the anterior ectosylvian gyrus. The high-frequency representation is relatively greater than the low frequency.
• Most cells have narrow tuning curves but others exist that show several minima (several f_c). In electrode tracks perpendicular to the cortical surface, tuning curves are very much alike with similar f_c values. This suggests a vertical columnar organization once more.

For these reasons and for others that will appear below it is nowadays considered that the two areas A and AI constitute a double system that assures a parallel treatment of auditory information contained in direct inputs from MGB, particularly from MGBv and MGBdp. [All is not absolutely clear, however, since, as we have seen, area A also receives projections from nuclei with a less tightly organized tonotopicity, in particular from MGBm. Yet no units of poor selectivity reappear in these particular cortical areas, at least under barbiturates].

Areas P (posterior) and VP (ventroposterior). Neurons in these regions have a similarly sharp frequency selectivity. In *P*, the tonotopic representation ranges from within the posterior ectosylvian fissure, then over the surface on the posterior ectosylvian gyrus. The zone corresponding to low frequencies is anterior and contiguous with AI and the higher frequencies range posteriorly (figure 3.32).

In *VP*, the low frequencies are found at the ventral boundary of the posterior ectosylvian fissure and high frequencies are situated in an extension of the region corresponding with area P, which is immediately dorsal.

Areas with poor frequency selectivity. The exact boundaries of these areas have yet to be defined. Sometimes described as a *nontonotopic surround*, the principal area is *AII*; another (dorsocaudal) is called *DP*; yet another, area *V*, is placed ventrally with respect to AII; the last, and least understood, is called *T*. Tonotopicity is less well defined than in the other areas we have just discussed (A, AI, V, and VP). We know also that the thalamic connections to these zones, where the tuning curves are most often wide, are generally quite distinct from those to the well-defined tonotopic cortical areas. Further measurements must be obtained before we can be more precise.

General Topography

Architectonic studies in primates have, insofar as the essentials are concerned, enabled a division of the auditory cortical receptive areas into regions that are distinguishable both cytoarchitectonically and by their connections from the immediately lower stage, the MGB.

Cortical regions. Cytoarchitectonically, the following areas are identifiable in the monkey and the human (figure 3.36):

• *Koniocortical areas* are characterized by their considerable graininess in layer IV. These are subdivided into median (Kam) and lateral (Kal) regions.
• *Parakoniocortical areas* with cytoarchitectonic properties a little different from the above and from one another are the internal (PaAi), rostral (PaAr), external (PaAe), and caudodorsal (PaAc).
• *Prokoniocortical areas* (ProA) and *parainsular areas* (PaI) are transition zones with the more medial insular zone.
• Other cytoarchitectonic regions less directly implicated in our present considerations are *retroinsular* (reI) and *posterior parietotemporal* (Tpt), together with *superior temporal* areas Ts3 and Ts2 (more anterior).

In monkey as in humans, the koniocortical areas Kam and Kalt are centrally placed in the areas to which auditory afferents project and are surrounded by a belt of parakoniocortical and prokoniocortical areas.

In the *macaque* the auditory areas occupy the dorsal part of the superior temporal gyrus (Pandya & Sanides 1973) and in *humans* the arrangement is essentially the same, except that:

• Area PaAc, lying caudodorsally, encroaches on the *posterior parietal operculum.* This has a certain interest in clinical neuropsychology in that a nontemporal, low parietal region is also concerned with auditory perception, contrary to the traditional opinion that limits the sensory auditory area in humans to the temporal cortex only, sometimes even to Herschl's gyrus only.
• The distribution of auditory areas spreads to two territories long distinguished in descriptive anatomy as Herschl's gyrus anteriorly and the planum temporale posteriorly (figure 3.36; Galburda & Sanides 1980).

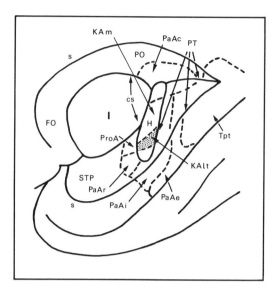

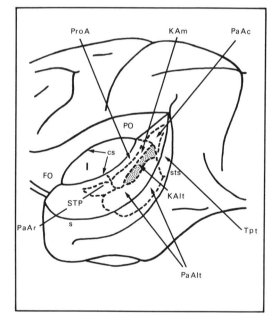

Figure 3.36
Subdivisions of auditory areas in the human (above) and monkey (below). In each case the diagram assumes that the sylvian fissure has been opened up to illustrate the extension of the auditory region towards the parietal operculum (PO) and inferior parietal lobe (area Tpt). STP, superior temporal plane; FO, frontal operculum; sts, superior temporal sulcus; H, Heschl's gyrus; PT, planum temporale; cs, circular sulcus; I, insula; s, sylvian fissure. Areas: KAm, medial koniocortical; KA, lateral koniocortical. PaAr, rostral; PaAi, internal; PaAe, external; PaAlt, lateral parakoniocortical; ProA, prokoniocortical. Tpt, parietotemporal. (From Galburda & Sanides 1980)

Thalamic projections. At the time of writing, the distribution of projections from the different areas of the thalamus to the different cortical areas seems to be much less well defined than in the cat.
The normally defined MGB divisions in the monkey are:

- *MGBpc* (parvocellular), which is lateral and has two subdivisions, *MGBpcA* anteriorly and *MGBpcP* posteriorly.
- *MGBm*, an anterodorsomedial magnocellular region.
- *MGBsg*, a dorsomedial suprageniculate nucleus.

The present specified projections of the thalamus to the cortex are:

- From MGBpcA to the true koniocortical areas, Kam and Kalt.
- From MGBpcP and MGBm to the peripheral surround of parakoniocortical and prokoniocortical areas (Mesulam & Pandya 1973).

Tonotopicity
A rather detailed investigation has been undertaken in the owl monkey. The cortical region responding to acoustic stimuli is situated on the dorsal and lateral surface of the rostral part of the superior temporal gyrus. The interest in this case is that multiple cortical areas have been discovered, characterized anatomically and to some extent electrophysiologically as well as by their connections with the MGB (Imig et al. 1977).
Six territories have been discovered, whose general characteristics show certain similarities to those discovered in the cat (figure 3.37; Fitzpatrick & Imig 1980).

- Two areas show strict tonotopicity, AI and another (rostral) area, R. In *AI*, low frequencies are rostrolateral and high frequencies caudomedial. In *R*, tonotopicity is apparently a repeat, with low frequencies rostral and high frequencies caudal.
- The surrounding belt probably comprises four physiologically distinct zones (not as yet studied in very great detail), where tonotopicity is much less clear, frequency selectivity much poorer, and response latencies relatively longer. These areas are called, respectively, *anterolateral* (AL), *posterolateral* (PL), *caudomedial* (CM), and *rostromedial* (RM) (Imig et al. 1977). To some extent these regions are distinguishable cytoarchitectonically (Fitzpatrick & Imig 1980) and by their connections with the MGB (Oliver & Hall 1978).

There is also some fine detail available for the macaque. The cochlea is projected onto the incurving superior temporal plane TI,

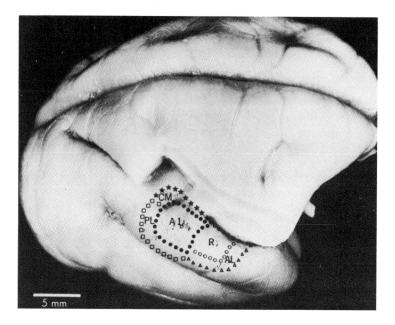

Figure 3.37
Photograph of the right hemisphere of the owl monkey, *Aotes.* Part of the parietal
operculum removed to show the superior temporal plane. Five auditory fields, with
their boundaries: AI, primary; R, rostral; CM, caudomedial; PL, posterolateral; AL,
anterolateral. The rostromedial field is not visible. (From Fitzpatrick & Imig 1980)

which is partly buried in the sylvian fissure. The projection occupies
the posterior two thirds of this convolution, the orientation of which
is practically horizontal (Merzenich & Brugge 1973). This sylvian area
comprises several contiguous zones, each to some extent tonotopically organized in a way that is more or less distinct depending on
the zone (figure 3.38).

AI is once again the area most thoroughly researched. It corresponds to a typical koniocortex region with a relatively well-
developed granular layer. Frequency representation is essentially the
same as those enunciated above for cat and owl monkey:

• The frequency band from 100 Hz to 32 kHz spreads from rostrolateral LF to caudomedial HF representations.

• Cells encountered along the length of an electrode track orthogonal
to the cortical layers show similar f_c, in other words, there is a columnar organization of frequency. Here, as probably also in the cat, it is
found that under anesthesia all the responsive cells seem to be confined to cortical layers II and IV.

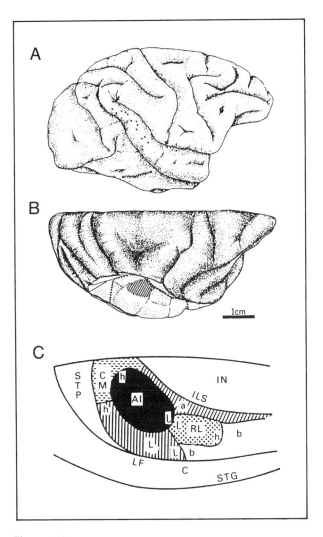

Figure 3.38
Cortical auditory areas in macaque. *A,* Lateral view of cortex; a, anterior and p, posterior poles. Arrows mark the boundaries of the superior temporal plane, where the
auditory areas are situated. It constitutes the lateral and inferior bank of the sylvian
fissure (s). *B,* Dorsal view of the temporal plane, uncovered by removing part of the
parietal cortex. The hatched area represents auditory area AI. *C,* Enlargement of the
auditory area of the superior temporal plane (STP). AI, auditory area I. Fields: RL,
rostrolateral; L, lateral; CM, caudomedial. IN, insula; SL limiting sulcus of insula; LF,
lateral fissure; STG, superior temporal gyrus. Note: Areas AI, RL, and L are tonotopically organized; h and l show high and low frequency limits. a, b, c, Areas of poor
tonotopic organization. (From Merzenich & Brugge 1973)

[We shall not deal in detail here with all animals that have been investigated. Suffice it to say that in the case of the American gray squirrel an area homologous with AI has been identified with a banded tonotopic frequency representation that is essentially the same as in the cat apart from the fact that low frequencies are represented anteriorly and high frequencies posteriorly (see figure 3.33). The area lies on a cytoarchitectonic region called *anterior temporal*. Remember also that one of the earliest signs of tonotopicity was found by Tunturi (1950) in the dog.]

Other fields have also been identified in the macaque around AI with varied arrangements of tonotopicity and which also correspond to different cytoarchitectonic structures than that of AI:

• There is a *rostrolateral* (RL) field in front of AI. But here the low frequencies are posterior (i.e., at the boundary with AI), with the high-frequency representation being anterior.
• In the *lateral field* (L), the tonotopic arrangement seems to be as in AI (low frequencies rostral, high frequencies caudal).
• A *caudomedial area* (CM) clearly responds to acoustic stimuli, but its organization has not apparently been examined in fine detail.

Homologous arrangements can clearly be seen in the owl monkey and the macaque. There are also at least approximate correspondences between their cytoarchitectonic divisions (see figure 3.36), for example:

• Between the AI areas which in each case are superimposed on the fields Kam and Kalt.
• Between the area R in one and RL in the other, in the field PaAr.
• Between the areas CM occupying zones ProA and PaAc.
• Between PL in one and L in the other, partly covering areas PaAc and PaAlt.

Similar homologous arrangements have been proposed between the cat and primates but they are much more uncertain (for example, between CM and AII or between PM and the sylvian bank SF in the old nomenclature, i.e., more or less area A in the new classification).

7.2 DETECTION OF THE CHARACTERISTICS OF SOUND SIGNALS

Apart from researching tonotopicity, it would be interesting to find out to what extent cortical cells detect particular parameters of an acoustic stimulus, whether concerned with its frequency, duration, or intensity.

In discussing frequency detection, there is no point in simply repeating the data already given above because, in the period since those tonotopic studies and the other investigations we shall mention, a new tack has been taken by various researchers who suspect that anesthesia may well be distorting the picture. Therefore, in addition to the traditional observations made using anesthesia, a corresponding series of investigations have been made on awake, alert animals. These represent a considerable step forward and have illustrated the extent to which responses become more complex and diverse than in the anesthetized state (but necessarily also become more difficult to analyze).

DURATION AND INTENSITY OF STIMULI

Temporal response patterns in cortical neural units are enormously variable in the awake, alert animal (Evans & Whitfield 1964). In these conditions, there are transient responses to tone pips but others that are sustained, and finally, other responses best described as complex combinations of excitation and inhibition. There seems to be no particular spatial distribution, laminar or columnar, for these various categories of response. In addition, response patterns can vary according to the frequency of the stimulus (figure 3.39).

As already pointed out, latencies in cortical cells depend on the cortical area they occupy; in particular they are smaller (20 ms) in A and AI than elsewhere in the cortex and particularly than in the posterior area P (Phillips & Orman 1984).

For a good number of cortical cells the discharge rate/stimulus intensity characteristic at a given frequency is nonmonotonic but shows a maximal value; in certain cases this curve can even be very sharp, indicating not only a preferred frequency but also a region of preferred sound intensity (the latter is seen often for frequencies near f_c). In these conditions a sound of a given frequency will generally only induce responses in a limited number of neurons as its intensity increases. But because of the sharpness of the response curve, these neurons will be particularly sensitive to variations of monaural intensity for frequencies around f_c.

Nevertheless, it must be remembered that much variability of temporal response patterns, particularly latencies and others such as the intensity/discharge rate characteristic, already exist at least to some extent at the next lower level: We cannot therefore rigorously attribute them to purely cortical neuronal processing mechanisms.

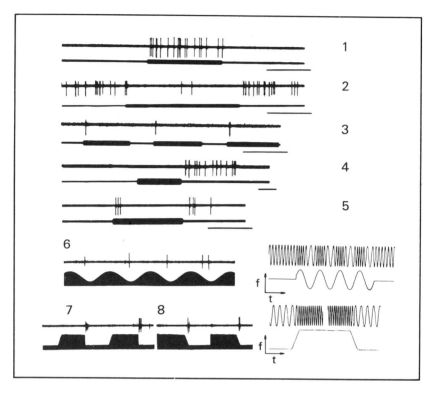

Figure 3.39
The various responses of AI cortical cells in the cat. 1 to 5, Responses to prolonged
stimuli: time bars = 0.5 s. 1, sustained excitation; 2, sustained inhibition; 3, ON
response; 4, OFF response; 5, ON-OFF response. 6 to 8, Responses to frequency
modulated sound: 6, sinusoidal modulation waveform; 7, 8, trapezoidal waveforms.
The insets on the right each show sound stimulus waveform above, frequency modulation waveform below. (From Evans & Whitfield 1964 and Evans 1982a)

STIMULUS FREQUENCY

It is in the fine structure of tonotopic arrangements and even more
in the shape of tuning curves that the greatest changes are seen in
experimental observations once the depth of anesthesia begins to be
reduced. If in a given restricted zone of cortex the f_c values of cortical
cells have every chance of being similar, the organization nevertheless does not show (even at this level, according to most researchers)
the precision of the columnar organizations seen in the visual and
somesthetic systems. A wide range of tuning curve widths is found
(figure 3.40), even in cells along a single radial electrode track (Erulkar

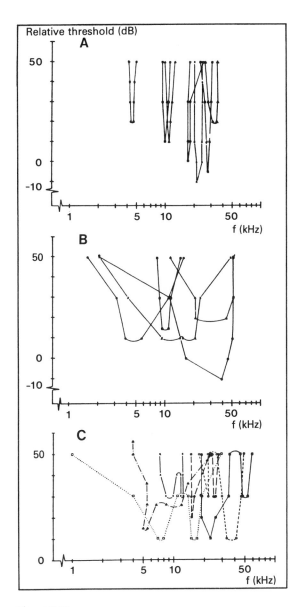

Figure 3.40
Tuning curves for auditory cortical cells in the cat. *A*, Narrow tuning curves. *B*, Broad tuning curves with single maxima. *C*, Tuning curves with multiple maxima. (From Abeles & Goldstein 1970)

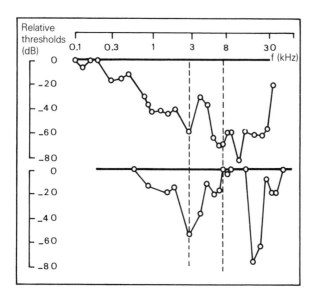

Figure 3.41
Complex tuning curves of auditory cortical units found in a single electrode penetration. *Above*, Very broad tuning curve. *Below*, Curve with multiple peaks. (From Oonishi & Katsuki 1965)

et al. 1956; Evans et al. 1965; Goldstein et al. 1968; Abeles & Goldstein 1970; cf. Goldstein & Abeles 1975).

It is also not rare to encounter cortical tuning curves with multiple minima corresponding to several f_c values (Oonishi & Katsuki 1965) and other curves for which the peak is so flat that it is difficult to ascribe any f_c value to the response (figures 3.40B, C and 3.41).

By analogy with what happens in the visual cortex, it might be expected that these cells with flat responses would be situated in an upper layer of the cortex, that they would be the result of convergent inputs from several cells situated in lower cortical layers showing multiple peaks, and that these multiple peak responses would themselves be the result of convergence of inputs from even lower cells with single peaks (e.g., from MGB). But this hierarchical organization has not been proved in recent experiments.

Finally, it should be mentioned that tonotopicity is particularly weak and hard to specify in the awake, alert animal, whether in cat (Evans & Whitfield 1964) or in *Saimiri* (Funkenstein & Winter 1973). This loss of tonotopicity may be the result of cortical mechanisms but it may also only be the result of modifications earlier in the pathway.

(We noticed above that the tonotopicity in MGB, at the thalamic level, also becomes less well marked with less anesthesia.)

The responses to complex sound stimuli are particularly interesting in cortical cells. Cells with special sensitivity to such stimuli have been found in many species. Thus many phasic cells have been found that are specially activated by sounds that are modulated in frequency or in amplitude and by more complex sounds (Whitfield 1957; Whitfield & Evans 1965; Swarbrick & Whitfield 1972; Sovijärvi 1975 in the cat; Tielen et al. 1969 in the dog; Katsuki et al. 1962 in the macaque). Some cells that are activated by complex sounds have zero response to pure tones; in other cases, their response to modulation and to complex sounds is not predictable from the pure-tone responses (cf. Whitfield 1980, 1982).

A notable example of this complexity is shown in the macaque and especially in the *Saimiri*, where responses to free-field stimulation are particularly easily elicited by sounds in the animal's vocal repertoire, which is known to be very rich (Newman & Wollberg 1973). Among these pattern receptors, some cells are also activated by simple sounds but other cells are not (figure 3.42).

One difficulty (but also an interesting observation) arises concerning the lability or relative constancy of responses to different complex sounds. As a general rule, most researchers agree that a considerable lability is seen in cat cortical cells that is quite as large as is observed in the monkey. When recording from *Saimiri* cortical cells for several hours subjected to a series of species-specific vocal stimuli, their response properties change. The intensity of the response to a given stimulus might change as much as the response pattern as does also the response selectivity, more or less, across the gamut of different stimuli provided (Winter & Funkenstein 1973; Newman & Symmes 1974; Manley & Müller-Preuss 1978; Glass & Goldberg 1979).

To summarize, the auditory cortex shows, particularly in the absence of anesthesia:

• A wide variety of responses following the usual experimental stimuli—clicks, tone pips, frequency-modulated sounds.
• Cells that preferentially respond to one or another of these stimuli and sometimes especially well to stimuli as complex as the species' own vocalizations. It has not been possible to extract any relatively simple law concerning the generation of these responses, and no universal explanation of them is available at the moment. Selectivity to complex stimuli not unnaturally stimulates speculation on the role

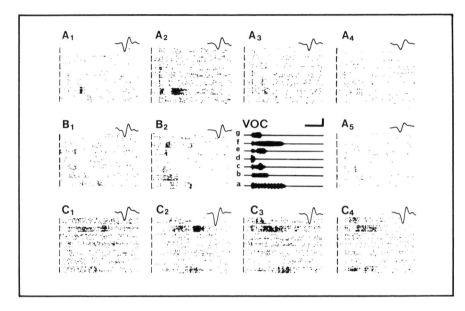

Figure 3.42
Responses of three auditory cortical cells (A, B, C) in *Saimiri* to seven types of species-specific vocalizations. VOC (center inset) shows the sound envelopes of the seven vocalization stimuli (a to g) respectively described as twitter, long peep, chirp, cackle, kecker, shriek, oink. Each stimulus presented 15 times in order a to g at zero time (vertical bars) in each dot display. Each dot generated by one action potential (illustrated above right in each diagram). The time base is 400 ms. The displays were recorded at the following times: A_1, 1707; A_2, 1753; A_3, 1848; A_4, 1933; A_5, 2025; B_1, 1715; B_2, 1808; C_1, 1511; C_2, 1605; C_3, 1837. Note that the same cell does not respond in the same way to the same cry at different times. (From Glass & Goldberg 1979)

of the cortex in the perception of biologically significant sound signals. There is no agreement yet, and some authors regard the complexity of such responses as being merely the secondary consequence of some alertness or emotion initiated by the stimulus.

Another problem concerns the significance of the multiplicity of auditory cortical areas. According to some authors, one should expect to find specialized regions for particular sorts of stimulus parameters, each area concentrating on a particular one. (In vision, this already seems to be justified by the data.) Insofar as the hypothesis has been studied in the auditory cortex, at present there is little to report, apart from A and AI enjoying similar response mechanisms and the posterior areas, P in particular, responding otherwise. Perhaps some of the new observations taking account of responses in the absence of anesthetic might add some more relevant detail.

It has been shown that many cells in the auditory cortex, in AI in particular, are stimulated from both cochleas and because of this may well be involved in sound localization mechanisms (Brugge et al. 1969; Brugge & Merzenich 1973). From the outset we find the same difficulty in discussing these results as was encountered for the IC, above—that is, how to encompass in any unified way the diversity of criteria that different research teams use to characterize the detailed operation of these cells in determining the parameters of lateralization. Some authors limit themselves to distinguishing EE and EI types; sometimes the classification is more complex, distinguishing three types (EE, EI, and EO) or specifying the dominant excitatory side (ipsilateral, contralateral, equidominant) or the type of interaction (summation, suppression, occlusion) with, finally, the introduction of further characteristics, as Rose initiated, such as specifying δt (the effective temporal disparity between binaural stimuli), and so on.

Only area AI seems at present to be well understood in this respect. Many neuronal types, particularly EI and EE, are clearly identifiable in this area. As discussed before, EE cells are excited from either ear, with a general facilitation if the stimulation is binaural. EI cells are normally excited from the contralateral ear with ipsilateral inputs being not alone excitatory but capable of diminishing any response from the contralateral input. Those, therefore, are two essential elements that we shall consider. In addition, other types have been reported; IE (with opposite laterality to EI) as well as EO (with purely monaural effects).

The EE and EI types of cells are not randomly distributed but show an orderly columnar arrangement according to their laterality parameters. In other words, an electrode penetration orthogonal to the cortical surface will encounter cells of essentially the same sort (for whatever selected criterion, EE, EI, or dominance).

An overall study of area AI (Middlebrooks et al. 1980) has shown that the columns of similar binaural reactions are arranged regularly in the rostrocaudal direction in AI (figure 3.43). In each isofrequency strip, oriented mediolaterally, are encountered successively a patch of type EI (near the boundary with AII), then more dorsally a patch of type EE, and a series of zones alternating between EI and EE up to a dorsal boundary, called DZ, with somewhat different characteristics. The result is that across AI there exist rostrocaudal bands of

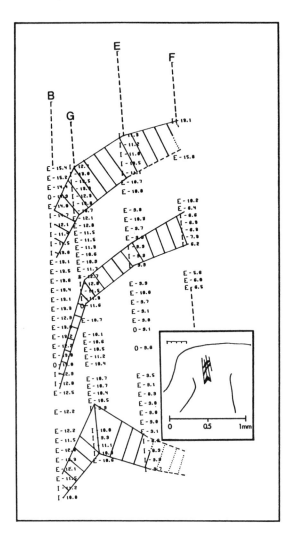

Figure 3.43
Cell-type mapping in the left auditory area AI of the cat. Inset shows cortical area mapped. The lines of letters show the types of response obtained in four systematic explorations (B, G, E, F) along iso-frequency lines in the mediolateral direction. To the right of each letter is the f_c for the cell encountered. The letter itself represents: E, an EE cell; I, an EI cell; O, a (rare) EO cell; asterisk, an IE cell. Boundaries are drawn to enclose EI cell regions which are hatched. They lie between separate EE regions. (From Middlebrooks et al. 1980)

binaural interaction, their surface map being therefore orthogonal to the isofrequency strips.

A more recent study (Middlebrooks and Zook 1983), using horse-radish peroxidase cell marking, analyzed the topological relationships between points in an isofrequency band representing at the same time a certain frequency and a certain lateralization (EI or EE) as well as the "points" on the isofrequency sheet in MGBv (lv or ov) that projected to them. The results are complicated. A given site on an EI zone receives inputs from many points on the isofrequency sheet and, conversely, a site on the isofrequency sheet projects to many points on the cortical isofrequency strip, while all of them belong to the same EI binaural classification. In other words, there exists a correspondence between an isofrequency sheet and its projection to the AI isofrequency strip of the same frequency such that there is simultaneously a convergence and a divergence, all within a patch dedicated to a given binaurality. Essentially the same type of arrangement is found for patches of EE cells. It is possible to conclude that the transfer of information from MGBv to AI does not imply any special emphasis on laterality (no more than its concern with frequency, for example). There is thus a sort of isomorphism established between MGBv and AI.

To complete this brief survey regarding adequate parameters for localization, some cells are found in the cortex that are sensitive to interaural time disparities δt, some to interaural intensity differences δI. Note, for one thing, that in the cortex the sensitivity to time disparity δt (for cells of low f_c) can in some cells be independent of frequency but in others be very frequency dependent and therefore more probably concerned with phase.

As in IC but unlike SC, there is no clear evidence for a mapping of sound space in the auditory cortex comparable with that seen for vision in the striate cortex and surrounding regions. We shall see, in section 9.1 below, how the above data and those obtained from lesions assist an understanding of coding mechanisms for the spatial attributes of sounds (Imig & Adrian 1977; Middlebrooks et al. 1980; Phillips & Irvine 1983).

However, cortical exploration does yield evidence for the existence of cells sensitive to movements of a source in a particular direction in space. These particular units respond to a stationary stimulus by an ON-discharge and an OFF-discharge. (Sovijärvi & Hyvärinen 1974).

8 CENTRIFUGAL ACTIVITY IN THE AUDITORY PATHWAYS

One of the most distinctive characteristics of the auditory system is the existence of an efferent system by which central regions can act peripherally even on the receptor cells themselves or on the cochlear nucleus, and exercise thereby a potential control of the initial message inputs to the CNS.

8.1 ORGANIZATION OF THE EFFERENT SYSTEMS

THE OLIVOCOCHLEAR BUNDLE

The best specified system, which demonstrates a variety of distinctive features peculiar to the nerve VIII (auditory and vestibular) pathway, is the olivocochlear bundle (OCB). It comprises neurons belonging to the superior olivary complex the axons of which reach and directly influence the cochlear receptor cells with connections at that level. The efferent olivocochlear fibers first travel in a branch of the vestibular nerve and are associated with the corresponding efferent vestibular fibers; they then abandon this nerve to join the auditory nerve via the *auditory-vestibular anastomosis*, which exists between the two nerves.

In the cat, the OCB contains between 1,300 and 1,800 axons, depending on the publication concerned. Some are myelinated, others nonmyelinated. More than half of these axons stay ipsilateral (58%), while 32% of them pass dorsally beneath the floor of the fourth ventricle to reach the contralateral eighth nerve and cochlea. One refers therefore to a *direct* and a *crossed* efferent path.

The detailed organization of the efferent system is, however, more complicated in the sense that the pathway innervating IHC is distinct from that innervating OHC, while each of these paths itself contains both direct and crossed components (figure 3.44) leading to the following distributions (Warr 1978, 1982):

• The (small) cell bodies of the nerve fibers innervating IHC are preferentially located in the lateral division of the olive in the dorsolateral and lateral periolivary clusters of nuclei. The lateral efferent systems are predominantly ipsilateral (86%) with only 14% of them crossing the midline (*lateral olivocochlear bundle*).

• The larger cell bodies that innervate OHC are situated more medially in the olivary complex (dorsomedial periolivary nucleus and medial nucleus of the trapezoid body). Their axons, constituting the medial efferent system, go predominantly contralateral (75%) with 25% ipsilateral (*medial olivocochlear bundle*). We shall not repeat here a description the tracts of these diverse types and their terminations on OHC and IHC (see section 3.4 of chapter 2).

The overall result is that stimulation, or interruption, of olivocochlear fibers near the midline, which therefore affects the crossed innervation, principally influences the olivocochlear control of OHC and affects that of IHC very little. We shall see that experimental neurophysiology has much exploited this happy situation. Finally, let us recall that the (internal spiral) fibers innervating IHC terminate as axodendritic (fiber to fiber) contacts, whereas those innervating OHC make axosomatic connections.

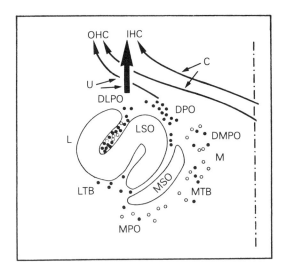

Figure 3.44
Position of the cells of origin of the olivocochlear bundle (principally determined by
HRP methods). Frontal section: L, lateral and M, medial. The interrupted straight
line shows the midline. LSO, MSO, DLPO, DPO, DMPO, MTB, LTB, MPO are the
subdivisions of the olivary complex. Filled and open circles show, respectively, the
cell bodies of the uncrossed and crossed OCB. The uncrossed OCB (U) has a considerable input from the lateral periolivary nuclei and mostly terminates on IHC with a
path from the medial periolivary nuclei serving OHC. The crossed bundle (C) also
provides an input from the contralateral medial nuclei which above all serves OHC.
Some lateral nuclei, crossed, outputs are directed to IHC. (Data from Pickles 1982,
after Warr 1975)

DESCENDING PATHWAYS

A considerable number of descending projections have also been
identified higher in the central nervous system (figure 3.45; Harrison
& Howe 1974). Corticothalamic neurons project from the auditory
cortical areas to the different divisions of the MGB. As already mentioned, these fibers make connections essentially with the distal parts
of the dendrites of the principal cells of the MGB. As for many other
thalamocortical projections, this auditory pathway is also generally
reciprocal; in each efferent case there is a corresponding ascending
afferent pathway. At least in the cat, apparently all the MGB nuclei
(including MGBd and MGBm) enjoy projections from the auditory
cortical areas, the most prominent of which, as mentioned above, are
the connections from A, AI, and AII. A and AI project to MGBlv,
MGBov, MGBdp, and MGBm with AI also sending efferents to POL.

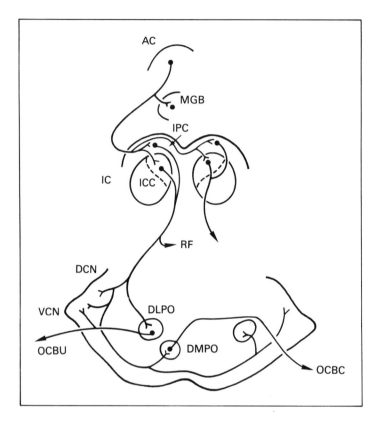

Figure 3.45
Descending pathways of the auditory system (much simplified diagram). AC, auditory cortex; MGB, medial geniculate body; ICP, peripheral area in inferior colliculus;
ICC, central nucleus of IC; RF, collaterals of reticular formation; DCN, VCN, dorsal
and ventral cochlear nuclei; OCBU, OCBC, uncrossed and crossed olivocochlear bundles. (From Harrison & Howe 1974b)

AII projects to MGBdc, MGBdl, and MGBm. The descending connections from A and AI are essentially "in register" with the ascending
tonotopicity (Pontes et al. 1975).

There are also descending projections from the auditory cortical
areas to the inferior colliculus. A detailed examination of these in the
cat shows the following organization: Areas A and AI project bilaterally (see above) to the dorsomedial part of the central nucleus of each
IC (ICCDM) and only ipsilaterally to the pericentral regions (ICP).
These efferent projections are organized tonotopically and are in register with the tonotopic organization of the cochlear representations

in these nuclei (Andersen et al. 1980a,b). Area AII projects to the pericentral nucleus ICP ipsilaterally in the lateral parts of ICP and bilaterally in its medial part. (This same study has little to add concerning any projections to ICX.)

Another efferent projection that is no doubt functionally important (remembering references above to the representation of visual space) is one that originates in the anterior ectosylvian fissure ("efa" in figure 3.32) anterior to AII and lateral with respect to A. Clarey and Irvine (1986) have shown this to provide an abundant projection to the superior colliculus and Meredith and Clemo (1989) show that it has a facilitatory action on the superior collicular responses to sound.

The inferior colliculus itself has an efferent output. Descending axons project to DCN and to certain of the olivary nuclei, in particular to the periolivary nuclei DMPO and DLPO. It is still a question where exactly these efferents originate in IC; perhaps they come from the lateral regions. As for the nuclei of the lateral lemniscus (NLL), there certainly exist descending efferent projections but, once more, these are poorly researched.

The olivary nuclei in their turn project efferents to the dorsal and ventral cochlear nuclei. Some of these are merely collaterals of the OCB. But others are more direct projections that pass along the acoustic striae. Their cells of origin are situated in the preolivary and periolivary nuclei, including also those from the trapezoid body. Some of these tracts make cholinergic terminations and others noradrenergic terminations in the CN.

In the brainstem, the descending tracts are separate from the ascending lemniscal afferents; this has been clearly demonstrated by physiological studies, as we shall see below.

One of the problems that remains to be resolved is to what extent the efferent neurons in successive levels make connections with one another and with the cells of origin of the OCB. Anatomically the facts are not very clear. Nevertheless, we are no doubt correct in speculating that the receptor cells may well be influenced from levels as high as the thalamus and cortex.

Some physiological experimentation also suggests the existence of another class of efferents with their origins, in this case, in the reticular formation. They reach the cochlear nuclei and possibly the cochlear hair cells themselves also. Anatomical data are somewhat lacking in this respect, and even the physiological results are still far from certain and a matter of much discussion, as we shall see.

Let us see what functional role can be ascribed to these various descending pathways. There are some results that are worth reporting, not all of them necessarily definitive or coherent.

INFLUENCE OF THE CROSSED OCB ON COCHLEAR RESPONSES

Essentially, these observations are achieved by stimulating the *crossed* OCB, at the level of its crossing the midline. Two types of experimentation predominate, one being the observation of global cochlear responses, the other looking at neuronal unit discharges in the cochlear afferents.

Desmedt and La Grutta (1963) and Desmedt (1975) measured response amplitudes at the round window following click stimulation. When the crossed OCB was repetitively stimulated electrically, a relative *increase* in the round cochlear microphonic amplitude was seen but also a very marked *diminution* in the peak amplitudes of the nerve responses N1 and N2. At its maximum value, this attenuation was equivalent to what would have occurred if the sound intensity had been diminished by 12 to 26 dB ("dB equivalents") while the *latency* of the response was not changed (figures 3.46 and 3.47).

More recent observations have studied the responses of single afferent fibers and their modification by repetitive electrical stimulation of the crossed OCB. Essentially, an inhibitory effect is confirmed by this method (Fex 1962; Kiang et al. 1970; Wiederhold 1970; Gifford & Guinan 1983; figure 3.48).

• The effect of OCB stimulation, once more, is equivalent to a diminution of intensity of the stimulus, from 1 to 25 dB depending on the afferent.
• The effect is frequency dependent and is maximal when the sound frequency is near the fiber's f_c.
• The greatest attenuation occurs for fibers with f_c between 6 kHz and 10 kHz. Those with $f_c < 3$ kHz are little affected.
• The attenuation in the fiber discharge is most marked at moderate acoustic stimulus intensities that are neither too weak nor too near the saturation plateau for the fiber.
• The effect shows up about 15 ms after the beginning of OCB stimulation, increases until about 50 ms thereafter, and can even continue for a while after stimulation ceases.

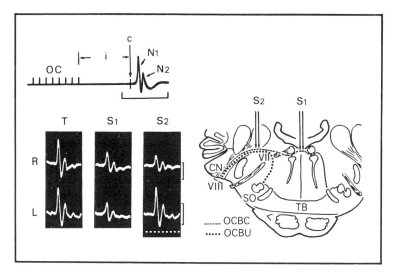

Figure 3.46
Electrical stimulation of OCB in the cat. *Above,* Stimulation scheme. The click sound stimulus (c) elicits responses N_1 and N_2 in the compound action potential of the cochlear nerve. This click is preceded (i = 15 ms), or not, by a train of electrical stimuli (OC) to the olivocochlear bundle. *Below*: T, responses at the round window of the right (R) and left (L) cochlea. S_1, same responses when C is preceded by 40 electrical stimuli at 40/s applied at S_1 (diagram on right). S_2, same responses with electrical stimuli applied at S_2 in diagram. (Ordinate bars 200 μV; abscissa bar 0.5 ms). The anatomical sketch is a frontal section at the bulbar level showing the approximate paths of the uncrossed OCBU and crossed OCBC olivocochlear bundles (after Rasmussen). CN, cochlear nucleus; SO, superior olive; TB, trapezoid body. (From Desmedt 1975).

Further experiments have been concerned with the effects of interrupting one or the other OCB, particularly the crossed OCB. From recent results it seems that the absolute threshold of a single fiber is not affected but that the tuning curve broadens in such a way that Q_{10dB} might be reduced by 30% with the "tail" of the curve at frequencies < f_c showing an increased sensitivity (Carlier & Pujol 1982). Other experiments (Bonfils et al. 1987a) have shown that interrupting the efferent pathway modifies the amplitude of the cochlear microphonic only if *all the fibers, direct and crossed, are interrupted* at the midline, that is, all the efferent innervation to OHC is ablated. The intact OCB therefore exercises a tonic facilitatory effect on OHC. Finally, Bonfils et al. (1978b) have found that section of the medial crossed OCB in the guinea pig—which does not change the magnitude of the acoustic nerve's compound action potential in response

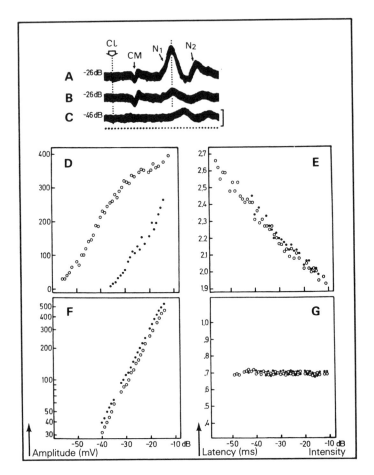

Figure 3.47
Effects of repetitive electrical stimulation of the olivocochlear bundle in the curarized cat after section of the middle ear muscles. *A to C,* Responses to clicks (C1) recorded at the round window. *A,* CM cochlear microphonic. N_1 and N_2 components of the auditory nerve compound action potential. *B,* With OCB stimulation preceding the click. CM is slightly increased, N_1 and N_2 are decreased but with no latency change. *C,* Without electrical stimulation of the bundle but with click intensity reduced by 20 dB. The components are smaller than in *A,* but this time the latency is increased. *D,* Amplitudes and *(E)* latencies of N_1 peak response to clicks as a function of click intensity in the presence (open circles) and absence (solid circles) of a maximal OCB electrical stimulation. Note: The latency is not changed but there is a diminution in amplitude that can be related to an "equivalent dB change" in sound level. *F,* amplitudes and *G,* latencies of CM, neither of which is changed by OCB stimulation. (From Desmedt 1975)

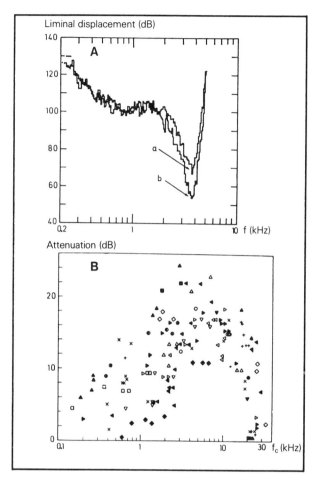

Figure 3.48
OCB stimulation and frequency response of the afferent nerve fibers. *A,* Effect of
crossed OCB stimulation on tuning curve of a cochlear fiber in the cat: liminal displacement of stapes, dB re 10^{-8} μm peak to peak as a function of frequency. b, without
and a, with OCB stimulation. *B,* Attenuation of nerve signal by OCB stimulation, in
"equivalent db of sound" at the peak of the tuning curve for a variety of experiments
(individual symbols) at a variety of f_c. (*A* from Kiang et al. 1970; *B* from Wiederhold
1970)

to a reference tone—does diminish the effect of forward or simultaneous masking, that is, the effect of the efferent input being intact must be to increase the masking effects.

How can these results be interpreted in terms of the mechanisms underlying efferent controls?

Dealing first of all with neuropharmacology, note that one of the synaptic transmitters of the OCB bundle pathway is acetylcholine, at least for OHC. A variety of data suggests that (1) acetylcholine is detectable in cochlear perfusates during OCB stimulation, (2) efferent terminals contain acetylcholinesterase and choline acetyltransferase, and (3) the effects of OCB stimulation are mimicked by infusion of cholinergic substances and are suppressed by atropine. One awkward observation, however, is that the effect of strychnine is not what one would expect for a purely cholinergic system but instead generates a powerful block, all of this suggesting that there may well be an additional mediator (perhaps GABAergic or glycinergic).

For IHC there are now good arguments in favor of an encephalinergic transmitter (Eybalin & Pujol 1984b; cf. Pujol & Lenoir 1985).

We have mentioned before the importance that now attaches to the OHC in cochlear mechanics. These cells can modify the mechanics of transduction by changes in their shape via their relationships with the tectorial membrane. These effects may well be significantly influenced by activity in the medial OCB which represents the major influence on the contralateral OHC. This effect has been clearly demonstrated (Brown et al. 1983) in the guinea pig, where stimulation of the crossed OCB (which innervates OHC) modifies the intracellular responses of IHC, even though the crossed OCB has no terminations on IHC cell bodies. Intracellular recording in IHC shows that crossed OCB stimulation diminishes the IHC receptor potential for frequencies near f_c for both weak and moderate sound intensities. We look forward to understanding one day exactly how the crossed OCB, by activating OHC, can influence what occurs in IHC.

At present, the elucidation of the mechanical role of OHC is not yet complete. Recent work on the turtle (*Pseudemys*) cochlea, which in contrast to the mammalian case contains only one sort of hair cell, also shows modification of hair cell responses by stimulation of their efferent innervation (Art et al. 1985).

Each hair cell has a tuning curve that is revealed, for instance, by measuring the intracellular receptor potential amplitude for a sound of fixed intensity but changing its frequency. This curve shows a quasi-linear decrease in sensitivity at each side of f_c. However, when the efferent pathway is repetitively stimulated electrically the following events occur:

• Hyperpolarization of the cells.
• Reduction of the receptor potential amplitude in the vicinity of the characteristic frequency.
• An increase in the response amplitude for frequencies $<f_c$.
• In contrast, a continuation of the sensitivity decrease for frequencies $>f_c$. The cell that originally behaved as a band selective filter now behaves more like a low-pass filter. Such a modification of the frequency response curve is not without its parallels seen after the selective destruction of OHC in mammals by kanamycin. [We do not wish to dwell on the interpretation in terms of ionic mechanisms that the authors give to their observations in this context].
• This effect probably involves a cholinergic link, being blocked by atropine and curare.

In the face of all these data, it still remains to be proved what the exact functional importance of efferent activity is, to what extent it is invoked by a sound input, and how it modifies sound perception. One way to attack these questions is to discover what aspects of efferent activation are provoked by acoustic stimulation. There are some results to report:

• OCB fibers can discharge (or change their spontaneous rate of discharge) under the effect of a sound input (mean latency 15 ms).
• In some cases it is possible to plot a tuning curve for the efferent fiber activity that is quite like that for afferent fibers (Cody & Johnstone 1982).
• Some observations suggest that sound stimulation to one cochlea can diminish the response to sound of the other cochlea or also that of the contralateral CN (all precautions having been taken to ensure that this cannot have taken place via a direct afferent-efferent coupling).

There have also been behavioral tests on awake animals, whereas all the above have taken place under anesthetic. In the cat, section of the OCB does not affect either the absolute or the differential threshold. In the monkey, the results are similar except for one positive effect. It is quite clear that although OCB section does not change the animal's sound discrimination in the absence of noise, operated animals do show deficits when the sound stimulus is applied in the presence of white noise, or at least of very wide-band noise (Dewson 1968).

In summary, one overall function of the efferent system to emerge from all these observations seems to be to improve the signal-to-noise ratio. We still need to reconcile this conclusion with the more analytical experiments reported above on the role of the crossed OCB.

ACTION OF THE OCB ON THE COCHLEAR NUCLEUS

Other investigations have examined the effects of OCB activity on the CN, a typical experiment consisting in stimulating an appropriate olivary nucleus and observing the effect on responses of CN neural units. Such experiments have shown the existence of very complex phenomena—some excitatory, some inhibitory—on both spontaneous and sound-induced activity in the CN.

One difference that has been demonstrated is between the effects of stimulating the principal olivary nucleus, which are predominantly facilitatory, and of stimulating the periolivary and preolivary nuclei, which are essentially inhibitory (figure 3.49; Comis & Whitfield 1968; Comis 1970). It is not clear whether these effects are the result of a direct action on the cochlear nucleus itself or only the reflection of a direct effect on the cochlear receptors. To that extent these results remain equivocal, but it is claimed that the results of olivary stimulation on a CN cell's *spontaneous* activity persist after destruction of the cochlea ipsilateral to that CN. This suggests a probable direct action on CN in this respect, not one occurring as a result of effects on the receptors. This action has also been shown to be cholinergic (figure 3.49). Nevertheless, another experiment reveals a variable effect that probably modifies the above conclusion. The action of strychnine is to suppress synaptic action at OCB terminals on receptor cells, as we have seen earlier. However, strychnine applied near the round window sometimes suppresses the inhibitory effect of OCB stimulation on the cochlear nucleus (suggesting therefore a peripheral involvement in that effect) but at other times it can have no effect (suggesting a direct effect on the CN itself).

Concerning functional aspects of OCB activity on the CN, recall that it is not possible to exploit sectioning the efferents that reach the CN. In this case, recourse has been taken to applying atropine locally, knowing that the terminals of the OCB in CN are cholinergic. Such an experiment in cat CN scarcely affects the absolute threshold but,

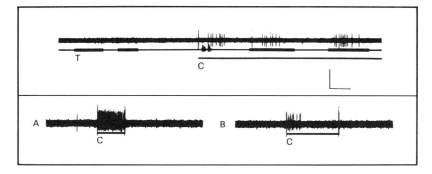

Figure 3.49
Olivary control of cochlear nucleus. *Above,* Olivary control of responses (upper) of CN. A sound T (11.25 khz, 10 dB suprathreshold) is presented (lower) twice before and twice during (C) OCB electrical stimulation at 100 μA. *Below,* Cholinergic nature of olivary stimulation's effect. *A,* Response of a VCN unit to electrical stimulation (C) of the ipsilateral olive at 40 μA. *B,* Same stimulus C, same neuron, but after local application of atropine. Time base 1 s. (From Comis & Whitfield 1968)

in contrast, increases thresholds in the presence of *noise* and therefore diminishes the capacity to distinguish signals in noise (Pickles & Comis 1973). A possible function of OCB activity is thus to *improve* the detection of signals in noise.

EFFECTS OF OTHER EFFERENT ACTIVITY

Stimulation of the descending pathways at the pontine or midbrain level, where there is no great confusion with the ascending lemniscal afferents, demonstrates a diversity of actions that sometimes increase, sometimes diminish responses measured at the round window. Such stimulation is also claimed by some researchers to show a reduction in CN click responses *without* round window responses being modified in any way. Other people have observed CN facilitation.

Effects of stimulating the reticular formation (particularly the mesencephalic) on global CN responses to click stimuli have also been studied in the cat. These effects have been correlated with those obtained by changing the direction or level of the animal's attention. Unhappily, these data have now been almost completely refuted as being attributable to various artefacts (e.g., contraction of middle ear muscles, changes in pinna orientation), so that the importance of such putative reticular controls on the CN has ceased to be taken seriously (Worden & Marsh 1963; Worden et al. 1964).

In summary, the study of these efferent effects is really the study of a set of very heterogeneous and badly coordinated experiments once more. Nothing in the data allows us to postulate realistically any incontrovertible function for these centrifugally invoked actions.

9 EFFECTS OF CENTRAL LESIONS ON AUDITORY PERCEPTION

Several times in the text we have deliberately refrained from mentioning the admittedly numerous observations (largely in cat and monkey but occasionally in other species) that have been made on the perceptual deficits (e.g., concerning frequency, intensity, sound localization) that might follow lesions at one or the other level of the auditory pathways. The brief review that follows summarizes a few of the more important results, first on cortical and then on subcortical lesions. Historically, many of the data have relied on postlesional measurements in humans.

9.1 EFFECTS OF AUDITORY CORTICAL ABLATIONS

In animals, one can in principle proceed by totally eliminating the auditory cortex, that is, the areas previously identified as auditory by other histological or physiological approaches (areas AI, AII, EP, SF, AIII, and INS for the cat, according to the old divisions in section 7.1, and in the monkey the auditory cortex itself plus its surrounding belt of nuclei).

In humans the situation is quite certainly less simple. The extent of the lesions seen is not necessarily well determined and most of them are not as extensive as total ablation of an area. For compactness in presentation, we will nevertheless discuss all types of observation together. Let us add that in animal behavioral work the experiments are carried out using training procedures with positive (rewarding) or negative (punitive) reinforcement; these studies exploit defined adequate sound stimuli that the animal must detect as merely existing or, alternatively, must distinguish as being different from another in intensity, frequency, duration, or direction, and so on. In human subjects, experimenters can often only assess deficits in auditory perception by talking to the subject.

To begin with, it is agreed that some auditory skills, listed below, are not affected by the absence of the auditory cortex:

- Detection of the onset of a sound stimulus
- Magnitude of the absolute threshold
- Discrimination between different intensities (differential intensity threshold)

In the case of animals, they may either retain their earlier training or, alternatively, retraining may be necessary. Nevertheless, the final result is a quasi-complete retention of the ability to carry out the variety of tasks above in the absence of a cortex. It is particularly remarkable that, in humans, there have been many observations on cerebrovascular accidents bilaterally affecting the superior temporal regions (where the auditory area is situated) that show rapidly recovering audiograms afterwards.

In contrast, there is quite a separate series of discriminations that are more or less severely impaired by the absence of an auditory cortex. Although this is also a matter of lesions in a variety of places, they are nevertheless all concerned with two sorts of processing, namely, with frequency or pitch discrimination, or with sound source direction finding.

DISCRIMINATION OF DIFFERENT TEMPORAL OR PITCH PATTERNS

Numerous experimenters have trained cats to discriminate different temporal changes in sound frequency or other acoustic patterns. Overall, postoperative discriminations have been found to be more or less severely deteriorated, allowing the attribution to the auditory cortex of a role in the *temporal patterning of sounds.*

In fact, this suggestion is essentially correct, but in many of its details there appear to be important differences that depend rather significantly on the type of task demanded of the animal. In many experiments this task is of the sort "GO—NO GO" with a positive stimulus S$^+$ to which it should respond and a negative stimulus S$^-$ to which it should not. Some examples will illustrate the problems.

Meyer and Woolsey (1952) used a protocol in which a "neutral" stimulus consisting of a series of identical 1-kHz tone pips was presented or alternatively a "positive" stimulus comprising the discrimination to be recognized: This was the same series of pips but ending with one of 1.1 kHz. No retraining in the task was successful postoperatively, suggesting that the cortex is indispensible. Operated animals responded in the same way to either stimulus (figure 3.50).

In contrast, Butler et al. (1957) made an apparently minor modification to this protocol. They had an uninterrupted series of pips at 800 Hz for the neutral stimulus followed by one alternating between 800 and 1000 Hz for the positive avoidance stimulus. No deficit was found in this case. Thompson (1960) and, notably, Neff et al. (1975) have suggested explanations for this apparent contradiction. In the

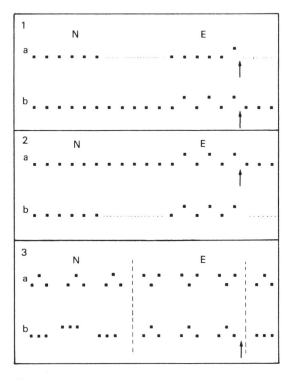

Figure 3.50
Protocols used in tests of frequency discrimination after ablation of all the auditory cortex in the cat. *1*, Sequences used by Meyer and Woolsey (a) and Butler (b). In (a) the neutral stimulus (N) is a sequence of short tone pips (squares) at 1 kHz and the positive (avoidance) stimulus (E) followed by a shock is the same sequence but terminating in a 1.1-kHz pip. The stimuli are separated by silence (small dots). Shock shown by arrows. In (b) the positive stimulus E (alternating 1 kHz and 1.1 kHz pips) is applied on a base of the negative stimulus N that is emitted continuously and not interrupted by silence. Discrimination is lost for case (a) but retained for case (b). *2*, Sequences used by Thompson (1960). In (a) the positive avoidance stimulus (E) is alternating pips at 1 kHz and 1.5 kHz and is applied on a, negative stimulus, base (N) of pips at 1 kHz. In (b) the stimuli are applied against a silent base. Discrimination is maintained in (a) but lost in (b). *3*, Sequences used by Diamond and Neff. Showing the neutral N and avoidance (E) stimuli with pips at 800 Hz and 1 kHz used in different patterns. In both (a) and (b) loss of auditory cortex abolishes discrimination entirely. (Data from Meyer & Woolsey 1952; Butler et al. 1957; Diamond & Neff 1957)

first case, each stimulus is in effect presented against a background of silence, implying that to respond to one or the other the animal needs to *identify* each stimulus. In contrast, in the second paradigm the acoustic baseline is effectively the negative constant signal and a changing rather than constant tone is the positive signal to be detected: This detection of a *change* makes the task much easier in cognitive terms. Cranford et al. (1976) have, however, cast doubt on the second set of results and also emphasized the importance of the exact procedure used in training. With certain precautions, these authors have effectively presented each of these last signals *against a background of silence* and have been able to train animals without an auditory cortex to discriminate between them, this time, however, after first training them against a neutral continuous stimulus.

Finally, an even more complex protocol to test discrimination between patterns of pips at these same frequencies (800 and 1000 Hz) but presented in a different temporal sequence (figure 3.50) was that used by Diamond and Neff (1957). They showed by using those stimuli that the auditory cortex has an essential role to play in the discrimination of tonal sequences that requires a certain retention in short-term memory of the arrangement of events within the sequence.

Logically one would expect the discrimination of even more complex sequences to be more easily deteriorated or abolished according to the difficulty in the discriminatory task. In keeping with this, Ploog (1979) observed that *Saimiri* are no longer able to discriminate different species-specific vocalizations after a less than complete ablation of the auditory areas. Hefner and Hefner (1986), studying the Japanese macaque, have confirmed the impossibility of recognizing species-specific cries after a bilateral ablation. They made an additional interesting observation, pointing out the predominant role of the left hemisphere in achieving such recognition (i.e., there is a cerebral lateralization of such recognition mechanisms).

The human situation is even more complicated, considering the much higher degree of lateralization and hemispheric specialization. Patients with unilateral or bilateral lesions of the temporal cortex have been presented with the Seashore Test of Tonal Memory in which sequences of three to five sounds are presented to subjects with instructions about the discrimination demanded. Subjects with right-sided lesions made significantly more errors than those with left-sided ones and significantly more errors than normal subjects (Milner

1962). This suggests a right-sided hemispheric specialization for "musical perception." In contrast, it is well known that left temporal lesions, probably only when they extend beyond the strictly primary auditory areas, bring with them deficits in understanding spoken language (Wernicke's aphasia). We shall not elaborate further on these phenomena, which are somewhat off the subject here.

The above data by no means exhaust the information on functions of the auditory cortex. Certain other tests, in particular using brief tones, will no doubt underline the importance of short-term memory, in which one or another cortical area will be implicated or appear to be indispensible. Some information exists already but is too incomplete to quote. Comparison with what is now becoming understood about the visual cortex suggests that in the future, certain functional specializations are likely to be found within the diverse auditory cortical areas. This will allow consideration of how parallel channels of different auditory information are set up and operate at this highest auditory level.

SOUND LOCALIZATION: AUDITORY SPACE

It is commonly considered that important deficits in the capacity to localize sound sources follow the ablation of certain auditory cortical areas. However, experimenters have not always agreed well with one another. One reason for this is known. Some researchers have been content to test the lateralization of sources, that is, to distinguish between a source to the left and a source to the right, whereas others have been concerned with investigating how well an animal can localize a particular source in azimuth and elevation among a number of point sources.

It is almost universally agreed that after complete ablation of the auditory areas, animals (cat and monkey in particular) show little or no deficit in their capacity to *lateralize* sources (right/left), whether of free-field stimuli or in more subtle tests of detecting intensity differences or temporal disparities between two stimuli applied dichotically from earpieces (e.g., Cranford 1979a,b).

Thus a monkey without auditory cortex can still indicate by pressing a button from which side a stimulus has arrived. Similarly, cats with similar lesions can be shown to recognize whether a series of clicks is applied at one side or the other by using a "GO—NO GO" type of training and "answering," or some other method that detects a discrimination.

In contrast, when animals are subjected to more refined tests implying precise *localization* of a source, the clinical picture is quite otherwise. It is clear that cats with a unilateral ablation of the auditory cortical areas have a significant and irreversible deficit of localization in the contralateral auditory hemifield. In contrast, their performance for the ipsilateral sound hemisphere remains normal (Jenkins & Masterson 1982).

A complementary series of experiments (Jenkins & Merzenich 1984) showed that (1) for this discrimination AI is necessary and sufficient, while the other areas do not seem to be essential, and (2) ablation of a restricted part of AI corresponding to *a certain frequency band* carries with it a deficit in contralateral localization *restricted to that same frequency band*. This is an important result, implying that auditory space is constructed by treating spatial information for each frequency within its own frequency channel. This conclusion recalls the data given above showing that each cortical isofrequency strip comprises distinct zones of different binaural characteristics (EI, EE).

FURTHER OBSERVATIONS

Not unexpectedly, experimental cortical lesions have thrown up a whole host of other observations. We can only list a few of them here:

"Auditory inattention" has been cited as a possible origin for some poor detection scores or, alternatively, a poor functioning of short-term memory could account for disabling appropriate responses, especially when it is a case of dealing with nervous events over a definite time (holding in memory the effect of one stimulus while inspecting the following one). This could be true for temporally ordered trains of stimuli or in the localization of sound when it is necessary to retain in memory the spatial position of the subject with respect to the source to which he must "point." (In these experiments the animal hears the sounds but is not usually freed until after a small delay.)

Decorticate animals cannot transfer into a real auditory space a training founded on a dichotic disparity simulating a virtual sound space (e.g., a disparity compatible with lateralization, say 500 μs). A real source with the real laterality that would produce the same disparity as had been trained for is not perceived as equivalent to the virtual source.

There are a few observations in humans that in essence confirm the animal data. Patients with a unilateral lesion localize sound poorly in the field contralateral to the lesion. After a bilateral auditory cortical lesion, that as far as can be seen is incomplete, sound localization and even lateralization show large deficits.

9.2 EFFECTS OF SUBCORTICAL LESIONS

There is an abundant literature describing in detail the effects of lesions at a whole variety of places in the auditory pathways: elimination of a cochlea; section of the commissures at the bulbopontine level (trapezoid body and dorsal acoustic stria); NLL lesions; transection of the brachium of the inferior colliculus (BIC), which essentially involves the IC afferent output to the MGB but also efferents from cortex to MGB; transection of the lateral lemniscus; lesions in the MGB; section of the intercollicular commissure; section of the corpus callosum.

Note first that some functions that are not affected by cortical lesions can be affected by one or other subcortical lesion:

• *Absolute threshold,* practically unaffected by cortical lesions, rises significantly after bilateral section of the lateral lemniscus, whereas IC lesions have less effect and BIC section only increases the threshold by 6 dB. Section of the commissures has no effect.
• *Simple pitch discrimination,* preserved after cortical ablation, is lost after bilateral transection of BIC.
• Intensity discrimination is moderately affected by IC lesions and more profoundly by BIC section (however, this conclusion needs reexamination).

Sound localization capacity has yielded the most interesting data (Jenkins & Masterson 1982). Notice, however, that it is best to be concerned with the localization of brief tones (such as clicks), since continuous sounds allow an animal to localize by sweeping the auditory field by head movements.

In the cat, elimination of one cochlea or section of one acoustic nerve practically abolishes all localization of brief tones such as clicks. However, some lateralization is still possible for continuous sounds: This allows the animal a small degree of monaural localization.

Unilateral lesions below or at the level of the superior olivary complex (TB, MSO, LSO) also generate large (*unilateral* or *bilateral*) deficits in localization of brief sounds.

Lesions above the olivary complex (lateral lemniscus, IC, MGB) produce localization deficits in the *contralateral* sound hemifield. Let us repeat again that these conclusions concern a finer localization than merely right/left lateralization, which is often hardly affected, and apply to very brief sounds such as clicks that do not give the opportunity for other ways of localizing such as exploiting head movements.

It seems that a lateralization of sound space begins to be coded at the level of the olivary complex. This is clearly in agreement with the electrophysiological work discussed earlier.

There will no doubt be more developments in lesion work to look forward to, inspired, for example, by the neurophysiological discoveries concerning a possible representation of auditory space in the superior colliculus reported above. A study of any localization deficits generated by lesions in that region might be rewarding.

9.3 AREAS FOR FUTURE STUDY

As some sort of conclusion to these physiological studies, we would like to draw attention to three particular aspects of the auditory system.

We have encountered one major difficulty throughout our study of the successive nuclei in the auditory pathways that we can in practice attribute to a certain repetition and redundancy in the investigation of these processing stages. This general impression probably hides a more fundamental problem: In contrast to what is known about the visual system, we remain fairly ignorant of which characteristics are really significant in each of the successive subcortical stages engaged in auditory information processing in the afferent pathways. Expressed another way, if we now agree that the old scheme proposed by Katsuki et al. (1959, 1962; i.e., that the sharpness of tuning curves progressively increases as an auditory pathway is ascended) is no longer tenable, it did nevertheless aim at finding a role for each of these stages, and at present we have no comparable theme with which to replace it.

Second, if we restrict discussion to the level of the auditory cortical areas, it remains very difficult to have any clear idea of the significant response patterns of the neural units at this final stage. Precise experimental conditions have been shown to be particularly crucial. Under anesthesia, responses seem to be almost simple, but in the awake, alert animal everything changes: The same cells give the impression of being detectors of complex temporal patterns of sound parameters (such as frequency). Yet any systematic sorting of these responses is forbiddingly difficult, even in the very heart of the first primary cortical area. The future will show whether any general law, or at least a guiding principle, can be found that will allow a rational classification of these response characteristics.

A third and final comment concerns the possibility that the auditory system has a duality in the organization of its pathways. In the visual system (see Buser & Imbert 1992), an initial hypothesis suggested the coexistence of mechanisms of position detection and of form detection for objects seen. This proved to be a fruitful preliminary signpost. A similar suggestion exists in audition: that one part of the cochlear nucleus (AVCN) together with the superior olivary complex form the early essential spatial detector; whereas a dorsal system (PVCN and DCN leading to ICC, MGB, and the auditory cortex) might, in contrast, be more dedicated to recognizing acoustic patterns. This may also prove to have been a useful preliminary signpost.

No doubt the future will have something to say about these three problems that we have just summarized.

10 PSYCHOPHYSICS OF HEARING AND NEUROPHYSIOLOGICAL STUDIES

In this discussion, it is difficult to suppress or ignore a certain number of unresolved problems when trying to establish parallels between research results from the neurophysiology of the auditory pathways with others from human psychophysics or from animal behavioral studies. We will not be able to resolve these problems here but will have to be content with pointing them out and discussing them.

10.1 PROBLEMS CONCERNING THE ABSOLUTE THRESHOLD

As described earlier, the absolute threshold as measured by behavioral methods in a given species (cat or guinea pig) is reasonably close to that determined by recording from auditory nerve fibers. There is some difference, however, since the behavioral threshold is about 10 dB smaller than the value found electrophysiologically. How can we explain this?

The most plausible hypothesis (but not necessarily correct) is that the subject can integrate the activity in a population of many nerve fibers, all of which might contribute to the behavioral threshold but in a way that is too subtle to be easily recognized in the *single unit* activity changes recorded electrophysiologically.

Another problem related to the above is to discover what it is in the frequency domain (low frequency in principle) in which phase locking is observed that provides the minimal criterion for perception. It could be locking itself (i.e., a certain sequential distribution of discharges) or, in contrast, an increase in the mean frequency of discharge. It is, in fact, quite conceivable that setting up a certain sequential pattern of discharge can happen without generating an increased mean discharge, each hair cell at low intensities being able to adapt its own spontaneous discharge pattern to the rhythm of the stimulus without also needing to augment the discharge rate. The answer is not known.

10.2 FREQUENCY DISCRIMINATION

Mechanisms for *frequency resolution* have already been discussed (chapter 2, section 7.2). There are ways of showing that the cochlea can act like the psychophysicists' picture of a series of band-pass filters with a bandwidth (critical band) varying with sound frequency. The *effective bandwidth* that can be defined for each acoustic nerve fiber in terms of its tuning curve is seen to behave in very much the same way.

This resolving power is no doubt in some way relevant to *frequency discrimination* mechanisms, determined by first hearing a tone of one frequency f and then another of frequency ($f \pm \delta f$) and perceiving them as different. This defines a differential threshold $\delta f/f$ which varies with frequency, as we have seen already. A question posed many times concerns how this discrimination is made. The mechanism could involve detecting that the place of maximal basilar membrane displacement is changed by the change δf or it could be a matter of detecting a change in nerve discharge rates. In truth there are arguments in favor of both mechanisms.

Proponents of the one solution can refute the other in the name of uncertainty due to the minuteness of the changes involved. Spatially, the differential threshold of 3 Hz at 1 kHz corresponds in spatial coding to a displacement of 18 μm along the basilar membrane, about the distance occupied by two hair cells. In the case of temporal coding, the same threshold corresponds to a periodicity change of 3 μs, whereas a single action potential lasts about 1000 μs with a variability in its duration of order 100 μs!

Since the experimental data demonstrate that coupling to the phase of sound waves does not happen above 5 kHz, it is tempting to adopt the eclectic position that for frequencies below 5 kHz temporal coding is exploited, whereas above that frequency, where temporal information becomes negligible, the discrimination becomes a matter of spatial coding.

However these parameters are finally discovered to be implicated in discrimination, it is probable that the mechanisms will use outputs from a large number of neurons. This in itself could in some way improve thresholds with respect to any that can be found by observing single neural units. However, crucial tests of the two hypotheses are still lacking.

10.3 FREQUENCY RESOLUTION OF INTENSE SOUNDS

Frequency coding in sounds of high intensity is another phenomenon that causes problems in comparing psychological and physiological data. It is difficult to see how the observed pitch discrimination, that surely must be related to frequency resolution, can be maintained over such a wide range of sound intensities (practically 100 dB) when tuning curves become so spread out and overlapping above a certain loudness level. How can one continue to understand a sound pattern as complicated as speech even when it is very loud?

In fact, the isodischarge curves of auditory nerve fibers retain a quite reasonable frequency bandwidth over a reasonably wide intensity range. But when sounds are generating neural saturation, where the discharge rate/intensity curve reaches a plateau, then there is very clearly a problem.

In the frequency range above 5 kHz where spatial coding of frequency needs to be invoked, we might explain the maintenance of frequency resolution by the intervention of *lateral inhibitory mechanisms* such as have been encountered in the cochlea (two-tone suppression) and in the central pathways where tuning curves are flanked by inhibitory zones.

In the frequency range below 5 kHz where phase locking (coding the periodicity) is thought to come into play, we might suggest the existence in the pathways of neurons that can conserve temporal coding in spite of saturation. Remember in particular the ON cells, those architipically phasic cells that include the "octopus" cells of the MGB.

The fact remains, however, that most individual units have a dynamic range no greater than 30 to 50 dB, and we still need to ask how so moderate a range can be transformed into the much larger dynamic range demanded by psychophysics. One (somewhat hypothetical) answer arises from the report of a small number (10%) of cochlear fibers with a much wider than usual dynamic bandwidth; maybe it is these that can operate appropriately at high intensities. Or perhaps we should consider the subset of fibers described as having the usual dynamic range (40 dB) but with thresholds 80 dB higher than the familiar, more excitable fibers. These would be capable of responding without saturation at high sound intensities.

Such a range of problems, like others we have mentioned in this text, will no doubt continue to stimulate the direction of research efforts to match the data of neurophysiology to the mechanisms demanded by psychophysics.

Appendix A

Notes on Deafness with a Peripheral Origin

1 TYPES OF DEAFNESS

Deafness related to peripheral deficits can be classified into two groups, conduction deafness (deafness due to poor sound vibration transmission to the cochlea) and sensorineural deafness (perceptual deficits).

1.1 CONDUCTION DEAFNESS

Transmission deficits are related to anomalies peripheral to the cochlea. They can be due to changes in the impedance transformation in the middle ear produced, for example, by immobilization of the ossicular chain or by a deficient transfer of sound pressure to the oval or round windows. Some of the many possible causes include: external meatus blockage by cerumen; blockage of ossicular vibration by an abnormal pressure at the tympanic membrane (barotrauma) due to either pus or fluid (effusion) in otitis media, or by adhesions at a wound; a loss of the tympanic membrane and/or ossicular chain (chronic otitis); or by pathological fixation of the stapes at the oval window.

[This last condition generates one of the most severe types of transmission deafness (otosclerosis); it is more common in women than in men and may thus have a hereditary component. It is a matter of progressive development of bony growth which immobilizes the stapes at the oval window, fixing the footplate to the bony frame of the window. Under these conditions, vibrations are no longer transmitted to the inner ear and in spite of the integrity of the round window, there can be no sound transmission into the cochlea.

Some transmission can be restored by a fenestration operation, which consists in opening another window into the labyrinth near the semicircular canal. The patient finds some return of hearing but this, of course, cannot benefit from the normal middle ear impedance transformation. Another possible intervention, stapedectomy, consists in removing the bony bridge that has grown between stapes and the oval window and replacing the stapes by an artificial mechanical link to the incus.]

Sensorineural deafness can arise either from retrocochlear acoustic nerve lesions or from lesions in the cochlea itself. Lesions to the nerve are in fact nerve blocks that usually arise from tumor growth (retrocochlear neurinoma of the auditory nerve). Deafness from this cause is sometimes accompanied by tinnitus and occasionally by problems of balance.

Most sensorineural deafness is, however, associated with cochlear lesions. Among the syndromes are the following:

• *Presbyacusis,* a biologically normal senescence of the ear from which there is no total escape but only greater or lesser degrees of hearing deficits.
• *Labyrinthitis,* difficulties often arising from vascular problems that are very varied in their etiology and which progressively involve the cochlea.
• *Degenerative deafness of hereditary origin,* generally associated with other malformations (e.g., retinitis, nephritis).
• *Ménière's disease,* associated with periodic and severe pressure changes in the endolymph which are accompanied by deafness, tinnitus, and vertigo.
• Deafness of *traumatic origin* (barotraumatic; aviator's deafness or deafness associated with diving or exposure to high winds; exposure to loud sounds or blows to the cranium).
• *Ototoxic deafness,* which can result from ototoxic properties in drugs such as quinine, antibiotics such as streptomycin, kanamycin, or gentamicin, among others.
• Deafness following *infectious* or *viral disease* (e.g., meningitis, mumps).

2 CLINICAL DIAGNOSIS OF DEAFNESS

2.1 BONE CONDUCTION AND AIRBORNE CONDUCTION

One of the problems in otological diagnosis is to distinguish between conductive and sensorineural deafness. A variety of audiometric tests are available, the principal techniques being those of Rinne and of Weber.

RINNE'S TEST

This classic, and entirely empirical, test consists in comparing the two routes for hearing in a particular ear, the usual air-conducted route (AC) and by bone conduction (BC).

A tuning fork is set into vibration by percussion and placed against the mastoid of the subject, who hears the sound by bone conduction and after a few seconds hears it no longer as the tuning fork's vibration amplitude decays. The tuning fork is now transferred, without being struck again, to the entrance of the external auditory meatus of the same side. A normal subject will once more hear the sound by the airborne route for another 15 seconds, more or less. The test is then said to be positive and the subject's hearing is normal.

In contrast, if the time of hearing the airborne sound is much shorter or nil, or even negative (with the fork heard better by BC than by AC), then there is a poor middle ear conduction. Transmission deafness can thus be detected by this global hearing test, the first step in diagnosis.

A normal positive Rinne result corresponds to a relative audiometric hearing loss of about 35 dB in BC compared with AC.

WEBER'S (LATERALIZATION) TEST

A driven tuning fork (frequencies between 250 and 8000 Hz) is placed on the middle of the forehead. The subject may hear the same sound intensity in each ear (*Weber indifferent* or *Weber negative*) and localizes the sound inside the skull. In contrast, if the Weber source is lateralized with the subject localizing the source near one ear, a lesion is probably present (figure A.1).

In transmission deafness, the patient tends to localize the source at the lesioned side. This apparently paradoxical response is understandable if we take into account that at the side where the middle ear is not effective it will not attenuate the vibrations carried by bone conduction. A more complex explanation holds that a certain attenuating phase change is produced by the healthy middle ear response which will not be produced by a damaged middle ear. If, on the other hand, the deafness is sensorineural, the source will be best perceived from the healthy side; this is easily understandable. The Rinne and Weber tests used together provide a good initial diagnostic tool.

2.2 TESTS BY THRESHOLD AUDIOMETRY

Clinical diagnosis uses, in addition, more quantitative tests, among which is plotting curves of a patient's auditory thresholds (audiogram; Hallpike 1976; Portmann & Portmann 1978). Clinical audiograms are, however, normally presented differently than a physiologist's usual plot. The reference level, taken as 0 dB, is plotted as

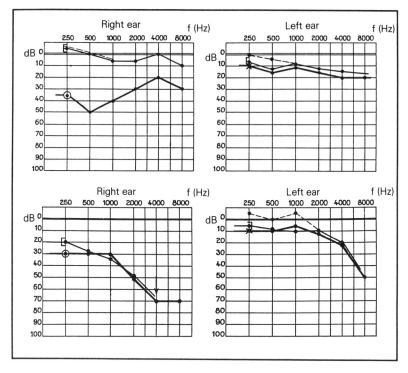

Figure A.1
Different tests for deafness. *Upper left,* Audiogram (right ear) for a unilateral right-sided transmission deafness. *Upper right,* The corresponding (normal) audiogram for the left ear. Rectangle, bone conduction (BC); Circle, airborne conduction (AC). In a Weber test the subject would lateralize the source to the right (affected ear). *Lower left,* Audiogram (right ear) for a pure unilateral right-sided neural deafness. *Lower right,* Right-sided (normal) audiogram. In a Weber test the subject would lateralize the sound to the left (unaffected ear). Note: In the audiogram plots the intensity of BC is automatically increased by 35 dB with respect to the intensity for AC so that in a normal audiogram the two curves are superimposed. (From Portmann & Portmann 1978)

a straight line as a function of frequency, parallel to the x-axis, that represents normal sensitivity (measured on young healthy subjects). Any negative deviation (in decibels) from this line represents a hearing loss (i.e., an increased threshold) that is evaluated (usually automatically in the audiometer) by comparing the subject's response with the normal audiogram. This plot makes it possible to detect anomalies more easily.

Another method adopted for clinical audiometry is to make the machine's reference for airborne and bone-conducted sensitivities coincide (by appropriate internal design of the audiometer circuits and assuming the mean normal bone conduction to be 35 dB worse than the normal air conduction case). Pure tone audiometric thresholds for BC and AC are then measured and certain characteristic differences between the two can be used to determine the type of deafness:

• In *transmission deafness*, the BC curve is effectively normal but the AC curve shows an approximately equal loss at all frequencies.
• In *sensorineural deafness*, the BC and AC curves both fall toward high frequencies and parallel one to the other.

Another source of diagnostic information (see figure 1.8), called *von Békésy's successive approximation method*, allows the subject to plot his or her own absolute auditory threshold curve. In measuring hearing loss with this technique, a new but absolutely essential procedure is introduced to avoid adaptation or fatigue of the responses, which consists in presenting discontinuous sounds to the subject by interrupting the sound output at a rate of 2.5/s. By this method, and again adopting the "horizontal" presentation of the normal standard response, useful conclusions can be derived by comparing the shape of curve "C" (continuous presentation) with that of curve "I" (presentation of interrupted, discrete sounds), as illustrated in figure A.2. For example, table A.1 shows how it is possible to differentially diagnose intracochlear deficits (in particular, Ménière's syndrome) from retrolabyrinthine lesions based on such comparison.

2.3 SUPRATHRESHOLD AUDIOMETRY

Suprathreshold measurements are also useful in diagnosis. Fowler (1937) introduced a test concerned with the interaural comparison of loudness, which permits the investigation of recruitment in the periphery (figure A.3). The measurement is simple in principle. A patient is exposed to two separate stimuli of the same frequency, one to each ear. The intensity of one is set to different values by the investigator. The patient adjusts the other until it is perceived as equally loud. Differences in the two intensities, often very clear, allow a differential diagnosis between conduction deafness, sensorineural deafness proper, and a retrocochlear lesion of the auditory nerve.

• In *conduction deafness*, the loss of sensitivity (30 dB in the examples illustrated) is equally maintained over the total intensity range (0 to 80 dB).
• If the deafness concerns the *receptors* themselves, the initial dispar-

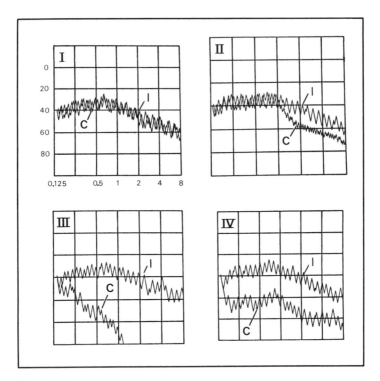

Figure A.2
Common types of curves obtained in von Békésy audiometry. C, continuous stimulation; I, interrupted stimulation. See text and table A.1. (From Hallpike 1976, after Jerger 1960)

Table A.1. Differential diagnosis of hearing loss by von Békésy's successive approximation method

Type of curve*	Response to stimulation*	Diagnosis
I	C and I similar	Normal or conductive deafness
II	C and I similar at LF; separate at $f > 1$ kHz	Ménière's syndrome
III	C and I widely separated; curve C falling steeply	Retrocochlear lesion
IV	C and I are parallel with 30 dB difference between them	Retrocochlear lesion

*See figure A.2 for key.

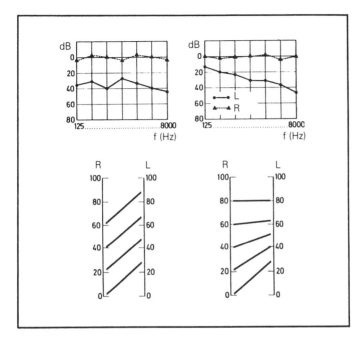

Figure A.3
Conduction deafness and neural deafness (see text). *Upper left,* Air conduction audiograms for left conduction deafness. *Upper right,* Air conduction audiograms for left ear neural deafness. Circles, left ear; triangles, right ear. *Below,* Corresponding plots for equalization of stimuli loudnesses between left ear (L) and right ear (R). Intensities perceived as equally loud are joined by the transverse bars. Any obliquity in these bars represents an interaural inequality. See text. (From Hallpike 1976, after Fowler 1937)

ity between the two intensities at the healthy and diseased ear for equal loudness (30 dB as before) diminishes as loudness is increased such that stimuli are approximately equal at high intensities (80 dB). This phenomenon is known as *recruitment* and originates at the cochlear level.

• Finally, with a *retrocochlear lesion* of the auditory nerve, the situation is similar to that for conduction deafness with the disparity maintained for all intensities. One or two examples of this are shown in figures A.3 and A.4.

2.4 IMPEDANCE AUDIOMETRY

Having discussed certain fundamental aspects of impedance and its measurement in the peripheral organ, we now describe some practical applications.

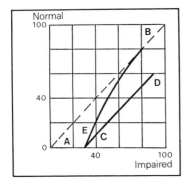

Figure A.4
Another way of presenting Fowler's test ("diagonal plot" of Steinberg & Gardner 1937). Ordinate, Intensities in dB suprathreshold for normal ear. Abscissa, ditto for affected ear. For equal loudness perception (normal) experimental points will lie on the line AB. For transmission deafness, curve CD would be typical (with no recruitment). For sensorineural deafness with recruitment the points would follow the curve EB. (From Hallpike 1976, after Steinberg & Gardner 1937)

The clinical apparatus used tends to be somewhat simplified compared with that used in research. It normally comprises an acoustic probe containing several narrow tubes. It fits closely into the ear canal and is introduced until its end is near the tympanic membrane. One tube leads a sound of frequency 200 Hz and known intensity to the vicinity of the eardrum; a nearby similar tube acts as a receiver to record the parameters of the sound wave reflected from the tympanic membrane. From these it is possible to measure the acoustic impedance at the tympanic membrane. A third tube permits the application of known steady air pressures (negative or positive) into the external auditory meatus, and the same pressure is exerted on the tympanic membrane (there being no leakage of air because of the tightly fitting probe). The measurements are made by a null-point bridge method.

In practice, in what is often called *tympanometry*, it is usually a matter of measuring the *compliance*, or suppleness, of the tympanic membrane. The test consists in plotting the variation of the compliance C with the pressure p, positive or negative, applied to the tympanum via the third tube. (C is normally maximal for $p = 0$ and decreases symmetrically to become effectively zero at a pressure of -200 or $+200$ mm of water). The curve of C as a function of p can show diagnostically useful characteristics:

• Compliance practically zero at all applied pressures, negative or positive; a rigid tympanic membrane or a middle ear filled with secretions
• Compliance abnormally low but with the plot being symmetrical (as in a normal ear) as the pressure is changed from high to low; otosclerosis
• Compliance very high; rupture of the ossicular chain

2.5 ELECTROPHYSIOLOGICAL TESTS

Electrophysiological tests developed more recently include electro-cochleography and recording of evoked potentials. We shall not discuss the former, which consists in recording the auditory nerve compound action potential via a transtympanic electrode; the interested reader will find a complete description in Aran and Portmann (1972). We will, however, deal in some detail with utilizing evoked potentials in appendix B.

2.6 SPEECH AUDIOMETRY

Speech audiometry is another test that nowadays plays an important part in diagnosis in parallel with the pure-tone audiometry that we have described above. To discuss it properly would need a long introduction and would also lead us far from basic auditory phenomena into the realms of congitive processes that we have deliberately chosen not to consider in this volume.

3 FURTHER COMMENTS ON HEARING DEFICITS

Detailed investigations have been conducted on certain other aspects of deafness. Loss of absolute sensitivity is most frequently observed at high frequencies; this has not yet been entirely accounted for. Also, some subjects, particularly those who have suffered exposure to high noise levels, experience a curiously local loss of sensitivity peaking at 4 kHz. No explanation has yet been given for this phenomenon except that the same sort of sensitivity deficit has also been seen in otherwise apparently normal cats.

Surprisingly, no apparent correlation has been established so far between the spontaneous otoacoustic emissions (discussed in the last chapter) that are observed in some subjects and the phenomenon of tinnitus that some of them suffer also (Rebillard et al. 1987).

Other deficits are certainly a matter of frequency resolution. A variety of relevant observations include the fact that the critical band (see chapter 1, 3.3, and chapter 2, 1.2) is much wider than normal in these patients. The critical band is widely regarded as a good measure of frequency resolution.

Various researchers have investigated the possibility of determining auditory tuning curves and their bandwidths psychophysically (Zwicker 1974) by methods based on masking. These seem to show, indirectly, some agreement with the tuning curves of the receptors. It has been observed also (figure A.5) that in sensorineural deafness

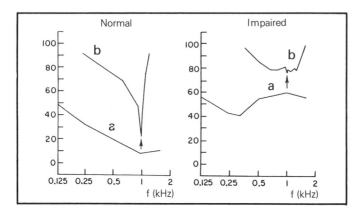

Figure A.5
Psychophysical tuning curves at 1 kHz (b) determined by forward masking for a
normal subject (*left*) and for another with sensorineural deafness (*right*). a, absolute
threshold audiograms. The arrows are positioned at the intensity and frequency of the
test tone corresponding to the absolute threshold. (From Nelson & Turner 1975).

these tuning curves so obtained lose the high sensitivity peak at the
place where normal hearing is also most sensitive (Nelson & Turner
1980). In contrast, the "wings" of the curve are not significantly affected. This sort of curve illustrates both the loss of sensitivity and
the concurrent loss of frequency resolution. Not only does the subject
"hear badly" but is also unable to perceive frequency differences
normally, this deficit no doubt often giving rise to poorer speech
comprehension as well.

Finally, it needs to be explained why recruitment occurs, that is,
why at threshold there might be a 40-dB deficit, say, in the loudness
of sound perceived via one ear compared with the other, whereas
this difference in subjective equality diminishes or even disappears
near 80-dB intensities. [It is also observed in practice that in those
suffering sensorineural deafness, the hearing and the discrimination
of intense sounds is better than would be predicted from the
audiogram measured at threshold (this being clearly relevant to the
provision of amplifying hearing aids).] An explanation might be as
follows: If loudness is related to the *total* amount of activity in the
acoustic nerve, then the observation that pathological psychophysical
tuning curves lose their sharp peak without much being affected at
their "wings" also implies that the relative loss of total activity is
greater near threshold (where only the sensitive peak is activated)

than at high intensities since at high levels there can be considerable summation in the more extensive flanks. These flanking regions are only significantly activated at high sound levels in normal subjects as well as in those with cochlear sensorineural deficits.

Finally, we turn to the data from animal experimentation that might help an understanding of deafness due to cochlear lesions (already discussed in some detail above). Ototoxic drugs such as kanamycin in carefully calibrated doses only affect outer hair cells in the medial and basal turns of the cochlea, without visibly modifying inner hair cells. Yet, after lesions of OHC it is the output from IHC (that serve 95% of the cochlear afferents) that lose their frequency selectivity precisely because their tuning curves lose their sharp peak in sensitivity, just as occurs in psychophysical tuning curves in subjects suffering recruitment. These and other observations suggest an OHC control of the sensitivity and selectivity of IHC in a way that we have broadly discussed but which is not yet known in detail.

To our knowledge, IHC lesions have rarely been reported. Some publications suggest that, although EM records show changes in the appearance of the IHC stereocilia after a prolonged exposure to high intensity levels of sound and that these are accompanied by an elevation of absolute threshold, yet there is no essential change in the frequency selectivity of these IHC.

We will not discuss here the attempts (that have shown variable effectiveness) to design hearing prostheses by exploiting electrical neural stimulation to alleviate sensorineural deafness.

Appendix B

Auditory Evoked Potentials in Human Subjects

Auditory evoked potentials, which follow stimulation by brief sounds like tone pips and clicks, have been the focus of a variety of detailed research. The apparatus most used is the general purpose one employed for recording EEG-evoked potentials detected at the scalp whatever the sensory modality in question. These machines are now highly developed and are aimed at extracting signals from a noisy electrical background by averaging techniques. Stimuli are applied successively and responses to them are individually selectively summated; usually several hundred stimuli are needed (if not more). These responses reflect an activity that is to some extent a global summation, spatially and temporally, from which instantaneous variations have been eliminated that might in some situations contain valuable data. However, the advantage of mean responses is that they can better provide some level of standardization so that, from one report to another, and from normal subjects to others, the data are readily extracted in an agreed form, classified, and listed with a largely universally accepted nomenclature by researchers in both clinical and basic science.

In the case of auditory evoked potentials, the presently agreed-on specifications include a number of details (figure B.1). Such potentials are often measured at the scalp between a point on the midline at the vertex with respect to some "indifferent" electrode. They show different components that are identified by the latencies with respect to the brief sound stimulus of the various peaks in the responses to it. It is customary to divide these responses into three types (Picton et al. 1974), short, mid, and long latency components.

1.1 SHORT LATENCY COMPONENTS

It has been clearly demonstrated by both animal and human experiments that the origin of these components is not cortical but in the brainstem. This is therefore a recording of far field potentials. Five successive peaks are usually recognizable, I, II, III, IV, V (and maybe

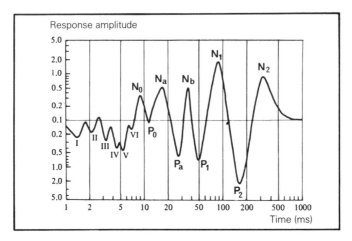

Figure B.1
Auditory evoked potentials in humans. Responses measured at an electrode on the vertex relative to a reference electrode over the mastoid apophysis or on the ear lobe. Computer average of responses to 100 successive clicks. Waves I to VI, short latency response components; N_0 to N_b, mid latency components; P_1 to N_2, long latency components. Upward deviations negative with respect to the reference (N) and downward deviations positive (P). (From Picton et al. 1974)

VI). The first is at about 1.5 ms after the stimulus and the rest occur within about the next 10 ms.

For monaural stimulation, I and V appear to come from a lateralized location, II and III from a bilateral source, and IV from a source located in the midline (Allen & Starr 1978).

Researchers have gone some way toward a more precise identification by exploiting observations from electrodes at a variety of different places on the scalp, or concentrating on the mastoid region, or even using intracranial measurements during neurosurgery (Hashimoto et al. 1981). This has been supplemented in animal preparations by measurements made after making local lesions in the auditory pathways, and although this has led to some general agreement in interpretation (listed below), there are nevertheless still arguments about detail (see, e.g., Møller et al. 1981).

I.   auditory nerve
II.   cochlear nucleus
III. superior olivary complex
IV. pontine regions
V.   inferior colliculus
VI. medial geniculate body

1.2 MID LATENCY COMPONENTS

These are varied in number; Picton et al. (1974) have five of them, identified by P or N depending whether their polarity is positive or negative with respect to the specified "indifferent" electrode. These components have a cortical origin (more precisely, from temporal cortex). There latencies are as follows, approximately: N_0, 10 ms; P_0, 12 ms; N_a, 16 ms; P_a, 25 ms; N_b, 36 ms.

1.3 LONG LATENCY COMPONENTS

These have a much longer delay: P_1, 50 ms; N_1, 80 ms; P_2, 160 ms; N_2, 300 ms, and sometimes a last positive component P_3 at 350 ms. These elements are clearly from some different origin, probably predominantly in frontocentral regions. (These later components are alternatively designed by a rounded-off mean latency; e.g., N200, P300, etc.).

Each of the three categories of components has both scientific and clinical relevance. The *early components* lend themselves to the study of thresholds and their psychosensory correlates. They can also determine whether particular neurological troubles are peripheral or brainstem, for example. Thus in the case of neurinoma of the acoustic nerve in the pontocerebellar angle, only the component I exists; in the case of a higher lesion in the brainstem, the three or four first peaks might be recorded. Similarly, in a conduction deafness, sufficiently suprathreshold stimuli might present peaks spaced out in the usual way. One can imagine the usefulness of these diagnostic methods in cases where verbal interrogation or other classic methods cannot be applied (young children, for instance).

Mid latency components are usually affected by cortical lesions, particularly in the parietotemporal regions.

The *longest latency components* are mainly interesting in neuropsychology in that they are significantly related to levels of alertness in the subject, to memory, to attention, or even to cognitive expectation of a stimulus.

References

Abeles M & Goldstein M (1970) Functional architecture in cat primary auditory cortex: columnar organization and organization according to depth. Journal of Neurophysiology. *33* 172–87

Ades H & Engstrom H (1974) Anatomy of the inner ear. In Keidel W & Neff W (Eds), Handbook of Sensory Physiology, Vol I (pp 125–158). Springer Verlag, Berlin

Aitkin L (1976) Tonotopic organization at higher levels of the auditory pathways. In Porter R (Ed), International Reviews of Physiology. Neurophysiology. II, Vol 10 (pp 249–279). University Park Press, Baltimore

Aitkin L (1979) The auditory midbrain. Trends in Neuroscience. *2* 308–310

Aitkin L & Dunlop C (1969) Inhibition in the medial geniculate body of the cat. Experimental Brain Research. *7* 63–83

Aitkin L & Prain S (1974) Medial geniculate body: unit responses in the awake cat. Journal of Neurophysiology. *37* 512–521

Aitkin L & Webster W (1972) Medial geniculate body of the cat: Organization and responses to tonal stimuli of neurons in ventral division. Journal of Neurophysiology. *35* 365–380

Aitkin L, Dunlop C & Webster W (1966) Click-evoked response patterns of single units in the medial geniculate body of the cat. Journal of Neurophysiology. *29* 109–123

Aitkin L, Anderson D & Brugge J (1970) Tonotopic organization and discharge characteristics of single neurons in nuclei of the lateral lemniscus of the cat. Journal of Neurophysiology. *33* 421–440

Aitkin L, Webster W, Veale J & Crosby D (1975) Inferior colliculus I. Comparison of response properties of neurons in central, pericentral and external nuclei of the adult cat. Journal of Neurophysiology. *38* 1196–1207

Aitkin L, Dickhaus H, Schult N & Zimmerman M (1978) External nucleus of the inferior colliculus: auditory and spinal somatosensory afferents and their interactions. Journal of Neurophysiology. *41* 837–847

Allen A & Starr A (1978) Auditory brainstem potentials in monkey (*M. mulatta*) and man. Electroencephalography & Clinical Neurophysiology. *45* 53–63

Andersen R, Knight P & Merzenich M (1980a) The thalamocortical and corticotha-lamic connections of AI, AII and the anterior auditory field (AAF) in the cat: evidence for two largely segregated systems of connections. Journal of Compara-tive Neurology. *194* 663–701

Andersen R, Roth G, Aitkin L & Merzenich M (1980b) The efferent projections of the central nucleus and the pericentral nucleus of the inferior colliculus in the cat. Journal of Comparative Neurology. *194* 649–662

Andersen R, Schneider R & Merzenich M (1980c) The topographic organization of cortico-collicular projections from physiologically identified loci in the AI, AII and anterior auditory cortical fields of the cat. Journal of Comparative Neurology. *191* 479–94

Anniko M & Wroblewski R (1986) Ionic environment of cochlear hair cells. Hear-ing Research. *22* 279–95

Aran J-M & Portmann M (1972) L'électrocochléogramme. Journal Français d'Oto-Rhino-Laryngologie. *21* 211

Art J, Crawford A, Fettiplace R & Fuchs P (1985) Synaptic hyperpolarisation and inhibition of turtle cochlear hair cells. Journal of Physiology. *360* 397–421

Arthur R, Pfeiffer R & Suga N (1971) Properties of "two tone inhibition" in pri-mary auditory neurones. Journal of Physiology. *212* 593–609

Bachem A (1937) Various types of absolute pitch. Journal of the Acoustical Society of America. *9* 146–151

Bachem A (1940) The genesis of absolute pitch. Journal of the Acoustical Society of America. *11* 434–439

Bachem A (1954) Time factors in relative and absolute pitch determination. Journal of the Acoustical Society of America. *26* 751–753

Baird I (1974) Anatomical features of the inner ear in submammalian vertebrates. In Keidel W & Neff W (Eds), Handbook of Sensory Physiology, Vol 1 (pp 159–212). Springer Verlag, Berlin

Barraud H (1968) Harmonie. In Encyclopaedia Universalis. Universalis, Paris

von Békésy G (1960) Experiments in Hearing. McGraw-Hill, New York

von Békésy G & Rosenblith W (1951) The mechanical properties of the ear. In Stevens S (Ed), Handbook of Experimental Psychology (pp 1075–1180). Wiley, New York

Bendat J & Piersol A (1966) Measurement and Analysis of Random Data. Wiley, New York

Blauert J (1983) Spatial Hearing: The psychophysics of Human Sound Localiza-tion. MIT Press, Cambridge, Massachusetts

de Boer E (1976) On the "residue" and auditory pitch perception. In Keidel D & Neff W (Eds), Handbook of Sensory Physiology. Auditory System: Vol 3 (pp 479–583). Springer Verlag, Berlin.

Bonfils P, Puel J, Orès S & Pujol R (1987a) Modulation of the masking phenomenon by the crossed part of the medial olivocochlear bundle. Archives of Otolaryngology. *244* 198–203

Bonfils P, Remond M & Pujol R (1987b) Variations of cochlear microphonic potential after sectioning efferent fibers to the cochlea. Hearing Research. *30* 267–272

Bonfils P, Bertrand Y & Uziel A (1988) Evoked otoacoustic emissions: normative data and presbyacusis. Audiology. *27* 27–35

Borg E (1972a) Regulation of middle ear sound transmission in the non-anaesthetised rabbit. Acta physiologica Scandinavica. *85* 175–190

Borg E (1972b) Excitability of the acoustic m. stapedius and m. tympani reflexes in the non-anaesthetised rabbit. Acta physiologica Scandinavica. *85* 374–389

Borg E (1973) On the neuronal organisation of the acoustic middle ear reflex. A physiological and anatomical study. Brain Research. *49* 101–123

Boring E (1942) Sensation and Perception in the History of Experimental Psychology. Appleton Century Crofts, Englewood Cliffs, N.J.

Botte MC & Scharf B (1980) La sonie. Effets simultanés de fatigue et de masque. Acutica. *46* 100–106

Bouasse H (1926) Traité D'Acoustique générale. Delagrave, Paris

Brillouin J (1958) Acoustique et musique. In Histoire de la Musique (pp 3–47). Gallimard Pléiade, Paris

Brown M, Nuttall A & Masta R (1983) Intracellular recordings from cochlear inner hair cells: effects of stimulation of the crossed olivocerebellar efferents. Science. *222* 69–72

Brownell W, Bader C, Bertrand D & Ribeaupierre Y (1985) Evoked mechanical responses of isolated cochlear outer hair cells. Science. *227* 194–196

Brugge J & Merzenich M (1973) Responses of neurons in auditory cortex of the macaque monkey to monaural and binaural stimulation. Journal of Neurophysiology. *36* 1138–1158

Brugge J, Dubrovsky N, Aitkin L & Anderson D (1969) Sensitivity of single neurons in auditory cortex of cat to binaural tone stimulation: effect of varying interaural time and intensity. Journal of Neurophysiology. *32* 1005–1024

Bruhat G (1940) Mécanique. Masson, Paris

Brunso-Bechtold J, Thompson G & Masterton R (1981) HRP study of the organization of auditory afferents ascending to central nucleus of inferior colliculus in cat. Journal of Comparative Neurology. *197* 705–722

Burns E & Ward W (1982) Intervals, scales and tuning. In Deutsch D (Ed), The Psychology of Music (ch. 8). Academic Press, London

Buser P & Imbert M (1982) Psychophysiologie Sensorielle. Neurophysiologie Fonctionelle II. Hermann, Paris

Buser P & Imbert M (1987) Vision. Neurophysiologie Fonctionelle IV. Hermann, Paris

Buser P & Imbert M (1992) Vision. Translated by RH Kay. MIT Press, Cambridge, Massachusetts. Originally published by Hermann, Paris, 1987

Butler R, Diamond I & Neff W (1957) Role of auditory cortex in discrimination of changes in frequency. Journal of Neurophysiology. *20* 108–120

Calford M (1983) The parcellation of the medial geniculate body of the cat defined by the auditory response properties of single units. Journal of Neuroscience. *3* 2350–2364

Calford M & Aitkin L (1983) Ascending projections to the medial geniculate body of the cat: evidence for multiple parallel auditory pathways through thalamus. Journal of Neuroscience. *3* 2365–2380

Calford M & Webster W (1981) Auditory representation within principal division of cat medial geniculate body: an electrophysiological study. Journal of Neurophysiology. *45* 1013–1028

de Candé R (1961) Dictionnaire de la Musique. Edition du Seuil, Paris

Carlier E & Pujol R (1982) Sectioning the efferent bundle decreases cochlear frequency selectivity. Neuroscience Letters. *28* 101–106

Clarey J & Irvine D (1986) Auditory response properties of neurons in the anterior ectosylvian sulcus of the cat. Brain Research. *386* 12–19

Cody A & Johnstone B (1982) Acoustically evoked activity of single efferent neurons in the guinea-pig cochlea. Journal of the Acoustical Society of America. *72* 280–282

Cody A & Russell I (1985) Outer hair cells in the mammalian cochlea and noise induced hearing loss. Nature (London). *315* 662–665

Colburn H & Durlach N (1978) Models of binaural interaction. In Carterette E & Friedman M (Eds), Handbook of Perception. 4. Hearing (pp 467–518). Academic Press, New York

Comis S (1970) Centrifugal inhibitory processes affecting neurones in the cat cochlear nucleus. Journal of Physiology. *210* 751–760

Comis S & Whitfield I (1968) Influence of centrifugal pathways on unit activity in the cochlear nucleus. Journal of Neurophysiology. *31* 62–68

Condamines R (1978) Stéréophonie. Cours de Relief Sonore Théorique et Appliqué. Masson, Paris

Corey D & Hudspeth A (1983) Kinetics of the receptor current in the bullfrog saccular hair cells. Journal of Neuroscience. *3* 942–976

Cranford J (1979a) Auditory cortex lesions and interaural intensity and phase angle discrimination in cats. Journal of Neurophysiology. *42* 1518–1526

Cranford J (1979b) Detection vs discrimination of brief tones by cats with auditory cortex lesions. Journal of the Acoustical Society of America. *65* 1573–1575

Cranford J, Igarishi M & Stramler J (1976) Effect of auditory neocortex ablation on pitch perception in the cat. Journal of Neurophysiology. *39* 143–152

Crawford A & Fettiplace R (1979) Reversal of hair cell responses by current. Journal of Physiology. *295* 56P

Crawford A & Fettiplace R (1980) The frequency selectivity of auditory nerve fibers and hair cells in the cochlea of the turtle. Journal of Physiology. *306* 79–125

Crawford A & Fettiplace R (1981) An electrical tuning mechanism in cochlear hair cells. Journal of Physiology. *312* 377–412

Crawford A & Fettiplace R (1985) The mechanical properties of ciliary bundles of turtle cochlear hair cells. Journal of Physiology. *364* 359–379

Crawford A & Fettiplace R (1986) Mechanical tuning in turtle cochlear hair cells. Hearing Research. *22* 91

Dallos P (1969) Combination tone $2f_1-f_h$ in microphonic potentials. Journal of the Acoustical Society of America. *46* 1437–1444

Dallos P (1986) Neurobiology of cochlear inner and outer hair cells: intracellular recordings. Hearing Research. *22* 185–198

Dallos P, Billone M, Durrant J & Raynor W (1972) Cochlear inner and outer hair cells: functional differences. Science. *177* 356–358

Dallos P, Cheatham M & Ferraro J (1974) Cochlear mechanics, nonlinearities and cochlear potentials. Journal of the Acoustical Society of America. *55* 597–605

Dallos P, Ryan A, Harris D, McGee T & Odzamar O (1977) Cochlear frequency selectivity in the presence of hair cell damage. In Evans E & Wilson J (Eds), Psychophysics and Physiology of Hearing (pp 249–258). Academic Press, New York & London

Dallos P, Sanchos-Sacchi J & Flock A (1982) Intracellular recordings from cochlear outer hair cells. Science. *218* 582–584

Danielou A (1959) Traité de Musicologie Comparée. Hermann, Paris

David E, Guttman N & van Berkeijk W (1959) Binaural interaction of high-frequency complex stimuli. Journal of the Acoustical Society of America. *31* 774–782

Davis H (1951) Psychophysiology of hearing and deafness. In Stevens S (Ed), Handbook of Experimental Psychology (pp 1116–1180). Wiley, New York

Davis H (1960) Mechanisms of excitation of auditory nerve impulses. In Rasmussen G & Windle W (Eds), Neural Mechanisms of the Auditory and Vestibular Systems (pp 21–39). Thomas, Springfield, Illinois

Davis H (1965) A model for transducer action in the cochlea. Cold Spring Harbor Symposium in Quantitative Biology. *30* 181–189

Davis H (1983) Active processes in cochlear mechanics. Hearing Research. *9* 79–90

Desmedt J (1975) Physiological studies of the efferent recurrent auditory system. In Keidel D & Neff W (Eds), Handbook of Sensory Physiology. Auditory System, Vol 2 (pp 218–246). Springer Verlag, Berlin

Desmedt J & La Grutta V (1963) Function of the uncrossed efferent olivo-cochlear fibres in the cat. Nature. *200* 472–474

Dewson J (1968) Efferent olivo-cochlear bundle: some relationships to stimulus discrimination in noise. Journal of Neurophysiology. *31* 122–130

Diamond I & Neff W (1957) Ablation of temporal cortex and discrimination of auditory patterns. Journal of Neurophysiology. *20* 300–315

Diamond I, Goldberg J & Neff W (1962) Tonal discrimination after ablation of auditory cortex. Journal of Neurophysiology. *25* 223–235

Doughty J & Garner W (1947) Pitch characteristics of short tones. I. Two kinds of pitch threshold. Journal of Experimental Psychology. *37* 351–365

Dünker J (1972) Zentrale Bahnsysteme und verarbeitung akustischer Nachrichten. In Gauer O, Kramer K & Jung R (Eds), Physiologie des Menschens. Vol 12 Physiologie des Hörens (pp 59–125). Urban & Schwartzenberg, München

Eldredge D (1974) Inner ear–cochlear mechanics and cochlear potentials. In Keidel W & Neff W (Eds), Handbook of Sensory Physiology, Vol 1 (pp 549–584). Springer Verlag, Berlin

Engström B (1983) Stereocilia of sensory cells in normal and hearing impaired ears. Scandinavian Audiology. Suppl. 19

Erulkar S, Rose J & Davies P (1956) Single unit activity in the auditory cortex of cat. Bulletin of the Johns Hopkins Hospital. *99* 55–86

Erulkar S, Butler R & Gerstein G (1968) Excitation and inhibition in cochlear nucleus. II Frequency-modulated tones. Journal of Neurophysiology. *31* 537–548

Evans E (1974) Neural processes for the detection of acoustic patterns and for sound localization. In Schmitt F & Worden F (Eds), The Neurosciences Third Study Program (pp 131–145). MIT Press, Cambridge, Massachusetts

Evans E (1975) Cochlear nerve and cochlear nucleus. In Keidel W & Neff W (Eds), Handbook of Sensory Physiology, Vol 2 (pp 1–108). Springer Verlag, Berlin

Evans E (1982a) Basic physics and psychophysics of sound. In Barlow H & Mollon J (Eds), The Senses (pp 239–250). Cambridge University Press, Cambridge

Evans E (1982b) Functional anatomy of the auditory system. In Barlow H & Mollon J (Eds), The Senses (pp 251–305). Cambridge University Press, Cambridge

Evans E (1982c) Functions of the auditory system. In Barlow H & Mollon J (Eds), The Senses (pp 307–332). Cambridge University Press, Cambridge

Evans E & Harrison R (1975) Correlation between outer hair cell damage and deterioration of cochlear nerve tuning properties. Journal of Physiology. *256* 43–44P

Evans E & Nelson P (1973a) The responses of single neurones in the cochlear nucleus of the cat as a function of their location and anaesthetic state. Experimental Brain Research. *17* 402–427

Evans E & Nelson P (1973b) On the functional relationship between the dorsal and ventral divisions of the cochlear nucleus of the cat. Experimental Brain Research. *17* 428–441

Evans E & Pick G (1972) Research strategy: simple vs complex stimuli. In Worden F & Galambos R (Eds), Auditory Processing of Biologically Significant Sounds. Neuroscience Research Program, Bulletin 10 (pp 10–14). Brookline, Massachusetts

Evans E & Whitfield I (1964) Classification of unit responses in the auditory cortex of the unanaesthetised cat. Journal of Physiology. *171* 476–493

Evans E & Wilson J (1973) The frequency selectivity of the cochlea. In Moller A & Boston P (Eds), Basic Mechanisms in Hearing (pp 519–551). Academic Press, New York

Evans E, Ross H & Whitfield I (1965) The spatial distribution of unit characteristic frequency in the primary auditory cortex of the cat. Journal of Physiology. *179* 238–247

Eybalin M & Pujol R (1984a) A radioautographic study of ^{3}H L-glutamine uptake in the guinea pig cochlea. Neuroscience. *9* 863–871

Eybalin M & Pujol R (1984b) Immunofluorescence with Metenkephalin and Leu-enkephalin antibodies in the guinea pig cochlea. Hearing Research. *13* 135–140

Eybalin M, Calas A & Pujol R (1983) Radioautographic study of sympathetic fibres in the cochlea. Acta Otolaryngolica. *96* 69–74

Fay R (1988) Hearing in Vertebrates. A Psychophysics Databook. Hill-Fay Associates, Winnetka, Illinois

Fedderson T, Sandel D, Teas D & Jeffress L (1957) Localization of high-frequency tones. Journal of the Acoustical Society of America. 29 988–991

Fex J (1962) Auditory activity in centrifugal and centripetal cochlear fibres in cat. Acta physiologica Scandinavica. Supplement. 189 5–68

Fex J & Altschuler R (1986) Neurotransmitter-related immunochemistry of the organ of Corti. Hearing Research. 22 249–263

Fitzpatrick K & Imig T (1980) Auditory cortico-cortical connections in the owl monkey. Journal of Comparative Neurology. 192 589–610

Fletcher H (1929) Speech and Hearing. van Nostrand, New York

Fletcher H (1940) Auditory patterns. Review of Modern Physics. 12 47–65

Flock A & Cheung H (1977) Actin filaments in sensory hairs of inner ear receptor cells. Journal of Cellular Biology. 75 339–343

Flock A & Strelliof D (1984) Graded and nonlinear mechanical properties of sensory hairs in the mammalian hearing organ. Nature (London). 310 597–599

Fowler E (1937) The diagnosis of the diseases of the neural mechanism of hearing by the aid of sounds well above threshold. Laryngoscope (St Louis). 47 289–300

Funkenstein H & Winter P (1973) Responses to acoustic stimuli of units in the auditory cortex of awake squirrel monkeys. Experimental Brain Research. 18 464–488

Galburda A & Sanides F (1980) Cytoarchitectural organization of the human auditory cortex. Journal of Comparative Neurology. 190 507–510

Garner W (1947) The effect of frequency spectrum on temporal integration of energy in the ear. Journal of the Acoustical Society of America. 19 808–815

Gerson A & Goldstein J (1978) Evidence for a general template in central optimal processing for pitch of complex tones. Journal of the Acoustical Society of America. 63 498–510

Gifford M & Guinan J (1983) Effect of crossed olivo-cochlear-bundle stimulation on cat auditory nerve fiber responses to tones. Journal of the Acoustical Society of America. 74 115–123

Glass I & Goldberg Z (1979) Lability in the responses of cells in the auditory cortex of squirrel monkeys to species-specific vocalisations. Experimental Brain Research. 34 489–498

Glendenning K, Brunso-Bechtold J, Thompson G & Masterton R (1981) Ascending auditory afferents to the nuclei of the lateral lemniscus. Journal of Comparative Neurology. 197 673–704

Goldberg J & Brown P (1968) Functional organization of the dog superior olivary complex: an anatomical and electrophysiological study. Journal of Neurophysiology. 31 639–656

Goldberg J & Brown P (1969) Responses of binaural neurons of dog superior olivary complex to dichotic tonal stimuli: some physiological mechanisms of sound localization. Journal of Neurophysiology. 32 613–636

Goldberg J & Brownell W (1973) Response characteristics of neurones in the anteroventral and dorsal cochlear nuclei of cat. Brain Research. 64 35–54

Goldberg J & Neff W (1961) Frequency discrimination after bilateral section of the brachium of the inferior colliculus. Journal of Comparative Neurology. 116 265–290

Goldstein J (1967) Auditory non-linearity. Journal of the Acoustical Society of America. 41 676–689

Goldstein J & Kiang N (1968) Neural correlates of the aural combination tone $2f_1 - f_2$. Proceedings of the Institute of Electrical and Electronic Engineers. 56 981–992

Goldstein M & Abeles M (1975) Single unit activity of the auditory cortex. In Keidel W & Neff W (Eds), Handbook of Sensory Physiology. Auditory system, Vol 2 (pp 199–218). Springer Verlag, Berlin

Goldstein M, Hall J & Butterfield B (1968) Single unit activity in the primary auditory cortex of unanesthetized cats. Journal of the Acoustical Society of America. 43 444–455

Greenwood D (1961) Critical bandwidth and the frequency coordinates of the basilar membrane. Journal of the Acoustical Society of America. 33 1344–1356

Greenwood D & Goldberg J (1970) Response of neurons in the cochlear nuclei to variations in noise bandwidths and to tone-noise combinations. Journal of the Acoustical Society of America. 47 1022–1040

Guinan J & Peake W (1967) Middle ear characteristics of anesthetized cats. Journal of the Acoustical Society of America. 41 1237–1261

Guinan J, Guinan S & Norris B (1972a) Single auditory units in the superior olivary complex. I. Responses to sounds and classification based on physiological properties. International Journal of Neuroscience. 4 101–120

Guinan J, Norris B & Guinan S (1972b) Single auditory units in the superior olivary complex. II. Locations of unit categories and tonotopic organisation. International Journal of Neuroscience. 4 147–166

Haas H (1951) Über den Einfluss eines Einfachechos auf die Hörsamkeit von Sprache. Acustica. 1 49–55

Hallpike C (1976) Sensorineural deafness and derangements of the loudness function: their nature and clinical investigation. In Keidel W & Neff W (Eds), Handbook of Sensory Physiology. Auditory System, Vol 3 (pp 1–35). Springer Verlag, Berlin

Harrison J & Howe M (1974a) Anatomy of the afferent auditory nervous system of mammals. In Keidel W & Neff W (Eds), Handbook of Sensory Physiology. Auditory System, Vol 1 (pp 283–336). Springer Verlag, Berlin

Harrison J & Howe M (1974b) Anatomy of the descending auditory system (mammalian). In Keidel W & Neff W (Eds), Handbook of Sensory Physiology. Auditory System, Vol 1 (pp 363–388). Springer Verlag, Berlin

Hashimoto I, Ishiyama Y, Yoshimoto T & Nemoto S (1981) Brainstem auditory evoked potentials recorded directly from human brainstem and thalamus. Brain. *104* 841–859

Hawkins J Jr (1976) Drug ototoxicity. In Keidel W & Neff W (Eds), Handbook of Sensory Physiology, Vol 3 (pp 707–748). Springer Verlag, Berlin

Hawkins J & Stevens S (1950) The masking of pure tones and of speech by white noise. Journal of the Acoustical Society of America. *22* 6–13

Heffner H & Heffner R (1986) Effect of unilateral and bilateral auditory cortex lesions on the discrimination of vocalizations by Japanese macaques. Journal of Neurophysiology. *56* 683–701

von Helmholtz H (1863) Die Lehre von den Tonempfindungen. Braunschweig Vieweg u. Sohn, Berlin

Hirsh I (1948) The influence of interaural phase on interaural summation and inhibition. Journal of the Acoustical Society of America. *20* 536–544

Holton A & Hudspeth A (1986) The transduction channel of hair cells from the bull-frog characterized by noise analysis. Journal of Physiology. *375* 195–227

Honrubia V & Ward P (1968) Longitudinal distribution of the cochlear microphonics inside the cochlear duct (guinea pig). Journal of the Acoustical Society of America. *44* 951–958

Honrubia V & Ward P (1969) Properties of the summating potential of the guinea pig's cochlea. Journal of the Acoustical Society of America. *45* 1443–1450

Horner K, Lenoir M & Bock G (1985) Distortion product otoacoustic emissions in hearing-impaired mutant mice. Journal of the Acoustical Society of America. *78* 1603–1611

Houtgast T (1972) Psychophysical evidence for lateral inhibition in hearing. Journal of the Acoustical Society of America. *51* 1885–1894

Houtsma A & Goldstein J (1972) The central origin of the pitch of complex tones: evidence from musical interval recognition. Journal of the Acoustical Society of America. *51* 520–529

Hudspeth A (1985) The cellular basis of hearing: the biophysics of hair cells. Science. *230* 745–752

Hudspeth A (1986) The ionic channel of a vertebrate hair cell. Hearing Research. *22* 21–27

Hudspeth A & Corey D (1977) Sensitivity, polarity and conductance change in the response of vertebrate hair cells to controlled mechanical stimuli. Proceedings of the National Academy of Sciences USA. *74* 2407–2411

Imig T & Adrian H (1977) Binaural columns in the primary auditory field (AI) of cat auditory cortex. Brain Research. *138* 241–257

Imig T & Morel A (1984) Topographic and cytoarchitectonic organization of thalamic neurons related to their targets in low, middle and high frequency representations in cat auditory cortex. Journal of Comparative Neurology. *227* 511–589

Imig T & Reale R (1980) Patterns of cortico-cortico connections related to tonotopic maps in cat auditory cortex. Journal of Comparative Neurology. *192* 293–332

Imig T, Ruggero M, Kitzes L, Javel E & Brugge J (1977) Organization of auditory cortex in owl monkey. Journal of Comparative Neurology. *171* 111–128

International Standards Organization (1961) Normal equal loudness contours for pure tones and normal threshold of hearing under free field listening conditions. R226. New York

International Standards Organization (1966) Method for calculating loudness level. R532. New York

Jenkins W & Masterton M (1982) Sound localization: effects of unilateral lesions in central auditory system. Journal of Neurophysiology. *47* 987–1016

Jenkins W & Merzenich M (1984) Role of cat auditory cortex for sound localization behaviour. Journal of Neurophysiology. *52* 819–847

Jerger J (1960) Békésy audiometry in analysis of auditory disorders. Journal of Speech Research. *3* 275–287

Jestaedt W, Wier C & Green D (1977) Intensity discrimination as a function of frequency and sensation level. Journal of the Acoustical Society of America. *61* 169–177

Johnstone B & Boyle A (1967) Basilar membrane vibration examined with the Mössbauer technique. Science. *158* 389–390

Johnstone B, Taylor K & Boyle A (1970) Mechanics of the guinea pig cochlea. Journal of the Acoustical Society of America. *47* 504–509

Johnstone B, Patuzzi R & Yates G (1986) Basilar membrane measurements and the travelling wave. Hearing Research. *22* 147–153

Jones L & Disterhof J (1983) The effect of auditory stimulus rate on ^{14}C-2-deoxyglucose uptake in rabbit inferior colliculus. Brain Research. *279* 85–92

Kachar B, Brownell W, Altschuler R & Fex J (1986) Electrokinetic changes of cochlear outer hair cells. Nature (London). *322* 365–368

Katsuki Y (1965) Comparative neurophysiology of hearing. Physiological Reviews. *45* 380–423

Katsuki Y, Sumi T, Ushiyama H & Watanabe T (1958) Electrical responses of auditory neurons in cat to sound stimulation. Journal of Neurophysiology. *21* 569–588

Katsuki Y, Watanabe T & Maruyama N (1959) Activity of auditory neurons in upper level of brain of cat. Journal of Neurophysiology. *22* 343–359

Katsuki Y, Suga N & Kanno Y (1962) Neural mechanisms of the peripheral and central auditory system in monkeys. Journal of the Acoustical Society of America. *34* 1396–1410

Kay RH (1982) Hearing of modulation in sounds. Physiological Reviews. *62* 894–975.

Kemp D (1978) Stimulated acoustic emissions from within the human auditory system. Journal of the Acoustical Society of America. *64* 1386–1391

Kemp D (1986) Otoacoustic transmissions, travelling waves and cochlear mechanisms. Hearing Research. *22* 95–104

Khanna S & Leonard D (1982) Basilar membrane tuning in the cat cochlea. Science. *215* 305–306

Khanna S & Tonndorf J (1971) The vibratory pattern of the round window in cats. Journal of the Acoustical Society of America. *50* 1475–1483

Khanna S & Tonndorf J (1972) Tympanic membrane vibrations in cats studied by time-averaged holography. Journal of the Acoustical Society of America. *51* 1904–1920

Khanna S, Tonndorf J & Walcott W (1968) Laser interferometer for the measurement of submicroscopic displacement amplitudes and their phases in small biological systems. Journal of the Acoustical Society of America. *44* 1555–1565

Kiang N (1965) Stimulus coding in the auditory nerve and cochlear nucleus. Acta Otolaryngologica. *59* 186–200

Kiang N, Moxon E & Levine R (1970) Auditory nerve activity in cats with normal and abnormal cochleas. In Wolstenholme G & Knight J (Eds), Sensorineural Hearing Loss (pp 241–268). Churchill, London

Kiang N, Watanabe T, Thomas E & Clark L (1965) Discharge patterns of single fibers in the cat's auditory nerve (Research Monograph 35). MIT Press, Cambridge, Massachusetts

Kim D (1986) Active and non-linear biomechanics and the role of the outer hair cell subsystem in the mammalian auditory system. Hearing Research. 22 105–114

Klinke R (1972) In Kramer K & Jung R (Eds), Physiologie des Menschens. Vol 12 Physiologie des Hörens (pp 19–27). Urban & Schwartzenberg, München

Knight P (1977) Representation of the cochlea within the anterior auditory field (AAF) of the cat. Brain Research. 130 447–467

Kohllöffel L (1971) Studies of the distribution of cochlear potentials along the basilar membrane. Acta Otolaryngolica. Supplement 288

Kohllöffel L (1972) A study of basilar membrane vibrations. Fuzziness detection: a new method for the analysis of vibrations with laser light. Acustica. 27 49–65

Kuijpers W (1969) Cation transport and cochlear function (PhD Thesis). University of Nijmegen. Nijmegen, The Netherlands

Lavine N (1971) Phase locking in response of single neuron in cat cochlear nucleus to low frequency tonal stimulation. Journal of Neurophysiology. 34 467–483

Legouix P (1974) Two tone inhibition. In Zwicker E & Terhardt E (Eds), Facts and Models in Hearing. Springer Verlag, Berlin

Legouix J, Remond M & Greenbaum H (1973) Interference and two-tone inhibition. Journal of the Acoustical Society of America. 53 409–419

Lewis R & Hudspeth A (1983) Frequency tuning and ionic conductances in hair cells of the bullfrog's sacculus. In Klinke R & Hartmann R (Eds), Hearing: Physiological Bases and Psychophysics (pp 17–22). Springer Verlag, Berlin

Liberman M (1976) Abnormal discharge patterns of auditory-nerve fibers in acoustically-traumatised cats (PhD Dissertation). Harvard University, Cambridge, Massachusetts

Liberman M (1980) Efferent synapses in the inner hair cell area of the cat cochlea: an electron microscopic study of serial sections. Hearing Research. 3 189–204

Liberman M (1986) Primary sensory input to the auditory central nervous system. Proceedings of the XXXth International Physiological Congress, Vancouver

Liberman M & Oliver M (1984) Morphometry of intracellularly labelled neurons of the auditory nerve: correlations with functional properties. Journal of Comparative Neurology. 223 163–176

Licklider J (1951) Basic correlates of the auditory stimulus. In Stevens S (Ed), Handbook of Experimental Psychology (pp 985–1039). Wiley, New York

Lim D (1986) Functional structure of the organ of Corti. A review. Hearing Research. 22 117–146

Lüscher E & Zwislocki J (1947) The decay of sensation and the remainder of adaptation after short pure-tone impulses on the ear. Acta Otorhinolaryngologica. *35* 428–445

Manley J & Müller-Preuss P (1978) Response variability of auditory cortex cells in the squirrel monkey to constant acoustic stimuli. Experimental Brain Research. *32* 171–180

Masterton R & Diamond I (1967) The medial superior olive and sound localization. Science. *155* 1696–1697

Masterton R, Jane J & Diamond I (1967) Role of brainstem auditory structures in sound localization. I. Trapezoid body, superior olive and lateral lemniscus. Journal of Neurophysiology. *30* 341–359

Meredith M & Clemo H (1989) Auditory cortical projection from the anterior ectosylvian sulcus (field AES) to the superior colliculus in the cat: an anatomical and electrophysiological study. Journal of Comparative Neurology. *289* 687–707

Merzenich M & Brugge J (1973) Representation of the cochlear partition on the superior temporal plane of the macaque monkey. Brain Research. *50* 275–296

Merzenich M, Knight P & Roth G (1975) Representation of cochlea within primary auditory cortex in the cat. Journal of Neurophysiology. *38* 231–249

Merzenich M, Kaas J & Roth G (1976) Auditory cortex in the grey squirrel: tonotopic organization and architectonic fields. Journal of Comparative Neurology. *166* 387–402

Mesulam M & Pandya D (1973) The projections of the medial geniculate complex within the sylvian fissure of the rhesus monkey. Brain Research. *60* 315–334

Meyer D & Woolsey C (1952) Effects of localized cortical destruction on auditory discriminative conditioning in cat. Journal of Neurophysiology. *15* 149–162

Middlebrooks J & Knudsen E (1984) A neural code for auditory space in the cat's superior colliculus. Journal of Neuroscience. *4* 2621–2634

Middlebrooks J & Zook J (1983) Intrinsic organization of the cat's medial geniculate body by projections to binaural response-specific bands in the primary auditory cortex. Journal of Neuroscience. *3* 203–224

Middlebrooks J, Dykes R & Merzenich M (1980) Binaural response-specific bands in primary auditory cortex (AI) of the cat: topographical organisation orthogonal to isofrequency contours. Brain Research. *181* 31–48

Miller A (1948) The reception of short bursts of noise. Journal of the Acoustical Society of America. *20* 160–170

Miller A & Garner W (1944) Effect of random presentation on the psychometric function: duplication for a quantal theory of discrimination. American Journal of Psychology. *57* 451–467

Miller J, Beaton R, O'Connor T & Pfingst B (1974) Response pattern complexity of auditory cells in the cortex of unanesthetised monkeys. Brain Research. *69* 101–113

Mills A (1958) On the minimum audible angle. Journal of the Acoustical Society of America. *30* 237–246

Mills A (1960) Lateralization of high-frequency tones. Journal of the Acoustical Society of America. *32* 132–134

Milner B (1962) Laterality effects in audition. In Mountcastle V (Ed), Interhemispheric Relations and Cerebral Dominance (pp 177–195). Johns Hopkins Press, Baltimore

Møller A (1963) Transfer function of the middle ear. Journal of the Acoustical Society of America. *35* 1526–1534

Møller A (1965) An experimental study of the acoustic impedance of the middle ear and its transformation properties. Acta Otolaryngolica. *60* 129–149

Møller A (1974a) Function of the middle ear. In Keidel E & Neff W (Eds), Handbook of Sensory Physiology, Vol 1 (pp 492–517). Springer Verlag, Berlin

Møller A (1974b) Acoustic middle ear reflex. In Keidel E & Neff W (Eds), Handbook of Sensory Physiology, Vol 1 (pp 519–548). Springer Verlag, Berlin

Møller A (1974c) Responses of units in the cochlear nucleus to sinusoidally amplitude-modulated tones. Experimental Neurology. *45* 104–117

Møller A (1978) Coding time-varying sounds in the cochlear nucleus. Audiology. *17* 446–468

Møller A, Jannetta P, Bennet M & Møller M (1981) Intracranially recorded responses of human auditory nerve: new insights into the origin of brainstem evoked potentials (BSEPs). Electroencephalography & Clinical Neurophysiology. *52* 18–27

Moore C, Casseday J & Neff W (1974) Sound localisation: the role of the commissural pathways of the auditory system of the cat. Brain Research. *82* 13–26

Morel A & Imig T (1987) Thalamic projections to fields A, AI, P and VP in the cat auditory cortex. Journal of Comparative Neurology. *265* 119–144

Morest D (1964) The neuronal architecture of the medial geniculate body of the cat. Journal of Anatomy. *98* 611–630

Morest D (1965) The laminar structure of the medial geniculate body of the cat. Journal of Anatomy. *99* 143–160

Morest D (1975) Synaptic relationship of Golgi type II cells in the medial geniculate body of the cat. Journal of Comparative Neurology. *162* 157–194

Morest D & Oliver D (1984) The neuronal architecture of the inferior colliculus in the cat: defining the functional anatomy of the auditory midbrain. Journal of Comparative Neurology. *222* 209–236

Moushegian G, Rupert A & Gidda J (1975) Functional characteristics of superior olivary neurons to binaural stimuli. Journal of Neurophysiology. *38* 1037–1048

Müller J (1838) Hanbuch der Physiologie des Menschen, Vol II. Hölscher, Coblenz

Nedzelnitsky V (1980) Sound pressure in the basal turn of the cat cochlea. Journal of the Acoustical Society of America. *68* 1676–1689

Neff W & Hind J (1955) Auditory thresholds of the cat. Journal of the Acoustical Society of America. *27* 480–483

Neff W, Diamond I & Casseday J (1975) Behavioural studies of auditory discrimination. In Keidel W & Neff W (Eds), Handbook of Sensory Physiology. Auditory System, Vol 2 (pp 307–400). Springer Verlag, Berlin

Nelson D & Turner C (1980) Decay of masking and frequency resolution in sensorineural hearing-impaired listeners. In van den Brink C & Bilsen F (Eds), Psychophysiological, Physiological and Behavioural Studies in Hearing (pp 175–182). Delft University Press, Delft

Nelson P, Erulkar S & Bryan J (1966) Responses of units of the inferior colliculus to time-varying acoustic stimuli. Journal of Neurophysiology. *29* 834–860

Newman J & Symmes D (1974) Arousal effects on unit responsiveness to vocalisations in squirrel monkey auditory cortex. Brain Research. *78* 125–138

Newman J & Wollberg Z (1973) Multiple coding of species-specific vocalisations in the auditory cortex of squirrel monkeys. Brain Research. *54* 287–304

van Noorden L (1982) Two channel pitch perception. In Clynes M (Ed), Music, Mind and Brain (p 251). Plenum Press, New York

Ohm G (1843) Über die Definition des Tones, nebst daran geknupter Theorie der Sirene und ähnlicher tonbildender Vorrichtungen. Annalen für Physik und Chemie. *59* 513–565

Oliver D & Hall W (1978) The medial geniculate body of the tree shrew *Tupaia glis*. II Connections with the neocortex. Journal of Comparative Neurology. *182* 459–494

Oliver D & Morest D (1984) The central nucleus of the inferior colliculus in the cat. Journal of Comparative Neurology. *222* 237–264

Oonishi S & Katsuki Y (1965) Functional organisation and integrative mechanism in the auditory cortex of the cat. Japanese Journal of Physiology. *15* 342–365

Osen K (1969) Cytoarchitecture of the cochlear nuclei in the cat. Journal of Comparative Neurology. *136* 453–483

Osen K & Roth K (1969) Histochemical localisation of cholinesterases in the cochlear nuclei of the cat, with notes on the origin of acetylcholinesterase-positive afferents and the superior olive. Brain Research. *16* 165–185

Pandya D & Sanides F (1973) Architectonic parcellation of the temporal operculum in the rhesus monkey and its projection pattern. Journal of Anatomy. *139* 127–161

Pfeiffer R (1966) Classification of response patterns of spike discharge for units in the cochlear nucleus: tone burst stimulation. Experimental Brain Research. *1* 220–235

Phillips D & Irvine D (1981) Responses of single neurons in physiologically defined primary auditory cortex (AI) of the cat: frequency tuning and responses to intensity. Journal of Neurophysiology. *45* 48–58

Phillips D & Irvine D (1982) Properties of single neurons in the anterior auditory field (AAF) of cat cerebral cortex. Brain Research. *248* 237–244

Phillips D & Irvine D (1983) Some features of binaural input to single neurons in physiologically defined area AI of cat cerebral cortex. Journal of Neurophysiology. *49* 383–395

Phillips D & Orman S (1984) Response of single neurons in the posterior field of cat auditory cortex to tonal stimulation. Journal of Neurophysiology. *51* 147–163

Philippot MP (1968a) Musique. In Encyclopaedia Universalis. Universalis, Paris

Philippot MP (1968b) Gamme. In Encyclopaedia Universalis. Universalis, Paris

Pickles J (1982) An Introduction to the Physiology of Hearing. Academic Press, London & New York

Pickles J & Comis S (1973) Role of centrifugal pathways to cochlear nucleus in the detection of signals in noise. Journal of Neurophysiology. *36* 1131–1137

Pickles J & Comis S (1976) Auditory-nerve fiber bandwidths and critical bandwidths in the cat. Journal of the Acoustical Society of America. *60* 1151–1156

Picton T, Hillyard S, Krausz H & Galambos R (1974) Human auditory evoked potentials. I Evaluation of components. Electroencephalography and Clinical Neurophysiology. *36* 179–190

Piéron H (1945) La Sensation. Guide de Vie. Gallimard, Paris

Plomp R (1970) Timbre as a multidimensional attribute of complex tones. In R Plomp & G Smoorenburg (Eds), Frequency Analysis and Periodicity Detection in Hearing (pp 397–414). Sijthoff, Netherlands

Ploog D (1979) Auditory agnosia after lesions of the superior temporal gyrus in monkey and man. In O Creutzfeld, H Scheich & C Schreiner (Eds), Hearing Mechanisms and Speech. Experimental Brain Research. Supplementum 2 (pp 351–357). Springer Verlag, Berlin

Pontes C, Reis F & Sousa-Pinto A (1975) The auditory cortical projections onto the medial geniculate body in the cat. An anatomical study with silver and autoradiographic methods. Brain Research. *91* 43–63

Portmann M & Portmann C (1978) Précis d'Audiométrie Clinique. Masson, Paris

Probst R, Lonsbury-Martin B, Martin G & Coats A (1987) Otoacoustic emissions in ears with hearing loss. American Journal of Otolaryngology. *21* 261–275

Pujol R & Lenoir M (1985) The four types of synapse in the organ of Corti. In A Altschuler, R Hoffmann & D Robbin (Eds), Neurobiology of Hearing: The Cochlea (pp 161–172). Raven Press, New York

Rayleigh J (1945) The Theory of Sound. Dover, New York (1st ed 1896)

Reale R & Imig T (1980) Tonotopic organization in auditory cortex of the cat. Journal of Comparative Neurology. *192* 265–291

Rebillard G (1987) Les autoémissions acoustiques. II Les auto-émissions spontanées: résultats chez des sujets normaux ou présentant des acouphènes. Annales d'otologie et de laryngologie (Paris). *104* 363–368

Redies H, Brandner S & Creutzfeldt O (1989) Anatomy of the auditory thalamocortical system of the guinea pig. Journal of Comparative Neurology. *282* 489–511

Rees A & Møller A (1983) Responses of neurons in the inferior colliculus of the rat to AM and FM tones. Hearing Research. *10* 301–330

Rhode W (1971) Observations of the vibration of the basilar membrane in squirrel monkeys using the Mössbauer technique. Journal of the Acoustical Society of America. *49* 1218–1231

Rhode W (1978) Some observations on cochlear mechanics. Journal of the Acoustical Society of America. *64* 158–176

Robles L, Ruggero M & Rich N (1984) Mössbauer measurements of basilar membrane tuning curves in the chinchilla. Journal of the Acoustical Society of America. *76* S35(A)

Rockel A & Jones E (1973a) The neuronal organization of the inferior colliculus of the adult cat. I The central nucleus. Journal of Comparative Neurology. *147* 11–60

Rockel A & Jones E (1973b) The neuronal organization of the inferior colliculus of the adult cat. II The pericentral nucleus. Journal of Comparative Neurology. *149* 301–334

Roederer J (1979) Introduction to the Physics and Psychophysics of Music (2nd ed). Springer Verlag, Berlin

Romand R (1978) Survey of intracellular recording in the cochlear nucleus of the cat. Brain Research. *148* 43–65

Rose J (1949) The cellular structure of the auditory region of the cat. Journal of Comparative Neurology. *91* 409–439

Rose J & Woolsey C (1958) Cortical connections and functional organization of the thalamic auditory system of the cat. In Harlow H & Woolsey C (Eds), Biological and Biochemical Bases of Behavior (pp 127–150). University of Wisconsin Press, Madison

Rose J, Galambos R & Hughes J (1959) Microelectrode studies of the cochlear nuclei of the cat. Bulletin of the Johns Hopkins Hospital. *104* 211–251

Rose J, Greenwood D, Goldberg J & Hind J (1963) Some discharge characteristics of single neurons in the inferior colliculus of the cat. I. Tonotopic organization; relation of spike counts to tone intensity and firing patterns of single elements. Journal of Neurophysiology. *26* 294–320

Rose J, Gross N, Geisler C & Hind J (1966) Some neural elements in the inferior colliculus of the cat which may be relevant to the localization of a sound source. Journal of Neurophysiology. *29* 288–314

Rose J, Brugge J, Anderson D & Hind J (1968) Patterns of activity in single auditory fibres of the squirrel monkey. In de Reuck A & Knight J (Eds), Hearing Mechanisms in Vertebrates (pp 144–157). Ciba Foundation Symposium. Churchill, London

Rose J, Hind J, Anderson D & Brugge J (1971) Some effects of stimulus intensity on the response of auditory nerve fibers in the squirrel monkey. Journal of Neurophysiology. *34* 685–699

Rose J, Gibson N, Kitzes L & Hind J (1974) Observations on phase-sensitive neurons of anteroventral cochlear nucleus of the cat: non-linearity of cochlear output. Journal of Neurophysiology. *37* 218–253

Roth G, Aitkin L, Andersen R & Merzenich M (1978) Some features of the spatial organization of the central nucleus of the inferior colliculus. Journal of Comparative Neurology. *182* 661–680

Russell I & Sellick P (1978) Intracellular studies of hair cells in the mammalian cochlea. Journal of Physiology. *284* 261–290

Russell I & Sellick P (1983) Low frequency characteristics of intracellularly recorded receptor potentials in mammalian hair cells. Journal of Physiology. *338* 179–206

Russell I, Cody A & Richardson G (1986) The responses of inner and outer hair cells in the basal turn of the guinea-pig cochlea and in the mouse cochlea grown in vitro. Hearing Research. *22* 199–216

Sachs M & Abbas P (1974) Rate vs level functions for auditory nerve fibers in cats: tone-burst stimuli. Journal of the Acoustical Society of America. *56* 1835–1847

Sachs M & Kiang N (1968) Two-tone inhibition in auditory nerve fibers. Journal of the Acoustical Society of America. 43 1120–1128

Scharf B & Buus S (1986) Audition I: Stimulus, physiology, thresholds. In Boff K, Kaufman L & Thomas J (Eds), Handbook of Perception and Human Performance. 1 (pp 14-1 to 14-71). Wiley, New York

Scharf N & Houtsma A (1986) Audition II: Loudness, pitch, localization, aural distortion, pathology. In Boff K, Kaufman L & Thomas J (Eds), Handbook of Perception and Human Performance. 1 (pp 15-1 to 15-60). Wiley, New York

Schouten J (1940) The residue and the mechanism of hearing. Proceedings of the Koningklijke Nederlandse Akademie van Wetenschappen. 43 991–999

Seebeck A (1841) Beobachtungen über einige Bedlingungen der Entstehung von Tönen. Annalen für Physik und Chemie. 53 417–436

Sellick P (1979) Recordings from single receptor cells in the mammalian cochlea. Trends in Neuroscience. 2 114–116

Sellick P & Russell I (1979) Two-tone suppression in cochlear hair cells. Hearing Research. 1 227–236

Sellick P & Russell I (1980) The response of inner hair cells to basilar membrane velocity during low frequency auditory stimulation in the guinea pig. Hearing Research. 2 439–445

Semple M & Aitkin L (1979) Representation of sound frequency and laterality by units in central nucleus of cat inferior colliculus. Journal of Neurophysiology. 42 1626–1639

Servière J, Webster W & Calford M (1984) Isofrequency labelling revealed by a combined 2-^{14}C-deoxyglucose, electrophysiological and horseradish peroxidase study. Journal of Comparative Neurology. 228 463–477

Shaw E (1974) The external ear. In Keidel D & Neff W (Eds), Handbook of Sensory Physiology. Auditory System, Vol 1 (pp 455–490). Springer Verlag, Berlin

Shepard R (1982) Geometrical approximations to the structure of musical pitch. Psychological Reviews. 89 305–333

Shower E & Biddulph R (1931) Differential pitch sensitivity of the ear. Journal of the Acoustical Society of America. 3 275–287

Sovijärvi A (1975) Detection of natural complex sounds in the primary auditory cortex of the cat. Acta physiologica Scandinavica. 93 318–335

Sovijärvi A & Hyvärinen J (1974) Auditory cortical neurons in the cat sensitive to the direction of sound source movement. Brain Research. 73 455–471

Spoendlin H (1970) Structural basis of peripheral frequency analysis. In Plomp R

& Smoorenburg F (Eds), Frequency Analysis and Periodicity Detection in Hearing (pp 2–36). Sitjoff, Leiden

Spoendlin H (1979) Anatomisch-pathalogische Aspekte der Electrostimulation des ertaubten Innenohres. Archives of Otorhinolaryngology. *223* 1–75

Steele C (1974) Cochlear mechanics. In Keidel W & W Neff (Eds), Handbook of Sensory Physiology, Vol 3 (pp 433–478). Springer Verlag, Berlin

Steinberg J & Gardner M (1937) The dependence of hearing impairment on sound intensity. Journal of the Acoustical Society of America. *9* 11

Sterkers O, Ferrary E & Amiel C (1988) Production of inner ear fluids. Physiological Reviews. *68* 1083–1128

Stevens S (1935) The relation of pitch to intensity. Journal of the Acoustical Society of America. *6* 150–154

Stevens S & Egan J (1941) Diplacusis in "normal" ears. Psychological Bulletin. *38* 548

Stevens S & Newman E (1936a) The localization of actual sources of sounds. American Journal of Psychology. *48* 297–306

Stevens S & Newman E (1936b) On the nature of aural harmonics. Proceedings of the National Academy of Science. *22* 668–762

Sun X, Jen P & Kamada T (1983) Neurons in the superior colliculus of echolocating bats respond to ultrasonic signals. Brain Research. *275* 148–152

Swarbrick L & Whitfield I (1972) Auditory cortical units selectively responsive to stimulus shape. Journal of Physiology. *224* 68–69

Tanaka Y, Asanuma A & Yanagisawa K (1980) Potentials of outer hair cells and their membrane properties in cationic environments. Hearing Research. *2* 431–438

Tartini G (1754) Trattato de Música secondo la vera scienza dell'armonia. Padua, Italy

Tasaki I & Spiropoulos C (1959) Stria vascularis as source of endochochlear potential. Journal of Neurophysiology. *22* 149–155

Tasaki I, Davis H & Legouix J (1952) The space time pattern of the cochlear microphonics (guinea-pig) as recorded by differential electrodes. Journal of the Acoustical Society of America. *24* 502–519

Terhardt E (1974) Pitch of pure tones: Its relation to intensity. In Zwicker E & Terhardt E (Eds), Facts and Models in Hearing. Springer Verlag, Berlin

Terhardt E (1979) Calculating virtual pitch. Hearing Research. *1* 155–182

Thompson R (1960) Functions of the auditory cortex of cat in frequency discrimination. Journal of Neurophysiology. *23* 321–334

Tielen A, Kamp A, Lopez da Silva F, Reneau J & van Leeuwen S (1969) Evoked responses to sinusoidally modulated sound in anaesthetised dogs. Electroencephalography & Clinical Neurophysiology. 26 381–394

Tonndorf J (1960) In Rasmussen G & Windle W (Eds), Neural Mechanisms of the Auditory and Vestibular Systems (p 21). Thomas, Springfield, Illinois

Tonndorf J (1976) Bone conduction. In Keidel W & Neff W (Eds), Handbook of Sensory Physiology, Vol 3 (pp 37–84). Springer Verlag, Berlin

Tunturi A (1950) Physiological determination of the boundary of the acoustic area in the dog. American Journal of Physiology. 162 395–401

Wallach H, Newman E & Rosenzweig M (1949) The precedence effect in sound localization. American Journal of Psychology. 57 315–336

Walliser K (1969) Zusammenänge zwischen dem Schallreiz und der Periodentonhöhe. Acustica. 21 319

Warr W (1975) Olivo-cochlear and vestibular efferent neurons of the feline brain stem: their location, morphology and number determined by retrograde axonal transport and acetylcholinesterase histochemistry. Journal of Comparative Neurology. 161 159–182

Warr W (1978) The olivo-cochlear bundle: its origins and terminations in the cat. In Naunton R & Fernandez C (Eds), Evoked electrical activity in the auditory nervous system (pp 43–63). Academic Press, New York

Warr W (1982) Parallel ascending pathways from the cochlear nucleus. In Neff W (Ed), Contributions to Sensory Psychology, Vol 7 (pp 1–38). Academic Press, New York

Watanabe T, Liao T & Katsuki Y (1968) Neuronal response patterns in the superior olivary complex of the cat to sound stimulation. Japanese Journal of Physiology. 18 267–287

Webster W & Aitkin L (1975) Central auditory processing. In Gazzaniga M & Blakemore C (Eds), Handbook of Psychobiology (pp 325–364). Academic Press, New York

Webster W, Servière J, Batini C & Laplante S (1978) Autoradiographic demonstration with $2(^{14}C)$ deoxyglucose of frequency selectivity in the auditory system of cats under conditions of functional activity. Neuroscience Letters. 10 43

Webster W, Servière J & Brown M (1984a) Inhibitory contours in the inferior colliculus as revealed by the 2-deoxyglucose method. Experimental Brain Research. 56 577–581

Webster W, Servière J, Crewther D & Crewther S (1984b) Isofrequency 2-DG contours in the inferior colliculus of the awake monkey. Experimental Brain Research. 56 425–437

Wersäll J, Flock A & Lundquist P (1965) Structural basis for directional sensitivity in cochlear and vestibular sensory receptors. Cold Spring Harbor Symposium on Quantitative Biology. *30* 115–132

Wever E & Bray C (1930) The nature of acoustic response: the relation between sound frequency and frequency of impulses in the auditory nerve. Journal of Experimental Psychology. *13* 373–387

Wever E & Lawrence M (1954) Physiological Acoustics. Princeton University Press, Princeton, New Jersey

White J & Warr W (1983) The dual origins of the olivo-cochlear bundle in the albino rat. Journal of Comparative Neurology. *219* 203

Whitfield I (1957) The electrical responses of the unanaesthetised auditory cortex in the intact cat. Electroencephalography & Clinical Neurophysiology. *9* 35–42

Whitfield I (1980) Auditory cortex and the pitch of complex tones. Journal of the Acoustical Society of America. *67* 644–647

Whitfield I (1982) Coding in the auditory cortex. Contributions to Sensory Physiology. *6* 159–175

Whitfield I & Evans E (1965) Responses of auditory cortical neurons to stimuli of changing frequency. Journal of Neurophysiology. *28* 655–672

Wiederhold M (1970) Variations in the effects of electric stimulation of the crossed olivo-cochlear bundle on cat single auditory-nerve-fiber responses to tone bursts. Journal of the Acoustical Society of America. *48* 966–977

Wier C, Jesteadt W & Green D (1977) Frequency discrimination as a function of frequency and sensation levels. Journal of the Acoustical Society of America. *61* 178–184

Wightman F (1973) The pattern-transformation model of pitch. Journal of the Acoustical Society of America. *54* 407–416

Wilson J (1980) Evidence for a cochlear origin for acoustic re-emissions; thresholds, fine structure and tonal tinnitus. Hearing Research. *21* 233–252

Wilson J (1984) Otoacoustic emissions and hearing mechanisms. Reviews of Laryngology. *105* 179–191

Wilson J & Johnstone J (1975) Basilar membrane and middle ear vibration in guinea pig measured by capacity probe. Journal of the Acoustical Society of America. *57* 705–723

Winer J (1984) Anatomy of Layer IV in cat primary auditory cortex (AI). Journal of Comparative Neurology. *224* 537–567

Winter P, Ploog D & Latta J (1966) Vocal repertoire of the squirrel monkey (*Saimiri sciureus*), its analysis and significance. Experimental Brain Research. *1* 359–384

Wood A (1944) The Physics of Music. Methuen, London

Woolf N, Sharp F, Davidson T & Ryan A (1983) Cochlear and middle ear affects on metabolism in the central auditory pathway during silence: A 2-deoxyglucose study. Brain Research. *274* 119–127

Woolsey C (Ed) (1982) Cortical Sensory Organization, Vol 3. Auditory Areas. The Humana Press, Clifton, New Jersey

Worden F & Marsh J (1963) Amplitude changes of auditory potentials evoked at cochlear nucleus during acoustic habituation. Electroencephalography & Clinical Neurophysiology. *15* 866–881

Worden F, Marsh J, Abraham F & Whittlesey J (1964) Variability of evoked auditory potentials and acoustic input control. Electroencephalography & Clinical Neurophysiology. *17* 524–530

Young E & Brownell W (1976) Responses to tones and noise of single cells in dorsal cochlear nucleus of unanesthetized cats. Journal of Neurophysiology. *39* 282–300

Zenner H (1980) Cytoskeletal and muscle-like elements in cochlear hair cells. Archives of Otorhinolaryngology. *230* 82–92

Zenner H (1986) Motile responses in outer hair cells. Hearing Research. *22* 83–90

Zurek P (1981) Spontaneous narrow band acoustic signals emitted by human ears. Journal of the Acoustical Society of America. *69* 514–523

Zwicker E (1974) On a psychoacoustic equivalent of tuning curves. In Zwicker E & Terhardt E (Eds), Facts and Models in Hearing (pp 132–141). Springer Verlag, Berlin

Zwicker E (1975) Scaling. In Keidel D & Neff W (Eds), Handbook of Sensory Physiology. Auditory System, Vol V.3 (pp 401–448). Springer Verlag, Berlin

Zwicker E & Feldtkeller R (1981) Psychoacoustique (trans. C Sorin). Masson, Paris

Zwislocki J (1978) Masking: experimental and theoretical aspects of simultaneous, forward, backward and central masking. In Carterette E & Friedman M (Eds), Handbook of Perception. 4. Hearing. Academic Press, New York

Zwislocki J (1984) How OHC lesions can lead to neural cochlear hypersensitivity. Acta Otorhinolaryngologica. *97* 529–534

Zwislocki J (1986) Analysis of cochlear mechanics. Hearing Research. *22* 155–169

Index